Asphalt

TO

Ecosystems

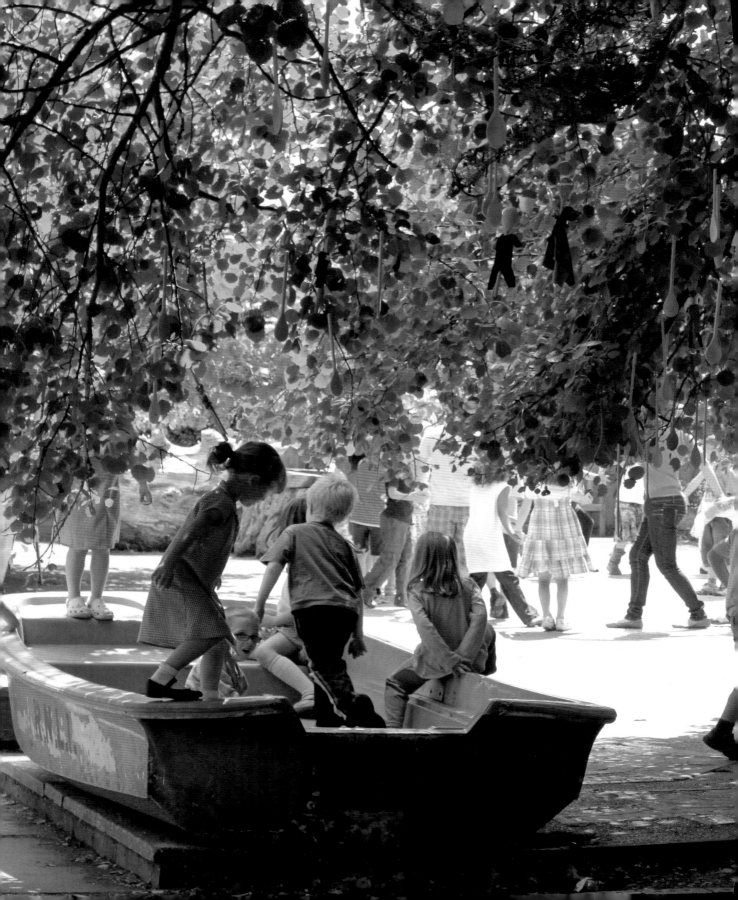

Asphalt

TO

Ecosystems

DESIGN IDEAS FOR SCHOOLYARD TRANSFORMATION

Sharon Gamson Danks

New Village Press • Oakland, CA

Published by
New Village Press
P.O. Box 3049, Oakland, CA 94609
(510) 420-1361
bookorders@newvillagepress.net
www.newvillagepress.net

New Village Press is a public-benefit, not-for-profit publishing venture of
Architects/Designers/Planners for Social Responsibility. www.adpsr.org

Printed in China

The printing papers used in this book are acid-free and the binding is
library quality.

Interior design and composition by Leigh McLellan
Cover design by Lynne Elizabeth
All photographs by Sharon Gamson Danks unless otherwise indicated
Frontispiece: Coombes School, England

ISBN-13 978-0-9766054-8-5
Publication Date: November 2010

Library of Congress Cataloging-in-Publication Data

Danks, Sharon.
    Asphalt to ecosystems : design ideas for schoolyard transformation /
Sharon Danks.
        p. cm.
    Summary: "Case studies from North America, Scandinavia, Great Britain,
and Japan demonstrate natural outdoor learning and play environments that
support hands-on interdisciplinary lessons and expand the possibilities for
schoolyard recreation, while nurturing healthy imagination and socialization"
—Provided by publisher.
    ISBN 978-0-9766054-8-5 (alk. paper)
    1. School grounds—Environmental aspects—Case studies. 2. Outdoor
learning laboratories--Case studies. I. Title.
    LB3251.D36 2010
    371.6'1--dc22   2010025517

Contents

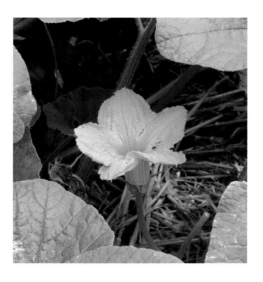

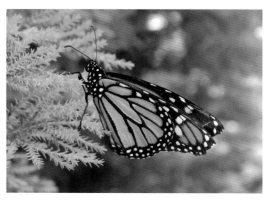

Foreword

On my first trip to San Francisco, by invitation from Sharon Danks, I had an unforgettable "aha!" moment about the future and potential of school grounds. It came as we were walking down the halls of LeConte Elementary School. We turned a corner and arrived at the door into the courtyard. "Farm" is all it said, causing me to do a double take as its mundane presentation seemed to suggest that farms at schools were as common as math and language arts. Proceeding into the courtyard, shock turned to delight at the sight of chickens and rabbits, grains and vegetables, and "Farmer Ben" surrounded by a clutch of students. The narrow space was teeming with life and learning and it was hard to imagine anyone remaining skeptical of the marriage of agriculture and academics.

That experience leads to an important question. What should drive the design of the outdoor learning environments at our schools? Creating opportunities for hands-on learning, the promotion of children's health, the construction of positive social environments, landscapes to connect with nature, the cultivation of healthy fresh food for student consumption, and the provision of spaces that facilitate a diversity of play are all options. Depending on where you live, this question may be answered quite differently.

On a recent trip to visit school grounds in Germany and England, I was struck by how many leading designers have made private spaces for children a top priority. Through North American eyes, it was a provocative choice. A self-perpetuating fear of liability has made such design choices sadly radical. However, witnessing the outcomes of this design goal—children seeking refuge, engaged in a variety of play experiences and participating in positive social interaction—was undeniably a positive experience for me.

Typically, these private places are pathways, or pockets, separated from busy areas by trees and shrubs. One example of this approach is at the Coombes School in England where a great number of the pathways are almost impassable for adults. Sue Humphries, former headteacher, commented on the design in this way: "The thing that's hardest to reproduce is the sense that you are in the wood. A real wild wood. If you do too much cutting and too much manicuring, you destroy that sense that you're among wild things that have a pattern of their own."

It seems to me that Humphries' point is crucial. In those moments when we realize that nature has a life and structure of its own, independent of the human hand, we are struck with a sense of wonder that begs further inquiry and exploration. It promotes interest in learning and a desire to know the natural world better. In our age, where childhood is predominately lived indoors, we need to carefully consider the design of buildings, landscapes and programs where children play and learn. It is necessary that these environments inspire and nourish an appetite for the natural and for the outdoors.

Consider this interesting footnote in Canadian educational history. Back in 1908, the Province of Ontario's Ministry of Education published a document entitled "Improvement of School Grounds" that reads as follows:

In neglecting so long to beautify schools and their surroundings, the people of Ontario have missed one of the best opportunities of implanting in the minds of the young a love for rural life and the beauties of nature as well as for the order and simple neatness which makes for so much in every day life in either town or country.

Where is the conversation about our "love for rural life" today? It would seem North American society has taken quantum leaps in distancing ourselves from rural life in the past 100 years—fewer personal connections to farms, greater anonymity of the source of the foods on our store shelves, and much less time in contact with the wild areas synonymous with rural life.

One of the most dramatic shifts in modern childhood in North America and many parts of Europe is the loss of freedom. Recent research in the UK by Natural England and the Royal Society for the Protection of Birds painted a dramatic portrait of how much has been lost in just four generations. The research documented the area that each generation of the same family roamed when they were eight years old. The oldest in the survey, great-grandfather George, walked up to six miles away from his home back in 1919, while, in 2007, little Ed was allowed to wander to the end of his block. Wow. It gives support to the idea that children are living under "virtual house arrest", one of Richard Louv's provocative descriptions of modern childhood.

It appears the outcomes of such dramatic loss of freedom are considerable. While the research is still emerging, the signs are clear: impaired social development, skyrocketing rates of childhood obesity, a diminished ability to develop a responsible approach to risk, and greatly reduced contact with the natural world.

The landscapes of childhood leave such deep impressions in our memories—places of refuge, freedom, discovery. Places that presented challenges that provoked a healthy mix of fear and joy. When I reflect back on my own childhood places, I discover key pieces of my identity that were forged by my experience in those early years—an appetite for adventure, a comfort with the unexpected, the creativity to make fun with whatever is at hand. And what was at hand? Nothing special for many of my generation: trees, water, sand, leaves, sticks, mud. But by today's standards, what was previously taken for granted has now become rare. One of the lessons that carries

forward is that modest pockets of nature can offer expansive palettes for play involving the opportunity to manipulate and interact with elements in the natural environment.

Almost 20 years ago, Wendy Titman, in the seminal research document on school grounds, *Special Places, Special People,* brought attention to the idea that a school ground is primarily experienced by a child as an expression of care by those who control the space—their teacher and parents. On a similar note, Alice Waters in her latest book, *The Edible Schoolyard: A Universal Idea,* states, "Beauty is a language: A beautifully prepared environment, where deliberate thought has gone into everything from the garden paths to the plates on the tables, communicates to children that we care about them."

Asphalt to Ecosystems comes at a time when there is unprecedented interest in transforming school grounds. There remains a strong need for practical how-to information that has stood the test of time in what is one of the most challenging public spaces to design. At this time, the vast majority of projects are led and carried out by visionary and motivated parents and teachers. Expertise is strongly needed to help the movement stabilize and mature so that more projects are successful and more schools can improve their outdoor spaces.

I first met Sharon when she came to learn more about school grounds in Toronto in 2001. It was one stop amongst many for her that included Japan, Europe and many locations in the U.S.A. Even at that time, Sharon projected a strong sense of understanding both the challenges and opportunities on school grounds, and her enthusiasm was overflowing. Traveling with her infant daughter at the time, one could tell right away that this work was something she was deeply committed to. That said, Sharon appears most comfortable when her sleeves are rolled up working on one project or another related to the transformation of school grounds. A practical approach is foremost in her mind and that is where this book will inevitably succeed.

Cam Collyer
Director, Toyota Evergreen Learning
Grounds Program, Canada

Preface

A seven-year-old girl stands in a courtyard garden with a paper cup in her hand. The two-story walls of the surrounding classrooms block out the noise from the nearby urban streets and make the courtyard a quiet space for the goats, chickens, and children within. The little girl reaches up into the lush row of fava beans in front of her and carefully removes plump snails from the leaves, placing them into her collecting cup. When the cup has several snails in it, she runs to find one of the black chickens that are contentedly roaming through the straw-covered ground in another part of the garden. A little boy scoops up a chicken in his arms and pets it while the girl feeds the snails she has just captured to the happy bird.

After observing this scene in the spring of 1998 at LeConte Elementary School in Berkeley, California, I walked over to the children to ask them more about what they were doing. The girl explained to me, simply and clearly, that the snails were harming their fava bean crop, so they had to be removed. Although the snails were a problem for the fava beans, the chickens loved to eat them so they were terrific chicken food. She added that her school also took the chicken droppings, composted them, and gave the compost to the soil, helping the fava beans to grow…and she *loved* fava beans so this type of garden work was important. From her explanation, it was obvious that the young girl, growing up in an urban area, clearly understood the complex ecological cycles that connected their tasty fava bean crop to the snails, the chickens, and the soil. This simple but excellent elementary school garden had succeeded in teaching complex, integrated ecological concepts in a manner that young students understood and will remember.

This first exposure to school gardening during graduate school resonated with me on a personal level because I had grown up with a home vegetable garden I enjoyed. It also sparked an ongoing professional interest that I have been exploring ever since. Soon after this experience, I had an opportunity to collaborate with the Ecological Design Institute and a fellow graduate student to lead a student-centered schoolyard design project at Lake Elementary School in San Pablo, California. Later, during my thesis research ("Ecological Schoolyards") for UC Berkeley's Department of Landscape Architecture and Environmental Planning, I was profoundly influenced by the work of Professor John Lyle from the Center for Regenerative Studies at California Polytechnic State University, Pomona.[1] His research examined university-level ecological design curricula and explored ways to make it more relevant to students by turning the campus into a hands-on experimental laboratory for green technologies and organic agriculture. After returning from a visit to the Center for Regenerative Studies, I decided to use my master's thesis to envision what John Lyle's design ideas would look like if applied to K-12 schoolyard campuses.

Over the next year and a half, I visited thirty K-12 schoolyards in California, Colorado, and Oregon that contained gardens, wildlife habitats, water systems, energy systems, and waste processing systems. I studied the ways in which the design of these outdoor learning environments, and the students' participation in the design and stewardship processes, shaped what students learned. At the time, most of these schools had narrowly defined outdoor education projects, generally led by one or two teachers in a single subject area. Paralleling Lyle's framework, my thesis argued that schools should try to broaden what they teach outdoors to show students the relationships among the various ecological systems in their midst. I also added "participatory design" as a key component for creating and sustaining these complex outdoor environments within the context of a K-12 school district.[2]

After completing graduate school in 2000, I was very fortunate to receive a Geraldine Knight Scott Traveling Fellowship from UC Berkeley to continue this research abroad. With this generous funding, I visited another 50 schools in Canada, England, Sweden, Denmark, and Norway in 2001, connecting with like-minded colleagues in each place. Schools in many of these countries have been working on onsite outdoor education projects for far longer than most American schools, and this was a chance to see projects that had matured over 10, 20, or even 30 years. This research also added depth to my conceptual framework for ecological schoolyards. To my previously developed themes of wildlife, water, energy, food, waste cycling and participation, I added green building practices, "creative play," and curriculum integration, equally vital parts of successful ecological schoolyards.

After I returned from my travels, I reconnected with a local organization called the San Francisco Green Schoolyard Alliance (SFGSA). This group of nonprofits and government agencies formed in 2001 to support each other's efforts to make San Francisco's schools a more "fertile" environment for the growing edible garden and nutrition education movements. My research abroad helped to steer this new organization, which had primarily focused on edible school gardens, toward a broader mission to create multifaceted school grounds.

While doing research in Sweden in 2001, I had participated in a wonderful schoolyard conference for teachers and community members that blended hands-on gardening instruction with green building techniques, lectures, workshops, and tours of successful local schoolyard projects. Four schools in the city of Lund in southern Sweden hosted the conference's events, and received the completed workshop products as permanent amenities for their schoolyards. The SFGSA decided to adopt this hands-on conference format as the first collaborative project for their member organizations; I was chosen to direct the event. Our conference was held in October 2002 and brought together individuals, organizations, and resources around the common goal of greening schoolyards in San Francisco. It was a highly successful way to launch the public face of the SFGSA and position the organization within the broader local environmental and education communities. Pleased with the results, the SFGSA asked me to lead a second, similar conference in 2004, and I co-directed their third conference in 2008. Another conference is planned for 2010.

Over the course of the three conferences, we held 55 workshops that trained over 600 people in hands-on techniques and curriculum ideas that they could then bring back to their own schools and neighborhoods. The nine San Francisco schools that hosted the workshops gained built-products from the events: outdoor classroom seating, pollinator gardens, tile mosaics, living willow play areas, solar-powered pond pump systems, an earth oven, recycled concrete retaining walls, small stormwater purification and irrigation systems, fruit trees and other garden features. These small contributions helped to strengthen the growing gardening and outdoor education practices at these schools, and encouraged other schools to follow their example.

In this same time period, I began to work as an independent consultant, helping schools around the San Francisco Bay Area expand their vision of a good schoolyard and connect their existing curricula to their landscape. I also partnered with the Trust for Public Land and other local organizations to lead participatory design projects in several urban schools in Oakland, California.

In 2005, I was hired to help the San Francisco Unified School District (SFUSD) plan their new bond-funded green schoolyard program for 16 elementary schools. I spent the next two years collaborating with the school district's architects and each school's "greening team" to help them imagine their grounds in a new light. At each of the schools, we began with the green schoolyard framework I developed and tailored it to fit their needs. Each project was founded on a participatory design process and structured to gather design ideas and site-specific curriculum connections from teachers, parents, and (when possible) students. All of the resulting schoolyard master plans include key gardening components, shade trees, and outdoor classroom spaces. Many also include wildlife habitat areas, ponds, water systems, solar-powered elements, natural and recycled materials, and artwork.

In 2007 I merged my consulting practice, EcoSchool Design®, with two like-minded colleagues to form a new design firm called Bay Tree Design, inc. (www.baytreedesign.com). Bay Tree Design specializes in ecological design, as it applies to schoolyards, public open spaces, edible landscapes, interpretative gardens, and children's spaces. Our collaborative firm blends environmental planning with landscape architecture, horticulture, and wildlife habitat expertise, which gives us the flexibility to approach each project we work on from a variety of angles.

In 2008, Bay Tree Design collaborated with CONCERN, Inc. and other national organizations based in Washington, DC, to create a model "Sustainable Schoolyard" exhibit at the United States Botanic Garden as part of their *One Planet-Ours!* exhibition. Our living exhibit, on display from May to October 2008, illustrated the ways in which a typical elementary school could use their schoolyard as a rich outdoor classroom for learning and play. It demonstrated the principles of ecological design and urban sustainability by integrating wildlife habitat features, edible gardens, renewable energy, rainwater harvesting, green building materials, student and community participation, creative play elements, and an outdoor classroom space. Components of the display, designed to be re-used after the exhibit ended, were donated to Brent Elementary School in Washington where they became useful elements of a real ecological schoolyard.[3]

At this writing, Bay Tree Design is working with SFUSD to help 27 elementary schools transform their "asphalt into ecosystems" using participatory green schoolyard master planning processes. Our work as "master planning strategists" enables each school to harness its community's creativity, skills, resources, and enthusiasm to create an ecological schoolyard that reflects its unique geographic location, community, ecology, and curricula.

🍃 Vision for this Book

Over the years I have continued to visit schools around the Bay Area and in other cities, such as Boston, Chicago, and Washington, DC, to expand my understanding of best practices for ecological schoolyards and to gather more ideas from successful schoolyard projects. I have also kept in touch with colleagues in Canada, Europe, and Japan and continue to be informed by their excellent work and ongoing research. I have personally visited more than 200 schools in eight countries and interviewed garden coordinators, school faculty, parents and students to understand their projects in detail. I have taken photographs of their work and documented their achievements. Through these experiences, I have gained an understanding of the design principles and programmatic factors that help ecological schoolyard programs succeed and

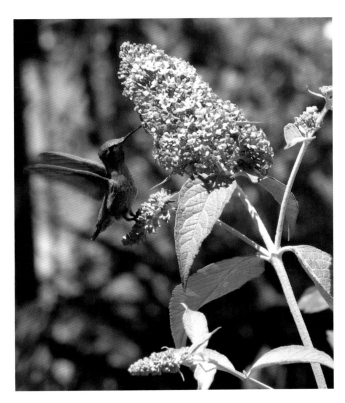

thrive. Now, I'm excited to be able to share this knowledge and experience with you.

This book presents compelling examples from my research and professional experience that I hope you, the reader, will find useful and inspiring. It documents the work of many wise garden coordinators, experienced teachers, dedicated parents, creative students, and other volunteers and professionals. I would like to thank them here for sharing their work with me, so that I can share it with you. As parents, teachers, school principals, school board members, school district staff, and community members interested in helping your local school prosper, I hope this book will lead you on a journey to create a fabulous schoolyard environment of your own. The case studies compiled in these pages demonstrate that all of these things are possible on school grounds, as they illustrate, too, how these rich environments help our children thrive. Visiting green schoolyards is the best way to experience them in action—but this book will give you a taste of that tour without leaving your chair.

1 *Why Transform Traditional Schoolyards?*

🍃 *Natural Systems Are Often Invisible in Today's World*

Most people today live in cities or their extended suburbs, disconnected from the natural systems that sustain us and generally unaware of how these systems function. Our immediate environment is filled with artificial materials and vast amounts of pavement that separate us from natural processes that occur all around us. For example, rainwater that falls in our schoolyards and neighborhoods is channeled into underground pipes that remove it from our view and make it inaccessible to plants almost as soon as it hits the ground. Local wildlife populations have been pushed to the edges of our communities and forced to make due with smaller and smaller habitat patches.

How did vital natural systems like these get so marginalized? Where are we headed if we maintain the current course? What can we do, on an individual and community-wide level, to change the ways we impact the surrounding environment? The answers to these questions are complex and multifaceted. It is clear, however, that we are now at an ecological turning point. We must begin to address these types of questions in fundamental ways.

Ecological schoolyards provide opportunities for students to build awareness about local ecology and their own neighborhoods. They help children notice the birds in the city, the butterflies that visit their flower gardens, the patterns falling rain makes on the soil. Green schoolyards help students mark seasonal changes with the turning of leaves in the fall, the migrations of wildlife, and the length of shadows on the ground, and, in so doing, make them better readers of their surroundings. Instead of learning about these natural processes from abstract descriptions in textbooks read in indoor classrooms, children experience them directly while getting their hands dirty to help improve their own environment. Many excellent, low-cost educational resources sit right outside the school doors, waiting to be tapped.

The green schoolyard movement addresses important environmental issues in ways that even young children can understand and participate in, enabling them to change their own corner of the world. While their individual actions may be small, together these projects can fundamentally improve the local environment and profoundly change the way that students experience the world.

🍃 *Schoolyards Are Uniquely Positioned*

Because they are responsible for educating our society's future leaders, schools are an ideal place to start this process of environmental renewal. When ecological schoolyards are incorporated into a school's curriculum, allowing children to make the connection between themselves and local natural systems, students learn that they have an impact on their environment and have opportunities to heal it.

Schoolyards are also an ideal place to address environmental issues because they are large public spaces with well-defined, dedicated communities of adults and children. They are found in almost every city and town, large or small, around the world. Schoolyards are conveniently located for use as outdoor classrooms and often function as public meeting places or parks after hours. These educational and social spaces provide good venues for the discussion and practice of ecological design concepts in which the wider community can observe and interact.

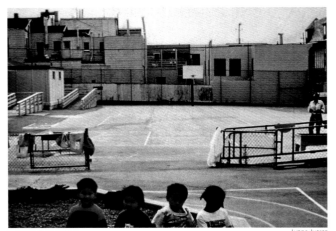

Ecological Schoolyards Address the Shortcomings of Traditional Design Patterns

Many ordinary schoolyards are characte2rized by a fairly predictable pattern of wide asphalt surfaces, large sports fields, and uninspiring commercial play equipment. Occasional trees sometimes dot the corners or edges of the playground, and foundation plantings of nondescript shrubs typically hug the buildings. A schoolyard found in New Jersey looks very much like a schoolyard in Ohio, Kansas, or California, despite the differences in climate, local history, and context. These types of schoolyards are ubiquitous, but are they really serving their communities well?

These common playground patterns—developed to promote organized sports games, regulate climbing "challenges," and minimize maintenance—offer few creative play spaces,

FIGURES 1.1 and 1.2 *These two photographs of Tule Elk Park Child Development Center in San Francisco, California, taken in 1991 and 2007 from a similar perspective, capture the degree of schoolyard transformation that is possible.*[1]

Lynne Juarez

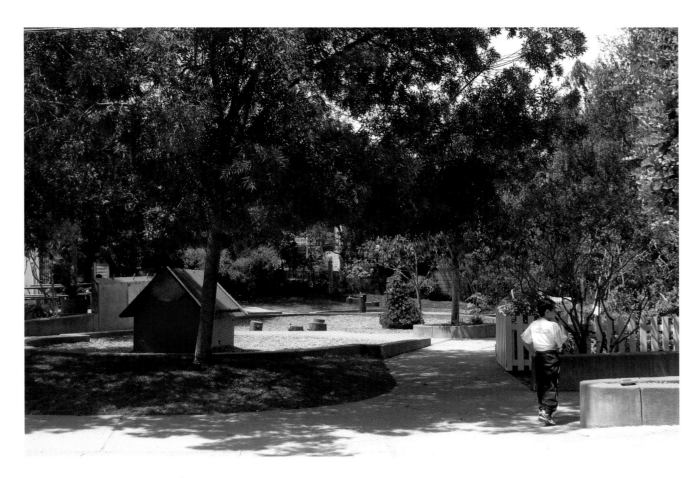

don't pique students' curiosity, and don't entertain children for very long. They can be problematic for local ecology, reducing rainwater infiltration, offering little wildlife habitat value, and relying on chemical inputs to maintain the grounds. Typical schoolyards have very little to add to academic lessons and frequently lack places where children and adults can sit quietly to talk to friends or colleagues. Many schoolyards are uncomfortable, providing little protection from the wind, sun, and rain. These spaces fall short of their potential, but most children and their school communities don't even know what they are missing. The fascinating ecology of their own neighborhoods has been hidden from them, robbing them of the wonder that might be kindled by a richer, more nuanced environment.

Ecological schoolyards however, are place-based so each one is unique and memorable. The trees and vegetation on green school grounds provide a variety of microclimates that make them more comfortable and inviting than ordinary schoolyard environments. They balance ball game areas and play structures with features that encourage imaginative play and self-expression, so children have many activities to choose from at recess. Their varied grounds are also ideally suited for lessons across the curriculum.

So, what does it mean, exactly, for a school to transform its grounds from a traditional arrangement into an ecological schoolyard? This paradigm shift has broad implications for topics from environmental sustainability, health, and maintenance to learning, play, and comfort.

Environmental sustainability

Many schools transform their traditional grounds into ecological oases with rich wildlife habitat, rainwater purification and storage capacity, the ability to treat greywater and blackwater flows from school buildings, and energy conservation and production capacity. Green schoolyards can also treat waste as a resource, produce some food for onsite consumption, and show students how all of these processes work. These experiences collectively teach students about ecological design and introduce environmental sustainability themes into their developing world view.

Variety

Traditional schoolyards are one-dimensional environments, geared almost entirely toward organized games and repetitive, physical play on climbing structures. They are generally the same from day to day, with little variation throughout the year. In green schoolyards, by contrast, ball games and play structures are complemented by a diverse range of other activities, from imaginative play to art projects. These activities occur in an ever-changing visual landscape that is designed to be continually growing, blooming, and shifting in some way. The seasons are often marked with plants that display spring flowers, summer greenery, fall color, and winter dormancy. These multilayered, nuanced environments attract birds, butterflies, and other wildlife that add interest and keep children engaged in their surroundings.

Educational value

Traditional schoolyards are not designed with outdoor education in mind, and are generally not conducive to outdoor instruction in their unaltered form. Most have limited seating, and it is likely to be lined up along a fence so children can observe athletic games, rather than grouped to facilitate conversation. Teaching props are also usually limited to occasional painted maps, number lines, or alphabets on the ground. These are useful items, but they are not very flexible or widely applicable on their own.

A well-designed ecological schoolyard is a valuable asset for teaching and learning. The varied plantings, topography, natural materials, and imbedded teaching resources in green schoolyards make these dynamic environments applicable to various grade levels and subjects—from science, math and history to language instruction, music and art. Many schools also teach nutrition, cooking, social studies, drama, renewable energy topics, and other subjects in their green schoolyard. To make outdoor lessons more effective and comfortable, schools frequently create special gathering places that allow small groups or an entire class to sit together.

Play value and behavior patterns

Most traditional schoolyards are designed to facilitate active play through adult-directed games with rules and physical play on climbing equipment. While these schoolyards generally meet the needs of physical education classes and provide some activities that children enjoy at recess, they do not satisfy the play needs of all of the children, all of the time. In recent years, climbing structures have also become increasingly limited, as a school's choices are constrained by ever changing safety regulations and fear of liability. At best, the resulting climbing apparatuses meet the physical play needs of the youngest children on the playground, leaving the older children without challenging play options. Most traditional schoolyards also lack features that encourage children to play imaginatively. Their fairly predictable layout and uninspiring asphalt and turf play surfaces do not create a sense of adventure or mystery that can be found in play spaces that are far less uniform.

Ecological schoolyards seek to balance space for traditional ball games and climbing structures with other play options that give children more control over their free time. They are wonderful places for student-directed, unstructured creative play. For young children, simple elements such as pinecones, leaves, twigs, or wood mulch on a garden floor can become play props that help to spur creative games.[2] In exploring an enriched schoolyard, children do not have to be asked to exercise. They simply see pathways before them and decide to run through them. If they find boulders in their environment, they will climb them so they may jump off onto the surrounding soft mulch. Children will hop and run and skip and jump if there are interesting places in the schoolyard to do these things, and if school rules do not prevent them from getting this exercise.

Research literature suggests that schoolyard "nature play" areas encourage collaborative and cooperative play, while also reducing aggression that often occurs on traditional playgrounds.[3] Along these lines, author Richard Louv has stated that if we want to end bullying at school, all schools should have green schoolyards.[4] Louv argues that traditional schoolyards, with their emphasis primarily on competitive sports and athletic ability, reward students who are the strongest and fastest and allow them to rise to the top of the playground social hierarchy. Their physical dominance seems to lend itself to bullying and other types of playground aggression in environments dominated by asphalt and playfields.[5] Authors Robin Moore and Wendy Titman also link aggression with barren asphalt-covered playgrounds.[6] My own anecdotal playground observations are consistent with their findings. I have observed that many children seem bored on asphalt playgrounds because they have limited play options. Perhaps bored children are more prone to cause trouble as a way to amuse themselves or add variety to their "play."

By contrast, the leaders who rise to the top of the playground social hierarchy in a green schoolyard or natural play environment, argues Louv, are typically those who are the smartest and most creative. These children make up games that engage other children and often encourage cooperative and collaborative interactions, completely changing the dominant dynamic in a play space. This finding suggests that the best way to end bullying may be to disempower the bullies by changing the physical and, thus, social landscape.[7]

Health

Standard schoolyards, designed to promote healthy physical activity through sports, may undermine health in other ways. With uninterrupted fields of pavement and grass, traditional schoolyards provide very little protection from the sun, exposing children to the harmful effects of ultraviolet rays as they play outside every day. In Canada, Australia, and many other places, this health concern is taken much more seriously that it generally has been to date in the United States. Green schoolyards in these countries often sport leafy green tree canopies, wide shade sails, and other shade structures that are specifically placed to help protect children from a higher lifetime risk of skin cancer.[8]

Asphalt and concrete surfaces in traditional schoolyards are also the source of many "knock and bump" injuries that result when children fall on the ground as they play. Research in Canada by Professor Janet Dyment suggests that green schoolyards are safer in this respect than traditional schoolyards because they tend to have more surface area covered by soft ground materials such as wood chips, sand, and grass, which result in fewer scrapes and bruises when children fall.[9]

In some green schoolyards, health is also actively promoted by including organic gardens with edible plants and tying the school's nutrition curriculum to hands-on outdoor lessons. When students cook and eat the vegetables and fruits they grow onsite, healthy eating patterns are reinforced.

Many green schoolyards are also managed organically or follow Integrated Pest Management (IPM) protocols, which reduce children's exposure to poisons such as pesticides, herbicides, and fungicides. Similarly, many of these schools avoid using pressure treated lumber and other materials that are potentially harmful to children's health and the environment. (See chapter 8 for more information on green materials.)

The increased vegetation and nature play in green school-yards, however, also have some potential health concerns that should be considered, including bee stings, allergies, and water safety issues.[10] Each of these concerns can be moderated by thoughtful design that, for example, places bee-attracting garbage cans away from children's play areas, selects plants that are not prolific pollen producers, and keeps ponds shallow.

Appearance

The land around a school building is the first thing that neighbors and visitors see when they visit a school. Most school districts feel that it is important to have a uniform "neat and clean" look, with good "curb appeal" to keep neighborhood residents and parents happy. Their vision of good curb appeal generally relies on the American suburban ideal of manicured lawns, accompanied by simple foundation plantings and a few trees.

Environments like these come at a social and environmental cost. They provide little enrichment for learning or play, and fail to reflect the local region or culture. In many school districts, these planted landscapes are heavily treated with herbicides, pesticides, and fungicides to keep them looking their "best," with the least effort. Such practices put harmful chemicals in close proximity to children, who like to explore these plantings on their hands and knees.

Schools can choose to modify their appearance to address the social and environmental shortcomings of the traditional approach while still retaining good curb appeal. There are many aesthetics that are "appropriate" for school perimeters, and it is important to find the right one for each school and its community. When developing the curb appeal aesthetic for a new green schoolyard project, consider questions like these: What is the existing perimeter landscape doing for the school now? What does it say about the school, and how can it project a message that is consistent with the school community's goals and identity?

If they are designed with multiple purposes in mind, highly visible spaces on school grounds can be aesthetically pleasing and useful at the same time. Perhaps the front of the school can be landscaped with flowering native plants that serve the science curriculum while also providing wildlife habitat. Native plants can be grown without the use of chemicals and, if well chosen, will use substantially less irrigation than typical lawn plantings. The addition of attractive fencing, seating, and other site furniture will "frame" the space, reinforce the appeal of the plantings, and welcome visitors to the site.

Community stewardship as the new primary maintenance model

An important benefit of the traditional "asphalt and lawn" schoolyard design model is that it simplifies maintenance tasks, which allows school districts to hire very few people to care for their overwhelmingly vast holdings. Paved asphalt playgrounds, free from vehicle traffic, require very little maintenance for decades. Large, open lawns require regular mowing, fertilization, and watering, but can be cared for by relatively inexpensive, minimally trained grounds-keeping staff. Foundation shrubs and sparse tree plantings also mean that there are few hedges to trim and a minimum amount of leaves to pick up in the fall. These are positive attributes for facilities departments, whose budgets are slashed regularly in many cities.

While it is true that almost any schoolyard configuration that does not rely on asphalt and lawn will be more work to maintain, substantial benefits for education and recreation make the extra work worthwhile. The solution is to distribute the responsibility for the increased maintenance to a wider network of people. In the traditional situation where the district is responsible for all of the landscape work on a school site, it is understandable that they would not be enthusiastic about increasing their responsibilities. If maintenance plans are approached as issues of "stewardship," instead, it is quite possible to empower children, teachers, and families to take on a portion of the increased work load. For example, areas of the schoolyard that are developed into outdoor classroom spaces with living gardens may be maintained, at least in part, by the classes that use them. Monthly or quarterly work parties, organized by the PTA, can accomplish larger tasks and help construct new focal points in the landscape. PTA groups may also decide to raise a small amount of money to hire their own supplemental specialty gardener to work a few hours each week to keep the yard looking its best. Other schools hire a garden educator who leads outdoor gardening classes and helps to maintain a portion of the grounds.

The keys to generating the level of community support that is necessary to maintain a schoolyard collaboratively are (1) broad community participation from the beginning and (2) designing and building the green schoolyard with teachers, parents, and students. It takes time to "grow" community "ownership" for a project, and that doesn't happen overnight. To maintain consistent participation and ongoing interest in the project, the school community should add new features to the yard each year, ensuring that it is never "finished." (See chapter 2 for more detailed coverage of this important topic.)

Sustained fundraising

Unlike traditional schoolyards that are built entirely from durable components, intended to last decades, green schoolyards often include components made from natural materials that are *designed* to wear out over time, allowing new members of the community to add their own "stamp" to the yard as the years pass. This phased construction and rebuilding philosophy means that green schoolyards will always need at least a small amount of funding on an annual basis to replace items that wear out and to add new elements. It is a good idea for the school's PTA to make a small annual financial allocation for this purpose. With community involvement, however, even small amounts of funding will go quite far as funds can be used primarily for purchasing building materials, plants, and other supplies, rather than paying for costly labor. Many school communities identify local businesses who donate plants, logs, lumber, boulders, mulch, and other simple building materials as they are needed.

Curriculum integration and use of the resources onsite

Ecological schoolyards provide valuable outdoor learning experiences for almost every subject taught at the school. However, they will only be able to reach their full educational potential if many teachers are interested in and involved with the project. Addressing this issue begins with ensuring that elements built in the green schoolyard are items that teachers want and need, and that a core group of teachers remain involved in the project as it develops over time.

Many teachers appreciate formal support and training to make the leap from teaching inside the classroom to outside in the schoolyard. Training can help teachers feel more confident about managing their class outside, and ensure that they are deeply familiar with the educational resources embedded in the schoolyard design.[11] One school I visited in Colorado commissioned an experienced teacher to write a handbook for their teaching staff to connect the particular plants and resources in their own schoolyard with the curriculum standards for each grade level. In California, the San Francisco Green Schoolyard Alliance and its partner organizations offer a variety of classes and conferences for teachers that encourage them to bring what they are already teaching outside. Numerous books and other written materials are also available to help teachers around the country make these connections so they, and their students, can make the most of their onsite resources.

Meeting needs of physical education classes

Another issue for many schools and districts is the desire to provide students with places to play organized sports and ball games, and designated space for physical education classes. These types of activities are extremely space intensive while only serving a small number of students at a time and filling a relatively small niche within the school as a whole. Meeting these needs on a small school site can be quite a challenge, even without the addition of green schoolyard features.

The green schoolyard design process involves asking the community to consider what they really need from their limited space, and finding ways to make each part of the yard serve multiple purposes. For example, a par course might be dispersed within the framework of a green schoolyard's nature play setting, or a school might choose to use ball courts that are smaller than regulation size or divide ball courts into half-courts. Because green schoolyards generally use the whole school site all the way out to the edges and disperse some of the active play features throughout the grounds, the overall result allows children to play in many more places and use the yard more effectively for physical education and recess than they can in traditional schoolyard layouts.

Liability and safety

Liability and safety are important issues for many schools and districts. School districts, large and small, generally feel comfortable purchasing commercial play structures because they already meet national safety standards. This arrangement also means that there is a clear corporate entity to share the legal liability, and potential legal cost, in the case of an injury on school grounds. However, it's important to remember that *safety and liability are not the same thing*—and play structures that are considered "risk free" by adults may not be meeting children's needs or holding their interest.

American culture is unusually obsessed with playground liability—in a manner that seems to be far out of proportion to actual risk of injury. Other countries around the world that value personal responsibility for one's actions see mild physical risk as a manageable and necessary part of healthy childhood play and development. Liability concerns and a sense of appropriate risk also vary by community within the United States. For example, some municipalities see shallow schoolyard ponds as safety demonstrations while others see only drowning potential.

Unusual schoolyard designs are not inherently more dangerous than asphalt and play structure paradigms, they are just a bit more complex to evaluate. Nature play environments can be designed to encourage imaginative play as well as safe, exciting physical play opportunities for all ability levels. Safety and liability issues are best discussed with the school community so that the group can agree on an acceptable level of perceived risk. Once a project has broad community support, it is generally easier for a school district to allow a school to try something new.

Vandalism and crime prevention

Vandalism is present on many school grounds, whether or not they green their schoolyard. As a green schoolyard project begins, it may be initially susceptible to damage as neighborhood vandals test the durability of new features on the yard. In some cases, they may be deterred if the community responds by quickly fixing the damage, as is usually recommended in the case of graffiti. It is a good idea for green schoolyards to have a small budget for paint, replacement plants, and other things that might be needed to make small, timely repairs that are due to vandalism or other types of wear and tear.

Increased community involvement and a sense of ownership for a schoolyard sometimes bring the school more respect in the eyes of bored neighborhood teenagers who might be tempted to harm school property. If they know that their parents and siblings are involved in a project, the potential vandals may be less likely to damage the school. Walls that are covered with tile mosaics, murals, or green plants also seem to

be less prone to graffiti than walls painted a solid color, which can beckon graffiti artists like a blank canvas.

In my experience, locking a green schoolyard or garden does not seem to improve its safety from vandalism. If anything, it may increase it by presenting an enticing challenge to teenagers looking for something to do. Once they gain entry to a forbidden space, they seem to feel a need to break something to prove they were there. To encourage more positive

FIGURE 1.3 *The garden gate at Cobb School in San Francisco connects Wallace Stegner's perspective to the school garden's rationale.*

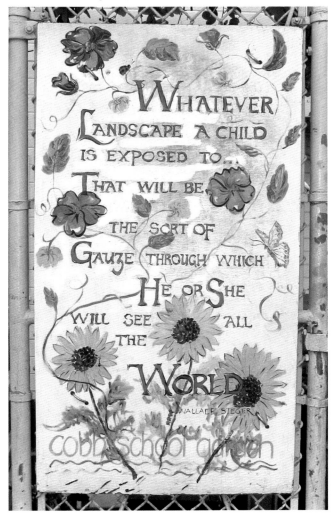

behavior, I encourage schools to welcome neighborhood children, and the rest of the community, into their yard when school is not in session by using signage that encourages visitors to enjoy themselves while also asking them to "please respect the students' work."

Well-Designed Ecological Schoolyards are Valuable Assets that Inspire Children

Ecological schoolyards may take many forms and are as different as the schools they serve. They create unique environments that speak to the school's local context. They help "repair" schoolyard ecology by restoring some of the natural diversity and ecological function that once existed before the school was built. They use native plant species to provide habitat for local birds, pollinating insects, and other wildlife. Areas freed of pavement once again allow rainwater to soak into the ground, recharging the ground water table.

Some ecological schoolyards display art installations and other design elements to reflect local history and culture. Well-designed green schoolyards present these themes in ways that students can interact with and appreciate. Children pick up on these small design details and the level of care that adults give to their school. They use this information to help form their view of themselves and to shape how they identify with their "place." Author Wendy Titman refers to this phenomenon as the "hidden curriculum" that is present on school grounds and councils that adults should pay much more attention to the subconscious messages we convey to children through the spatial design and maintenance of their environments.[12] Renowned environmentalist Wallace Stegner once expressed a similar philosophy saying, "Whatever landscape a child is exposed to early on, that will be the sort of gauze through which he or she will see all the world afterwards."[13] (Figure 1.3 on the previous page)

Schoolyard landscapes may be shaped into almost any form that is desired by a creative and passionate school community. Ecological schoolyards bring teachers, parents, students, and other stakeholders together to transform schoolyard asphalt into living ecosystems, in a process that strengthens social bonds, fosters biological diversity, provides educational resources, improves ecological functions, and makes the schoolyard enjoyable. Why would we settle for anything less?

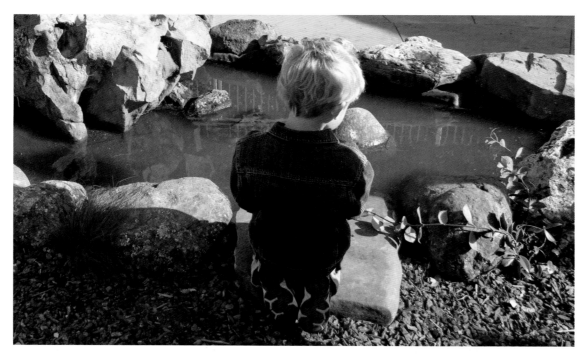

FIGURE 1.4
The pond at Rosa Parks School in Berkeley, California, is a lovely place for children to relax and to look for fish.

2 Project Launch:
Designing Your Dream Schoolyard and Building the School Community to Make It Happen

How do Ecological Schoolyards Come About?

Green schoolyard projects spring forth at schools around the world in a wide variety of ways. On my travels to over 175 schools in seven countries during the last ten years, I spoke with green schoolyard project leaders, garden coordinators, school principals, and others to find out how they began their work and what keeps their projects going over time. Their answers were varied, but a few patterns emerged.

Sometimes green schoolyards start with a modest project idea, like a small garden, that is developed and built by an individual teacher, parent, or principal and connected to the curriculum. When others at the school see that the project is interesting and effective, it gains momentum and grows as they join in the fun. These projects are usually funded by the school community or through small grants.

In other cases, schoolyard renovations may be started by the school or district in response to needed repairs or modernization work. Preparations for this work sometimes launch a discussion about how best to renew the grounds, allowing green schoolyard themes to enter the conversation. For example, schools preparing to repave their playground may decide to remove some of the asphalt in order to add plantings and outdoor classroom space. This type of project sometimes receives a portion of the renovation funding.

Ecological schoolyard projects may also be initiated by outside groups, such as nonprofits or government agencies, seeking to promote a particular agenda that is in line with their own work—wildlife habitat, stormwater management, renewable energy generation, edible gardening—particularly where these topics intersect with larger urban planning issues. The community group that initiates this type of project may also fund it.

Successful, Long-Lasting, Ecological Schoolyard Programs Start with Community Building and a Master Plan

The design and implementation of a successful green schoolyard is an ongoing, iterative process with many steps that are best accomplished over a number of years. The most effective approach to create a sustainable, large-scale green schoolyard project is to follow a comprehensive, participatory planning process that includes all of the potential stakeholders, to produce a master plan drawing (map) that illustrates the community's consensus about the schoolyard's future.

The process of creating a schoolyard master plan is as important as the product, because it draws the community together around the common goal of developing the yard and helps them take "ownership" of the project. Ecological schoolyard environments may be quite elaborate and often need dedicated, ongoing stewardship. If the schoolyard design is created with widespread community involvement, the school community will frequently volunteer to take responsibility for its development and maintenance. Projects that don't foster community ownership at the outset have a hard time getting parents and teachers involved at a later date, so they often end up underutilized and generally require paid staff to keep them well maintained.

Green schoolyard master plans should be thought of as living documents—intended to illustrate a community's consensus about the general direction for their schoolyard project as it develops over time, while leaving the details open to interpretation as each phase of the project is constructed. School communities are inherently dynamic. Teachers, principals, and other school staff come and go through the years as their careers develop, and students continually grow older and "age out" of the school, making room for new staff and students each fall. Curriculum standards, teaching methods, and school budgets also shift over time, changing the school's internal priorities and budget allocations from year to year. Because green schoolyards exist amidst this ever-changing social landscape, they should always be considered works in progress

and allowed to continually adapt to the shifting needs of their resident populations.

🌿 Who Should Be Included?

Students, teachers, school staff, custodians, administrators, parents, family members, and neighbors are all schoolyard

---

🌿 Rules of Thumb for Starting and Sustaining Green Schoolyards

The following general, and essential, rules of thumb will help you get your green schoolyard off the ground and set it up for long term success. If you follow these principles, I guarantee the project will run more smoothly.

1. *Start with buy-in from the principal.* If the principal is enthusiastic about the green schoolyard, things will generally proceed efficiently: he/she can ask teachers to participate and give students permission to engage in the design process. If you want to start a green schoolyard project at a school with a reluctant principal, "make the case" by introducing examples of successful projects that are similar to what you wish to create, or show him/her resources such as this book.

2. *Form a green schoolyard committee to oversee the project's development.* Creating a green schoolyard is a time intensive project. It is definitely too much work for one individual to take on alone for any length of time, and requires community support to move forward. A green schoolyard committee should include parents/family members, teachers, and other stakeholders who are in direct communication with the principal. When the committee has formed, assess the group's skills to understand what the group is realistically capable of—and what kinds of skill sets are still needed to make the project successful. For example, the committee should have a well-organized leader, at least one person who likes to build things, at least one person who is knowledgeable about local horticulture, and at least one teacher who can help connect the schoolyard to the curricula.

3. *Discuss new ideas with the school faculty before engaging parents.* School faculty members spend all day at school. They should have input on what will happen to their work and teaching environments before parents are consulted. Their help is also needed to make the most of the yard's educational features.

4. *Make initial inquiries to the school district to see what's possible.* It is useful to get a feel for the school district's flexibility before moving too far into the design process. The principal can often suggest the best way to proceed and whom to contact first to ensure success. If the district is reluctant to support a large schoolyard renovation, ask to start with a small project to demonstrate that your group is capable and follows through well, before taking on larger tasks.

5. *Allow enough time to give careful thought to your schoolyard master plan.* Most schoolyard design processes take one or two semesters to complete. Public meetings with parents and teachers proceed about once a month over the course of the school year—with time in between spent gathering the community, conducting related research, sketching out ideas, and reviewing the plans.

6. *Allow project participants to "get their hands dirty" as soon as possible.* It is often hard for enthusiastic parents and teachers to wait a semester or more to start working on the schoolyard. Understandably, they want to see change happening before their eyes while they talk about it more abstractly at community meetings. Encourage them to develop small, portable, or temporary projects that improve the schoolyard. For example, adding

---

stakeholders. They are the main users of the school site, and I also consider them the central creative forces in green schoolyard projects. Due to their close familiarity with the site, they also understand the schoolyard's microclimates and pros and cons of how the space is currently being used.

The school principal is vital to the ecological schoolyard design process. He/she sets the tone for the project, engages the school's faculty, and carves out time for the students to participate in the design, construction, and ongoing site stewardship.

It is wise to invite school district officials, such as facilities department staff, into the discussion from the beginning so the project develops within their permitted guidelines. If district officials understand the green schoolyard's goals, and see that the community is engaged in the project, they will

large pots with mature plants, portable play houses, or moveable benches to the yard quickly improves its appeal and function, but their position can be shifted as the project develops.

7. *Dream big, but start small. Plan to implement the project slowly, over time.* Set short- and long-term goals for the green schoolyard. Allow the project to grow at a manageable speed by completing one task each semester. Fully finish each project that you start, and "make it shine" so the whole community is proud of it. Working at a measured pace will allow teachers to incorporate new projects into their curriculum, give the community time to learn how to properly maintain the yard, and keep fundraising needs manageable. It may also inspire other school community members to join the committee.

8. *Thoroughly document the design, construction, and stewardship process.* A community design process is an important milestone in a schoolyard's development. Since the community changes over time, and not everyone at the school can be involved in it consistently, document each step in the process and display your progress prominently for all to see. Photographs and written descriptions of the project are also very useful for raising money to support the project's implementation.

9. *Institutionalize the green schoolyard program.* Create a support network at the school that will keep things going year after year. The Green Schoolyard Committee is the center of this network, but it should extend to include other members of the school community and neighborhood.

10. *Never "finish."* Because school communities are constantly in flux, it is very important to keep the *current* community actively involved. A master plan creates a framework that allows project participants to continually add to the site over time, fostering a sense of "ownership" for the yard and allowing it to grow and change as needed. Continued project growth keeps the green schoolyard alive, maintains the community's interest, and deters vandalism. Schools that green their grounds all at once and then pronounce the project "finished" often have a much harder time sustaining their living schoolyard over the years—particularly after the last of the project's creators have left the school. This is quite a different concept from a traditional schoolyard or park design process that seeks to complete a permanent installation as quickly as possible and leaves it unchanged for 20–30 years.

11. *Plan for stewardship from the beginning.* Green schoolyards involve more maintenance than asphalt and lawn, so it is important to plan for that added maintenance from the very beginning. Think of green schoolyard maintenance as "stewardship" and empower students, teachers, and family members to be primary caretakers for the yard. If groundskeepers are involved, make sure they feel supported and are trained in any special tasks the site requires.

12. *Raise money* to start the project and work to secure a consistent funding source to support ongoing maintenance and expansion efforts.

13. *Do not give up.* Be persistent, flexible, and creative.

be more likely to approve designs that fall outside traditional approaches. Working closely with the school district also will improve communication about schoolyard maintenance and help the community and district reach agreement about how they can each ensure the project's success.

School communities often engage professionals to help them move through the design process more smoothly. Urban planners, landscape architects, and architects hired by the school may act as consensus builders or translators, transforming the school community's verbal discussions into master plans and illustrative drawings of the desired physical changes to the schoolyard. These designers help schools make specific decisions about their implementation priorities, the size and shape of each element in the master plan, and which construction materials and methods to use. Licensed landscape architects may create plans for irrigation, grading, and drainage, and advise schools on plant selection. They can also ensure that the planned schoolyard improvements comply with federal requirements for disabled access, playground safety standards, building codes, and other school district standards.

Participatory Schoolyard Design

There are many ways to lead a successful schoolyard design process, and I have experimented with various methods to engage school communities over the years. Because each school is different, it is important to make sure the process is flexible. If one approach doesn't work, try another. For example, some schools choose to include students in the design process, while others don't have time to take their students out of class to participate. In some schools, many faculty members collaborate on the green schoolyard's development and want schoolyard elements to be tailored to their curricula. At others the process is led by parents focused on improving play options for their children. All of these social configurations can be successful, but the goal is to involve as many people as possible over the duration of the project, and to aim for an end product that is multifaceted so it will continue to engage and delight the school community for many years to come.

When I lead schoolyard design processes, I feel that my primary role is to act as a catalyst—harnessing the creative ideas, site-specific curriculum, and talents of the school community to help them create a schoolyard design that better

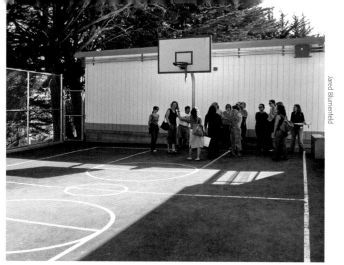

FIGURE 2.1 *The school principal and Sharon Danks lead a group of parents and teachers on a site walk at Rooftop School in San Francisco, California, to evaluate each part of the yard for its "greening" potential.*

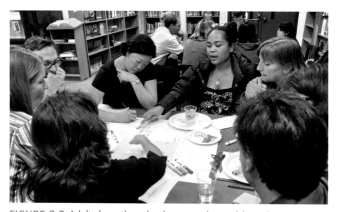

FIGURE 2.2 *Adults from the school community participate in a design workshop at Grattan School in San Francisco, California.*

serves the learning and play needs of their students, and makes their yard comfortable and ecologically-sound. I feel that the central goals of a green schoolyard design process should be (1) to create a Green Schoolyard Master Plan (schoolyard map and short written description) that communicates the direction that future schoolyard improvement projects will take, and (2) to engage teachers, students, and family members in this process so that they will actively support, use, and maintain the schoolyard improvements as they are built in the coming years. To accomplish these goals, I use the approach below.[1]

STEP 1: *Project kick-off and research*

The first phase of the schoolyard master planning process usually includes three components that ensure that all necessary information about the site and the school community is gathered and that a core group of supporters is formed.

- The project organizer convenes an initial set of meetings with the principal, teachers, parents/family members, and students to introduce them to the wide range of green schoolyard possibilities. I accomplish this step using a slideshow of successful projects to help the group "think outside the box" and expand their knowledge about what's possible. (This book could be shown to the school community for that purpose, too.) At this stage, the stakeholders should write a mission statement for their green schoolyard, develop goals, and create a list of schoolyard design features they would like to add to their grounds.

- A Green Schoolyard Committee, composed of key stakeholders, should be established to spearhead the development and future stewardship of the green schoolyard.

- The project organizer, a design professional, and/or members of the Green Schoolyard Committee should conduct site research to explore the schoolyard's existing physical conditions such as sunlight, wind, water availability, and other factors, and gain a detailed understanding of how the school community currently uses the grounds. (Figure 2.1) There are also many rich educational opportunities for students if they take part in this research. (See sidebar, page 19.)

STEP 2: *Design workshops*

After the school community is engaged in this project and site analysis research is complete, the next step is design. I recommend scheduling one design workshop for parents and teachers, and at least one other workshop for a group of 30 students, selected to include representatives from each class. At these workshops, participants work in small groups to explore their ideas for the schoolyard. They apply the goals, objectives, and list of site features they brainstormed earlier in the design process by drawing these concepts onto maps of the grounds. After each small group has created their own draft site plan, they then share their ideas with each other and begin to explore the pros and cons of each potential spatial arrangement. (Figure 2.2) Children's design workshops are typically shorter but may follow a similar pattern, as described later in the chapter. (See sidebar, page 19.)

STEP 3: *Master plan*

After the workshop(s), the project organizer/designer reviews the school community's drawings to distill their overall themes and understand what the school community envisions for each area of the schoolyard. Next, these ideas are combined into a draft master plan for the school grounds. The school community then reviews the master plan and discusses potential alternate design options. The final master plan is usually approved by the principal and school community after several rounds of review and revision. The level of detail in a master plan drawing is usually sufficient to show the location and approximate size and shape of the project elements, and indicates some basic material choices if they are known, but it is not detailed enough to use for construction. (Figure 2.3 on the next page)

STEP 4: *Green schoolyard implementation planning*

With a completed master plan in hand, the school community is ready to discuss their priorities for implementing the plan and to select their first project. Schools often choose to divide their master plans into phases to manage costs, maximize the community's participation, and allow time to realize each step creatively and thoughtfully. This is also a good time to explore fundraising opportunities and plan for future maintenance needs.

STEP 5: *Design development and construction document preparation*

With the first project chosen, it is time to make decisions about the size and shape of each element that will be built, and to select which construction materials and methods to use. Many schools choose to maximize the impact of their scarce funding resources by opting to build and plant the simplest parts of the green schoolyard themselves. This is often feasible and desirable for small- to medium-scale parts of the project and may use a "design-build" method that allows volunteers to work out the project's details as they install them.

If the initial building phase will be extensive or complex, requires precision, or involves the use of heavy machinery or skilled labor, it is wise to employ a professional contractor to implement those portions of the project. Professional contractors need detailed construction drawings, created by licensed landscape architects or architects, to guide them in their work. These technical drawings show the exact locations of project

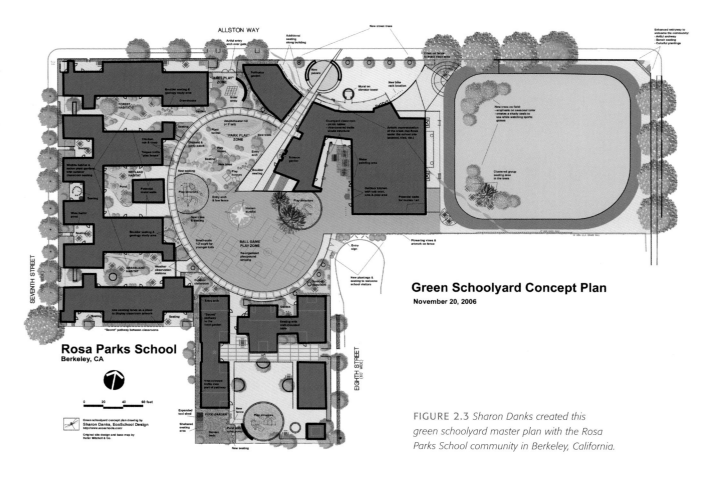

ALLSTON WAY

SEVENTH STREET

EIGHTH STREET

Rosa Parks School
Berkeley, CA

0   20   40   60 feet

Green schoolyard concept plan drawing by
Sharon Danks, EcoSchool Design
http://www.ecoschools.com/

Original site design and base map by
Keller Mitchell & Co.

Green Schoolyard Concept Plan
November 20, 2006

FIGURE 2.3 *Sharon Danks created this green schoolyard master plan with the Rosa Parks School community in Berkeley, California.*

elements and how those elements are built and/or installed. Construction documents typically include drawings such as a precise layout plan; a grading and drainage plan; a planting plan; and any necessary design details required to construct special elements such as ponds, benches, or outdoor classroom spaces. Many school districts and permitting agencies also require construction drawings before they grant approval to begin a major construction project.

STEP 6: *Construction management*

Additional professional oversight, beyond the original set of working drawings, is often required during construction whether the project is built by contractors or on community workdays. Sometimes a portion of the design is changed during construction in response to something unforeseen during the design process—unmapped underground utilities, for example, or changes in the budget that occur during the course of the

project. Having a design professional to oversee the construction process may eliminate costly mistakes or miscommunications.

STEP 7: *Repeat*

After the first project is finished, revisit the master plan and start planning the next phase of the green schoolyard's implementation (Step 5). Repeat each year, adding depth and detail to the yard.

Trying a Schoolyard Design Process without Professional Help

Some schools choose to work on their design process without outside professional assistance if their budgets are low or if their green schoolyard project is not very large, complex, or technical. It is more challenging to run a project this way, without someone being paid to coordinate it, but it is possible.

If this is the course you prefer, try to follow the steps described above: seek permission from the principal, gather your team of school stakeholders, begin your site research, and start to build community around the idea of a green schoolyard. Try to recruit professionals who might donate their services by contacting their local chapters and describing your needs or by enlisting the help of professionals within your school community. Design processes can be run on a shoestring if your school community has talented volunteers willing to contribute their time. It is also a good idea to do some fundraising to buy supplies for the classrooms involved in the design process and for seed money for the initial construction projects. (Figure 2.4)

Make sure that the master plan the group creates fits the needs of the school community and is feasible for the volunteers' skill set. Work closely with the school and district to ensure that the design meets their safety and accessibility standards; move slowly and carefully to give them the time they need to review the project at each stage.

For assistance with the design process in more detail, I recommend using the guidebook *All Hands in the Dirt*. This

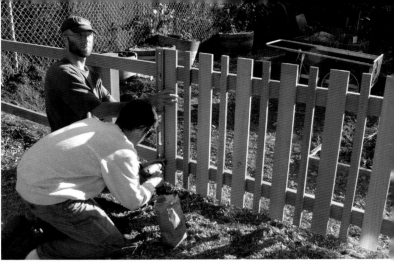

FIGURE 2.4 *Parents at Rosa Parks School in Berkeley, California, construct a simple and attractive redwood fence for the school garden using design-build methods.*

step-by-step guide published by the Canadian organization, Evergreen, includes surveys for gathering information, tips for reaching out to your school community, and key questions to ask throughout the design process. It can be accessed on their website for free and can be purchased in print.[2]

🌺 The Schoolyard Design Process as an Educational Tool

The schoolyard design process not only "builds community" around a green schoolyard project, but can also serve as an educational resource for teachers.

Schoolyard site analysis research for students

Students are capable researchers who have the ability to explore and record information about their schoolyard's existing conditions for use during the design process. They can learn to read maps and then practice their skills by creating thematic site analysis diagrams that illustrate sunny and shady areas of the yard; water sources and wet places (spigots, downspouts, rain barrels, seasonally moist areas and wetlands); topography (hills and valleys in the schoolyard); "favorite things on the playground" (things to keep); "least favorite things on the playground" (things to change).

Teachers may also ask students to map existing plants on school grounds and list animals they have seen onsite to create a flora and fauna "before studies" of their grounds. Many schools start their schoolyard design process with bare asphalt and sports fields that support insects, birds, and squirrels—but not much else, so the changes a green schoolyard brings can be dramatic and gratifying to document. Signs to look for at the beginning might include ant hills, beetles or other crawling insects, bird and squirrel nests. By repeating this study year after year, students will document changes in schoolyard ecology in a meaningful way.

Students can also use maps and aerial photographs to explore the neighborhood's environmental history, and observe how it has changed over time. This type of inquiry may be connected to oral history lessons if students interview older members of the community about the neighborhood's past. Students' research findings may then be included in the design for the schoolyard, bringing some of the neighborhood's past into its future. *(continued on the next page)*

Older students may engage in more complex studies of the schoolyard by discussing water cycles and the school's location within its watershed (see chapter 5); studying solar geometry using shadows that shift on the playground over the course of a day (see chapter 9); or testing the nutrient levels of the soil to see if they are adequate for plant growth.

Schoolyard research can also be a good segue into career discussions. Teachers can invite available parents or local community members—cartographers, soil scientists, geologists, water resource experts, landscape architects and planners—to share their work with students, relating their jobs and career paths to the schoolyard design process.

Schoolyard design exercises

When the green schoolyard project reaches the design phase, teachers have further opportunities to engage students in creative thinking skills and art projects.

Student design workshops can be held either at the beginning of the planning process, when the adults are doing similar brainstorming work, or after the general spatial decisions and project parameters have already been defined by the adults. Student design workshops usually begin with a description of the task at hand and an introduction to what might be possible at their school with the aid of photographs or other visuals. Once that introduction is delivered, students typically work in small groups to collaborate on design ideas. As each small team of students presents their vision to the larger group, the adults should take notes—what is verbally expressed may not be immediately clear from the drawings. (Figure 2.5)

While it is best to allow creative ideas to flow, unconstrained by adult perspectives, some student ideas may need editing. For example, requests for amenities such as swimming pools, ice rinks, and zoos are fairly difficult to implement on most school grounds, while suggestions for a bench shaped like a dragon, a reading nook in the form of a fairy castle, climbing holds put on a bare concrete wall, or the school's name spelled out in flowers, are more easily translated to a schoolyard context.

Some schools use design contests, based on drawings or scale models, to gather student input. The resulting student

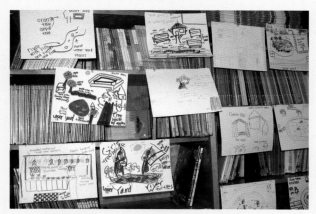

FIGURE 2.5 *Students can express their schoolyard design ideas by drawing on a map of their school grounds, or by creating illustrative, annotated drawings of key features they desire (as shown here).*

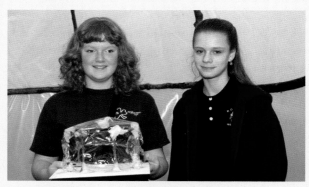

FIGURE 2.6 *These students at Rowe Middle School in Milwaukie, Oregon, won a contest to design a greenhouse for their school's "Naturescape." The resulting structure, shown here in model form and as the backdrop for the picture, was created using recycled plastic sheeting and tree branches.*

design ideas often help to make the schoolyard unique and memorable. (Figure 2.6)

Ultimately, the best student design process is the one that the school feels is most likely to result in a real, visible contribution from the students. Including students in the design phase empowers them, shows respect and recognizes them as creative, thoughtful individuals. This affirmation from adults helps to build students' self-confidence and acknowledges that their contributions are important for shaping their environment.

4 *Schoolyard Wildlife Sanctuaries*

Schoolyard wildlife areas are a particularly important and engaging way to connect students of all ages to the natural world. They illustrate that "the environment" is not just the rainforest in a far away place—it is something that surrounds us all in our local neighborhoods. Wildlife sanctuaries, large or small, enrich their school's curricula while providing refuge for a variety of species. They allow students to see that wildlife can exist in urban and suburban areas and even thrive with a little help. Wildlife areas can be connected to the curriculum in countless ways, including nature observation in science classes, sketching practice in art classes, and population estimates/counts for math classes.

The strongest projects provide well-rounded habitats that fulfill the basic needs of wildlife—consistent food sources, clean water, shelter, and areas where they can rear their offspring.[1] Successful schoolyard wildlife sanctuaries also provide places for students to observe visiting birds, animals, and insects while leaving the creatures relatively undisturbed. They are peaceful havens for quiet reflection where flora and fauna are nurtured, changes happen slowly following ecological cycles, and planting schemes mimic natural patterns. The psychological advantages of having wild places in the schoolyard are significant.[2] Who can put a price on the value of filling a child's life with fluttering butterflies and other fascinating creatures?

❧ *Reflections of Local Context*

Schoolyard wildlife zones spring from their surrounding ecosystems and site conditions and are as varied as their geographic locations. The finest ones focus on attracting native species using indigenous plants. They are influenced by local climate and microclimate, elevation, rainfall, and other key factors such as the amount of human development nearby. Habitat projects in rural, suburban, and urban schools typically have differing amounts of space available, and varying levels of access and proximity to nearby core wildlife populations.

The physical form of schoolyard wildlife areas is usually determined by the shape and size of the available land, the types of wildlife the habitat is designed to attract, the budget for the project and the range of people involved in the design process. Schools in spacious rural or suburban settings may create or restore large habitat areas or connect their projects to relatively undisturbed ecosystems nearby. For example, some schools convert perpetually damp parts of the schoolyard into successful wetland environments. Others choose to replant native prairie grasses on school lands that were previously cleared of this vegetation. Schools with nearby creeks may use their onsite plantings to enhance local riparian restoration work. Many of these large wildlife zones may support such animals as deer, raccoons, rabbits, opossums, and migratory birds. These large-scale projects are often designed to look like "natural" habitats, rather than gardens, and include various food and nectar plants to attract birds, butterflies and other pollinators. In this case, plant and tree placements are often arranged to mimic patterns found in natural ecosystems.

Most schools have little available land, so they develop smaller schoolyard wildlife areas, instead. These demonstration-size gardens are found tucked into tight spaces around the school buildings, in previously underutilized corners of the schoolyard, or nestled in quiet interior courtyards. The overall aesthetic of smaller habitats is generally closer to a "wild garden" than a naturally occurring ecosystem. Although larger areas make a more significant contribution toward supporting local wildlife, even modest habitat patches will assist small creatures and provide a dynamic outdoor resource for the school. Small wildlife gardens, including container gardens, often attract a variety of birds, squirrels, chipmunks, and pollinators, such as hummingbirds, bees, and butterflies.

A habitat patch's physical form may also be affected by the timing of its creation—before, during, or after the school was built. Until recently, most urban and suburban school sites were graded and stripped of their original vegetative cover in favor of more "modern" lawns and asphalt. More work is required to turn these "blank slates" into habitats that serve classroom and wildlife needs. In recent years it has become increasingly popular to retain natural landscape features when building a new school; some new campuses include well established wildlife zones as a result of these preservation efforts.

The following examples range from small to large, urban to rural, and cover different parts of the globe. They include habitat areas for creatures that buzz, fly, swim, crawl, and scamper. Some of these case studies reflect well-developed, extensive habitat restoration work, while others are less complex yet quite effective. All of these examples bring students into contact with plants and animals from their local environment in a straightforward manner, making science and other lessons more relevant while also deepening students' understanding and appreciation of their neighborhood's ecology.

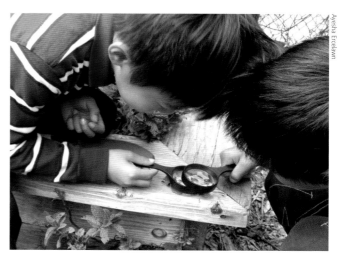

FIGURE 4.1 *Tule Elk Park Child Development Center in San Francisco, California, provides magnifying glasses to children at recess to make their bug hunts even more interesting.*

🍃 *Small-Scale Schoolyard Wildlife Sanctuaries*

Schools of all sizes and contexts can create useful habitat zones for pollinators, birds, and aquatic creatures. Even schools in urban areas, with small schoolyards and a neighborhood covered with asphalt, can attract hummingbirds, native bees, butterflies and other insects if they provide the right combination of plantings and microclimate. Most schools can also attract and support bird populations by using appropriate plantings, shelter, and water sources, and by creating ponds to nurture small aquatic creatures, as well. (Figure 4.1)

Habitat for pollinators

Because they play a key role in plant reproduction and food production, pollinators are extremely important to the health of our ecosystems and agriculture. Schools can help nurture and support local pollinators by providing the right habitat for them.

Flowering plants and "bee nesting blocks" encourage non-aggressive native bees to take up residence at Salmon Creek School in Occidental, California, and make the bees' lifecycle more visible to students. Bees typically fill the nest blocks during the spring and summer, when female bees enter the holes to create brood cells and lay their eggs. The mother bee leaves food for her offspring and then seals off each chamber. The bee pupae typically mature over the course of a year and emerge the following spring. Unlike commercially raised honey bees, the native bees in Sonoma County, where Salmon Creek School is located, do not produce honey or beeswax that people can harvest. Instead, they ensure that the productive and beautiful organic garden onsite is well-pollinated, helping to create bigger harvests of fruits, vegetables, and herbs.[3] The garden coordinator has noticed many types of native bees using the box since its installation in 2004.[4] (Figure 4.2)

The butterfly garden at LeConte School in Berkeley, California, is installed along an undulating perimeter fence. (Figure 4.3) This creative linear garden separates the neighborhood's sidewalk from the schoolyard, provides bright flowers for the school and neighborhood to admire, and fills the surrounding area with the multicolored wings of many types of local butterflies. Some of the garden's plants include passion vine to attract gulf fritillaries (Figure 4.4); fennel to attract anise

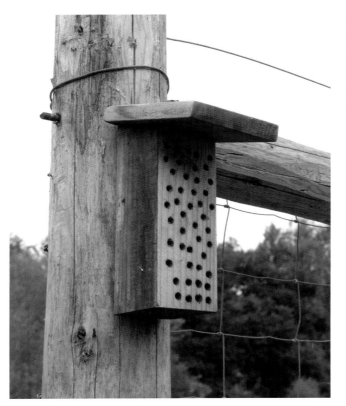

FIGURE 4.2 *This bee nesting block at Salmon Creek School consists of a block of wood drilled with holes approximately 5/16" in diameter, capped with an over-hanging "roof" that shelters the block from direct sunlight and rain. The holes in the wood mimic naturally occur-ring nesting places used by solitary wood- and tunnel-nesting bees, such as leafcutters and mason bees.*

FIGURE 4.4

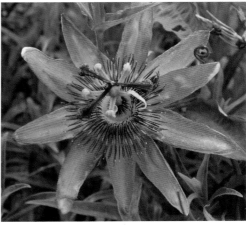

FIGURE 4.3

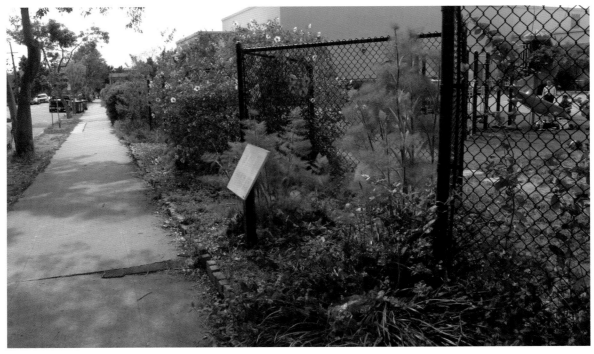

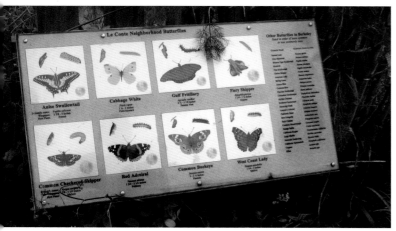

FIGURE 4.5 *LeConte School's butterfly garden includes an interpretive sign along the sidewalk to help students and neighborhood residents appreciate and learn from the garden.*

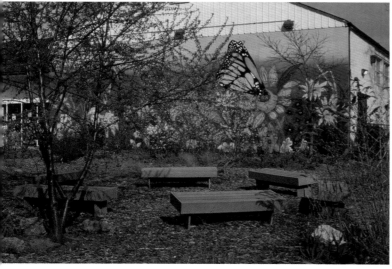

FIGURE 4.6 *A dramatic, colorful mural greets visitors to Humber Valley Village School in Ontario, Canada, and sends a strong message about the school's interest in wildlife habitat. The mural brightens the school's front entrance and is a vibrant backdrop for the adjacent outdoor classroom and butterfly garden, bringing the site to life even when the plants are dormant in the cool seasons.[5]*

swallowtails; field mustard to attract cabbage whites; grasses to attract fiery skippers; mallow to attract common-checkered skippers and west coast ladies; pellitory to attract red admirals, and plantain to attract common buckeyes. (Figures 4.5)

Bird habitat

Birds are present near most schools but do not always spend time in the schoolyard. Providing food is one of the easiest ways to attract birds. Some schools use feeders filled with seeds specific to the bird species they wish to invite. Feeders are somewhat controversial among bird enthusiasts, however, because they often attract aggressive or invasive types like blackbirds, cowbirds, and pigeons that are already well adapted to urban environments. Feeders can also spread disease among bird populations, and they attract cats that may prey upon birds that eat in the same location every day.

The best way to feed birds is to grow native plants that produce seeds, berries, nuts, and fruits, and to create conditions that encourage birds to forage on their own. Plantings take a little more work to set up than feeders, but they provide the added benefits of shelter for the birds and aesthetic appeal for the school community. Some birds, such as towhees and thrashers, are ground feeders who look for worms, pill bugs, and other insects in the soil—and virtually all bird species need insects to feed their young. To provide these food sources, add an under-layer of leaf mulch to your garden to help insects thrive.[6]

Wild birds also seek out water sources for drinking and bathing, so it is a good idea to provide shallow birdbaths (with the water changed regularly), schoolyard ponds, or other sources of accessible fresh water onsite. Moving water is more likely to attract birds than still water.

Providing food and water will often be enough to get neighborhood birds to visit your schoolyard. If you want the birds to stay, however, you will also need to offer them shelter, so they will feel safe from predators and be able to find places to raise their young. Vertical layers of trees and shrubs offer cover and nesting sites to various species. Grow both deciduous and evergreen plants to provide cover year-round. Birds prefer the plants they have evolved with, and so do the insects that they rely on for food, so grow as many native trees and shrubs as possible. Brush piles made from dead sticks and other plant debris are also good places for birds to forage and seek shelter.

Nesting places also vary among bird species. Cavity nesters, such as bluebirds and owls, prefer to nest in a tree hole—or a nesting box—and each species has its own housing preferences. To successfully attract a particular type of cavity-nester, first make sure that that species is likely to live in your neigh-

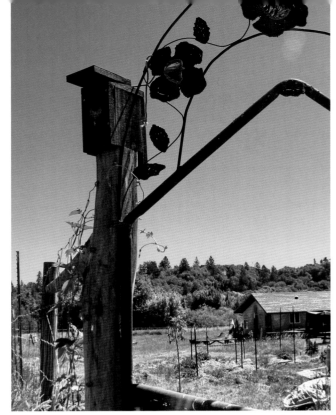

FIGURE 4.7 *This bluebird nesting box at Salmon Creek School rests on top of an 8-foot tall post that is part of the garden's deer fence.*

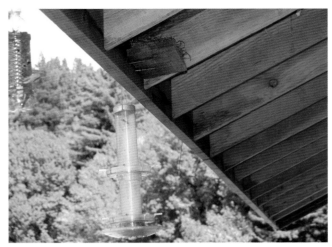

FIGURE 4.8 *This small, thoughtfully-built shelf on the underside of the garden building's eves at Salmon Creek School has been successful in attracting a nesting pair of black-capped phoebes.[9]*

borhood and prefers the type of habitat you have onsite. Then create a birdhouse that has the right size opening for the target bird, appropriate interior dimensions, and the correct placement in the landscape. Some birds, such as purple martins, are particular about the exterior "look" of their bird houses, and won't live in them unless they meet their aesthetic criteria. Avoid assisting invasive birds such as house sparrows and European starlings, which often take over the nests or nest materials of other less common birds.[7] All nest boxes require annual maintenance to keep them clean, so plan for maintenance from the beginning, if you choose to go this route.

At Salmon Creek School, mentioned above, students planted bird-attracting vegetation, added feeders, and built bird houses and nesting platforms to encourage many different types of birds to live in their schoolyard. At least ten different types of birds now visit the yard on a regular basis, including red-winged and Brewer's blackbirds, goldfinches, turkey vultures, and several species of warblers, swallows, and woodpeckers.[8] (Figures 4.7 and 4.8)

Aquatic creatures: Schoolyard ponds and wetlands

Ponds are an important, and frequently overlooked, wildlife resource that can be added to school sites of any size. They are high quality educational resources that allow teachers to show their students "miniature ecosystems" with everything from microscopic aquatic organisms to larger plants, animals, insects and fish. They can be studied in science classes or become the subject of writing assignments, visual arts lessons, and informal observations during recess. Ponds often act as "child magnets" at play time, capturing children's imaginations and instilling a sense of wonder, as children flock to their edges to observe fish, frogs, dragonflies, and other creatures found there.

In our overly litigious culture, many schools avoid ponds because they are afraid of liability. The decision to have a pond on a school site should be made by the school community, in collaboration with its school district, and should comply with local codes about water safety. That said, it is important to remember that *safety and liability are not the same thing*. Often, the *perceived* risk of having a pond is far greater than the *actual* risk. The educational benefits of this type of rich learning environment are substantial, and can be reaped by the whole school community. Some communities, comfortable with this level of risk and its educational reward, create large ponds on their elementary school grounds—while also teaching their students to respect the water and act safely at its edge. Other schools, even with older children, may only allow a small pool of water in a raised bed—behind a tall locked fence.

If a school decides to have a pond, there are many ways to improve safety without diminishing the value of the resource to the school community or the wildlife it supports. The first issues to consider are placement and security: Should the pond go out on the schoolyard or inside a protected courtyard? Should it have a tall locked fence around it, or just a visual border that alerts the community to its presence, so people don't fall in by accident? Each of those questions typically requires a community debate to resolve—and any of these choices can work.

Many schools also consider whether to put the pond in a raised bed, above ground level, or dig it into the ground. From a wildlife perspective, a ground level pond in an area near wildlife plantings is the most desirable choice, because it allows small creatures to visit the edge of the water and come and go as they please. To keep this type of pond as safe as possible, many schools decide to keep the water shallow, under two feet deep, so that it only reaches a child's knee or waist level. It is also important to design the pond with gradually

sloping edges, so that a person (or an animal) who accidentally falls into the water can easily walk out. (Figure 4.9)

If an in-ground, schoolyard pond is deemed too risky at a given school, the next best thing is to build a pond in a raised bed or in a locked school courtyard. Ponds of these types can also be effective teaching tools, but they will probably not develop ecosystems as complex as ponds connected to the surrounding landscape. Improve their habitat value and richness by adding a range of plantings around the perimeter to provide some shade and cover for the aquatic creatures. After the pond is installed, fill it with wildlife-safe water such as rainwater or tap water that has had the chlorine or chloramine removed. (Many pet stores carry a water treatment chemical that is made for this purpose.) In many places, untreated tap water will kill pond life.

After the physical design characteristics of the pond have been established, select a method to keep the pond water free of mosquito larvae to avoid mosquito-related health concerns. There are several easy ways to accomplish this. One technique is to have a pond pump system to keep the water moving and make it less appealing for mosquitoes to lay eggs there. Self-sufficient solar pond pump systems make this a straightforward and inexpensive task.

It is also helpful to place fish in the pond to eat mosquito eggs or larvae. Tiny, "guppy-like" fish such as *Gambusia affinis* can often be purchased from pet stores or obtained from local mosquito abatement offices.[10] These fish can often live self-sufficiently in schoolyard ponds, requiring little regular care beyond maintenance of adequate water levels. They are not compatible with local ecosystems, however, so do not add them to natural water bodies. They are only appropriate for man-made, self-contained ponds. *Gambusia* also inhibit tadpoles and nibble frog eggs, so it would be difficult to have frogs and mosquito fish in the same pond. If there are local fish species in your area that can live in a pond and eat mosquito larvae, it is preferable to use them instead of non-native *Gambusia*.

If the pump system and fish are not successful (which is somewhat unlikely) and wiggling mosquito larvae are observed in the pond, consider using mosquito dunks to prevent mosquitoes from breeding. These tablets generally contain a bacteria that kills mosquitoes but is not harmful to humans, fish, or wildlife. They can often be purchased at local hardware stores.[11] If you are considering adding a chemical of any type

FIGURE 4.9 *Sometimes children do get a little bit wet in schoolyard ponds—but it's not a big deal. If it happens frequently, the solution is to ask them to bring a change of clothes...or shoes!*
Sandra Koike

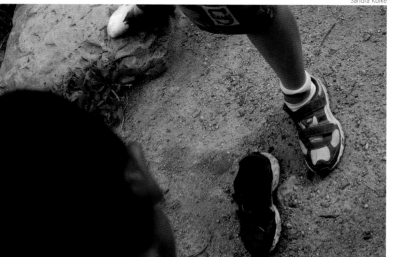

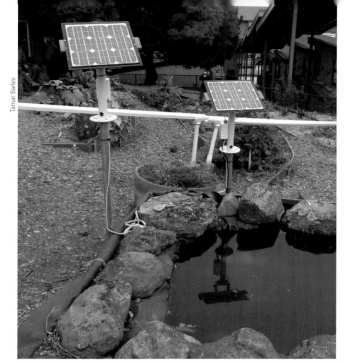

FIGURE 4.10 *The solar panels for the pond pump system at Alice Fong Yu School were reclaimed from their previous use as power sources for highway telephones and given a new life in this location.*

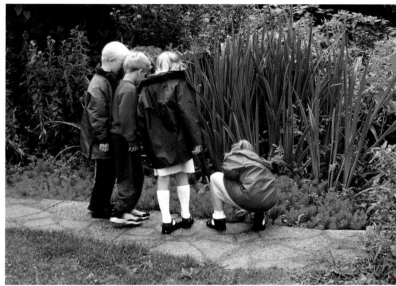

FIGURE 4.11

to your pond, read the label carefully. Do not use any products that may be harmful to children or aquatic creatures. Be sure to avoid any chemicals in the adjacent planted areas, as well, so the water quality stays high.

The best way to ensure pond safety in the schoolyard is to talk with the students before and after the pond is installed. Instruct them in safe behavior when they are next to open water, and establish a set of ground rules for water-side activities. Some schools find that their ponds are so popular that they need to establish a system for taking turns at the water's edge to make the experience enjoyable for everyone.

Students at Alice Fong Yu Alternative School in San Francisco, California, enjoy a small pond built in a raised bed in their hillside garden. A black plastic pond liner retains the water, and attractive rocks were added to mask the edge of the liner and hold it in place. The pond is approximately 3 feet wide and 6 feet long, with water about 12 inches deep. It is home to many tiny pond creatures, including *Gambusia affinis,* that the students study in their science and garden classes. The schoolyard and garden are surrounded by a chain link fence, so the school has not installed any additional barriers near the

pond. The raised pond is easy for a class to gather around to take part in lessons.

When the pond was first installed at Alice Fong Yu School, a local organization helped to mount two solar panels near the pond to power the small pump system that keeps the water moving. Children at the school love to make the water stop and go by tilting the panels on their rotating mounts, or by covering the surface with their hands. When these beloved panels were stolen in 2006, the school replaced them with a single, larger panel that serves the same purpose.[12] (Figure 4.10)

Cowick First School, in southwest England, created a small pond in the late 1980s. Pond creatures abound in the shallow water and are thoroughly enjoyed by students during informal play times when they crowd around to hunt for frogs and tadpoles, watch dragonflies perch on plants near the water's edge, or spy on other pond-dwelling creatures. Teachers connect their curricula to the pond for lessons ranging from scientific studies to art classes. (Figure 4.11)

As in the United States, safety and liability are important concerns for schools in England, where fences are usually required around open water. The school community at Cowick, however, felt that it was important to make their pond accessible to students and wildlife at all times; they chose to reduce the safety risks through an innovative design approach. The 10-foot diameter pond is shallow (only 1-2 feet deep) so anyone who falls in can climb out easily. The school planted a dense, prickly blackberry thicket around the back of the pond to keep children from approaching the water from behind. The front of the pond is demarcated by a low hill at the edge of the playfield that stops children from running into the water accidentally. A sign in a child's handwriting, atop the hill, warns students of the pond's presence with the words "Danger, Pond." These simple safety precautions, and the children's common sense,

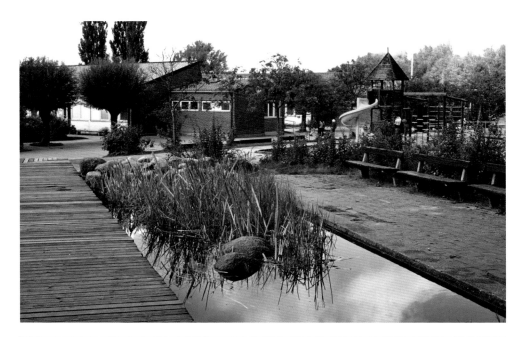

FIGURE 4.12 *Palett School, in southern Sweden, has a rectangular pond surrounded by a wooden deck that makes it easy for students to access the water from every side. The pond's plantings and rocks provide cover for fish and other aquatic life.*

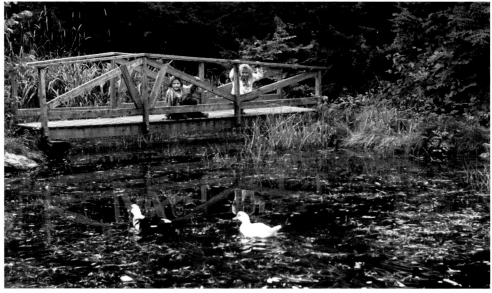

FIGURE 4.13 *Bergen Steiner School in Norway has a large in-ground pond that predates the site's use as a school. Children are allowed to play near the pond and can observe ducks, fish, frogs, and other wildlife there. A bridge across the water is a particularly nice place to sit and enjoy the view.*

have made the pond a useful and exciting resource for the school for many years.[13]

Sagano School in Kyoto, Japan, has a beautiful recirculating pond and "creek" that is accessible to students for academic studies and for nature play at recess. The manmade environment is home to diverse native plants and local wildlife, including fireflies. Each year during the first week of June, the school hosts a firefly viewing party for 1,000 students, families, and community members. In July, the banks are roped off to protect the fireflies and allow them to burrow into the ground to complete their lifecycle.[14] (Figure 4.14)

Sherman School, in the heart of urban San Francisco, California, installed a pond in 2007 as part of a large schoolyard renovation project. The pond, 15 feet in diameter and 12 inches deep, includes a dramatic 20-foot long waterfall that cascades down a hill. (See Figures 5.13 and 12.47) A powerful recirculating pump keeps the water moving so mosquitoes do not lay eggs there. In addition, the pond is stocked with goldfish and koi that eat the insects that land in the water. The school finds that it has to restock the fish quite often, as local herons and other birds come by for a tasty snack from time to time!

Sherman's pond is surrounded by large, smooth, granite boulders and a wide variety of smaller rocks. The rocks create a clear edge and keep the children from accidentally falling into the water. The school has established behavioral guidelines to help students interact with the water in a safe manner. For example, students are allowed to lie down on the rocks and put their hands in the water, but they may not stand on them or jump from them. They are also asked to respect the pond creatures and may not throw things into the pond.[15] (Figure 4.15)

The pond at Sherman School has quickly become one of the schoolyard's centerpieces. Its popularity inspired the school to build a second pond nearby. Students flock to both ponds at recess and are delighted when their teachers announce that they will be visiting them for a lesson. Teachers and administrators from other schools also come by for tours of this schoolyard to learn how to create something similar on their own school grounds.

🍃 *Native Plant Gardens—Educational Microcosms of Surrounding Native Landscapes*

Every geographic region has its own palette of naturally occurring plants that are adapted to local microclimates. In many

FIGURE 4.14

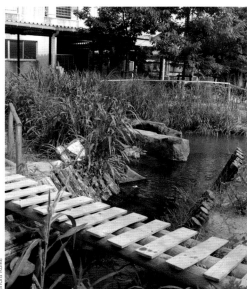

FIGURE 4.15

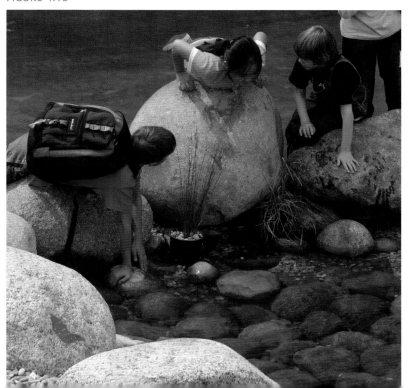

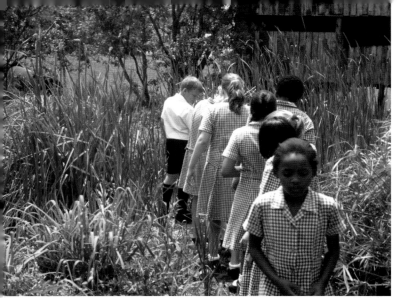

FIGURE 4.16 *Students shown in their native plants garden at Epworth Co-educational Primary School in South Africa.*

Mary Jackson

urban and suburban areas, this native plant palette has been removed in favor of paved surfaces and a preference for more uniform plant species, chosen to fit a narrow aesthetic. By planting flora that is indigenous to a given area, and by grouping the plants according to their natural plant communities, we can begin to reverse this trend. Native plant gardens create a microcosm of our local habitats, and, if planted wisely, also serve some of the same ecological functions as naturally occurring plant communities.

Schoolyard native plant gardens vary in size and shape and by region and microclimate. By their nature, they are adapted to local rainfall patterns, so they conserve water and are generally easy to care for once the plants are established. Many flowering native plants are useful for attracting pollinators, a wide variety of beneficial insects, and birds. Native plant gardens are also easily incorporated into curricula at many grade levels.

Students at Epworth Co-educational Primary School in KwaZulu-Natal, South Africa, planted a large indigenous plant garden (Figure 4.16). Students also participated in raising some animals in their classrooms and cared for other animals onsite.[16]

Ulloa Elementary School in San Francisco, California, created an inviting coastal dune garden in 2002 to showcase native plant communities found along the nearby sandy shores of the Pacific Ocean. The garden was built on a previously underutilized area between the school building and the sidewalk, adjacent to the school's main entrance. It was developed through the

hard work of dedicated teachers and the volunteer assistance of a member of the California Native Plant Society. The vibrant, low-water garden features plants that are adapted to the seasonally dry climate of this region and has fairly low maintenance requirements. Over the years the school has used log stumps, in different configurations, to create a flexible outdoor classroom space for academic use. The mature garden is an attractive public face for the school, brightening its main entrance.[17] (Figures 4.17 and 4.18)

At the heart of Rowe Middle School in Milwaukie, Oregon, sits a vibrant courtyard haven for wildlife and students called "the Naturescape." Over a six-year period, hundreds of students (and many adult volunteers) participated in the design, construction, and maintenance of the Naturescape, led by a dedicated art and ecology teacher. The space became a microcosm of the nearby Willamette Valley forest ecosystem and a demonstration site for sustainable building materials and techniques.

When the project began, science classes conducted a baseline study of the limited plant and wildlife diversity onsite to document potential changes over time. Math classes measured the courtyard and made scaled maps of the available space. Local landscape architects showed the art classes how to use these maps to draw their design ideas and worked with students to refine their ideas into a single landscape plan. Students then built a clay model of the plan to explain their concepts to the school community. A local master gardener helped the ecology class select native plants and other professionals assisted students with construction.

Students in the popular Naturescape class acted as the courtyard's stewards. Over a six year period, classes came out several times a week to tidy up, embellish existing structures, and dream up new things to add to the maturing landscape. The Naturescape class built something new in the courtyard each semester. Some of the projects improved outdoor seating and work areas, whereas others enhanced the wildlife habitat value of the site or other ecological systems such as energy or water flows. All of the projects used environmentally-friendly building materials. Students also decided to use hand labor and hand tools for all construction projects to conserve energy and avoid fossil fuels.

Other student-built projects include a cob bench; a solar-powered recirculating stream and pond; raised beds; a hand-

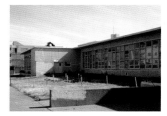

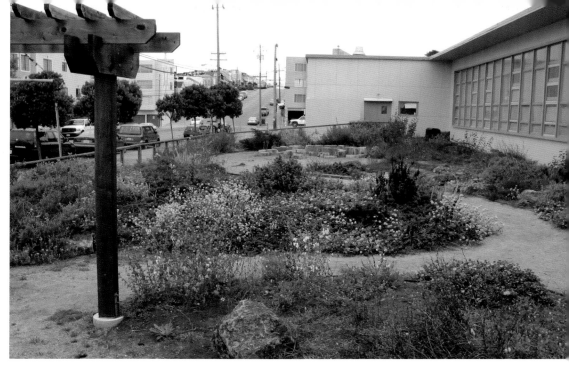

FIGURES 4.17 and 4.18 *Ulloa's "coastal classroom" before the garden was created (May 2002) and at 2 years old (July 2004).*

tiled birdbath; a student-designed domed greenhouse (see chapter 2, Figure 2.6); art pieces; and a large "Diversity Bench," crafted from the branches of twenty different kinds of trees. The students also built a snaking 22-foot long table with legs along one side that extend upward to hold birdhouses and feeders.

Rowe Middle School's courtyard Naturescape successfully brought a piece of Oregon's Willamette Valley forest into the school in a manner that is beautiful, educational, and useful to local wildlife. The students involved in this project fully understood the ecological cycles in their midst and learned about ecological design through its direct application to their own learning environment.[18] (Figure 4.19)

The "Habitat" at Crest View Elementary School in Boulder, Colorado, is a wetland restoration project that turned a perpetually damp area of the schoolyard into a vibrant learning environment, a thriving wildlife habitat, and a great place to play. The project features a small, meandering prairie slough filled with water creatures. An abundance of native trees, shrubs, and smaller plants give this suburban schoolyard a wild feel. To make the wetland accessible to the students, the site includes small bridges, a "floating" boardwalk, an amphitheater, and enough dirt pathways and large boulders to satisfy an elementary school student's urge to "tramp through the wilderness" and climb "tall mountains."[19]

FIGURE 4.19 *A December rain falls softly in the courtyard Naturescape at Rowe Middle School in Milwaukie, Oregon.*

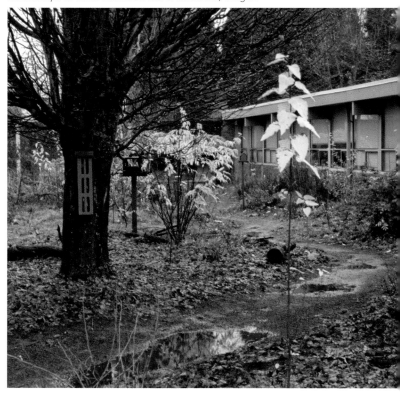

Boulder, Colorado, crisscrossed by creeks and rivers, is rich in groundwater fed by snowmelt and rainfall. The geology and hydrology underlying Crest View's campus provide the moisture that keeps the Habitat wet year-round. Before the school was built in the 1950s, the land was a horse pasture with a wetland running through it. When the school and surrounding neighborhoods were developed, extra dirt from the construction projects was dumped into the wetland. The material largely filled the depression that had been there, but did not succeed in drying it out. For more than thirty years, this part of the schoolyard was damp and muddy.

In 1989 and 1990, a local restoration ecologist/school parent proposed that Crest View could turn this problematic, soggy area into an asset by making it an outdoor teaching environment.[20] The resulting Habitat is designed to showcase many different plant communities from the local ecosystems. More than 2,000 native plants—from willows and chokecherries to tall grass prairie species and ponderosa pines— are concentrated in one small area. A prairie cord grass wetland, native to the Platte River, is also represented in the Habitat for its social and historical significance to the Native Americans of this region.

The Habitat is built into a hillside that protects it somewhat from cold winter breezes. The hillside also blocks the view of the neighborhood, creating a more "wild" landscape, while also making it easier for teachers to unobtrusively monitor the children in the "wilderness" from above.

Wildlife that visit or live in the Habitat include dragonflies, butterflies, praying mantises, and other insects; crawdads, fish, and other water creatures; snakes, foxes, raccoons, mule deer, frogs, and other small mammals and amphibians; pine juncos, redwing blackbirds, western meadowlarks, gold finches, mallards, and many other bird species. The pond is stocked annually with mosquito fish to keep the mosquito population in check. (Figures 4.20 and 4.21)

An extensive nature study area and garden covers more than one third of the school grounds at a primary school in the heart of Tokyo, Japan. Founded in 2002, the goal of this "biotope" (as schoolyard nature projects are called in Japan) is to recreate an environment similar to what existed before Tokyo became a large city. Adjacent to the school's extensive edible garden, this biotope includes over 4,000 plants from 50 native woodland and wetland habitats. Students track seasonal changes through the use of spring flowers, summer greenery, fall leaf colors, and winter's bare branches.

The most prominent landscape feature, a grassy mound, is the source of a recirculating "spring." Water bubbles up from the spring and tumbles down a short series of waterfalls as it travels to the pond. Well designed pathways circle the site's perimeter, and weave through its center, to allow children access to all parts of the nature study area.[21] (Figures 4.22–4.25)

FIGURE 4.20 *The 1.25-acre wetland is located on Crest View School's property line, nestled between the classroom buildings and an adjacent city park.*

FIGURE 4.21 *Students at Crest View enjoy looking for water creatures at recess.*

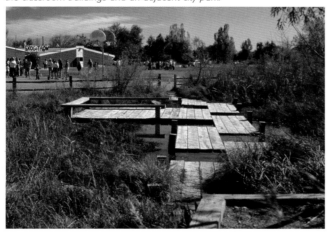

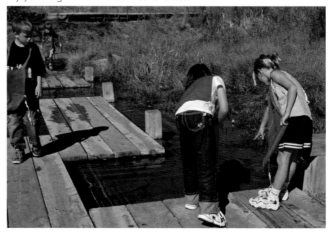

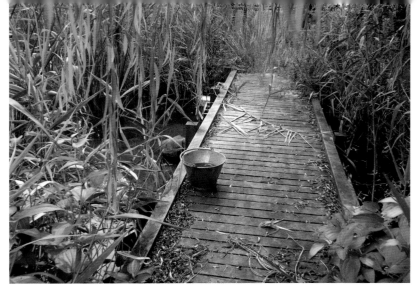

FIGURES 4.22 and 4.23
In this Tokyo schoolyard, children have free access to the water's edge and the center of the pond via a wooden bridge and a viewing platform.

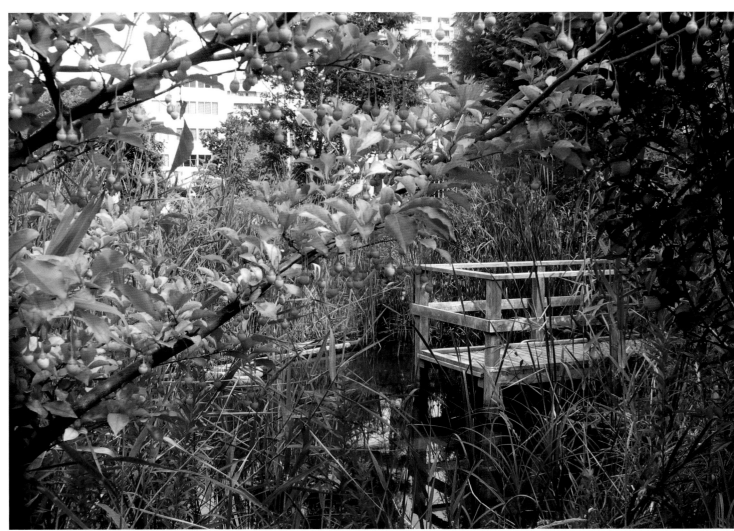

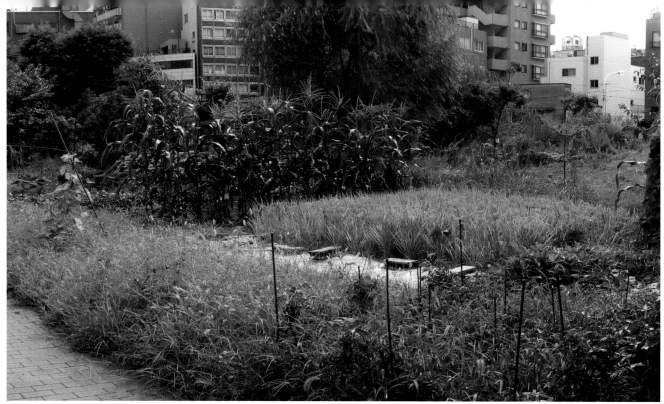

FIGURE 4.25 *An edible garden in the Tokyo schoolyard includes a large rice paddy (center) and row crops, such as taro, corn, tomatoes, bell peppers, decorative gourds, and eggplants. Shiso, lavender, and other herbs help to further expand the schoolyard's culinary offerings and provide additional food sources for pollinators.*

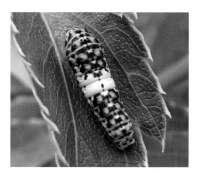

FIGURE 4.24
Many of the plants in this urban Tokyo schoolyard were specifically chosen to attract butterflies, dragonflies, and other small creatures.

🍃 Habitat Restoration Projects— Large-Scale Efforts

All of the preceding projects have great educational merit and are excellent demonstrations of ecological concepts. They are teaching tools that make students more aware of local plants and animals and clearly illustrate how students can improve local wildlife habitat. Many of those projects also attract a noticeable amount of wildlife and make modest contributions to their local ecosystems.

Some schools go beyond these admirable accomplishments to create environments on a much larger scale. These schools seek not only to achieve the educational and ecological goals mentioned above, but to surpass them by creating restored landscapes that are large enough to support wildlife *populations*—rather than individuals.

Schoolyard habitat restoration work, unlike the native plant gardens discussed above, seek to replicate the original plant palette that might have been found onsite, rather than to create a microcosm of what occurs nearby. Their primary goal is ecological improvement, rather than demonstration, but the educational value of these sites is clear. (Figures 4.26–4.28)

The United Anglers of Casa Grande, at Casa Grande High School in Petaluma, California, is a student-run organization dedicated to the restoration of nearby Adobe Creek and its native, endangered fish populations. Each year twenty student Anglers in grades 9–12, with the help of their dedicated teacher and several enthusiastic volunteers, commit themselves "to heal a stream, repair its habitat, and save a species from extinction."[23] Founded in 1983, the program has transformed a dry, barren,

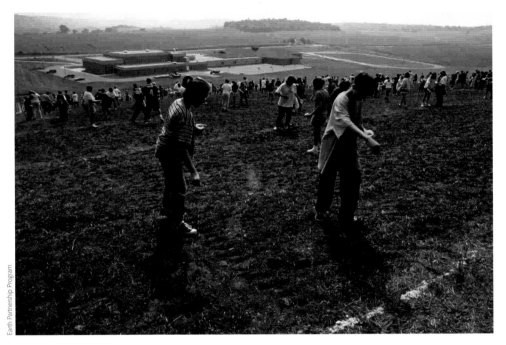

FIGURES 4.26–4.28 *Lodi Middle School, Kennedy Elementary School, and Oregon Middle School in Wisconsin are some of the many schools in the Midwest that are restoring prairie habitat on a large scale on their grounds. These images vividly depict the processes of planting schoolyard prairie grasses, maintaining the habitat through the use of controlled burns, and actively using the mature landscape with school classes.[22]*

Earth Partnership Program

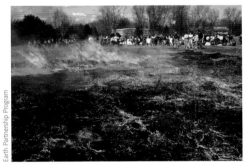

Earth Partnership Program

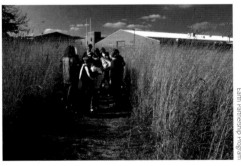

Earth Partnership Program

seven-mile stretch of Adobe Creek into a clean, water-filled riparian corridor, home to spawning endangered salmon and steelhead trout. They now nurture salmon and trout from egg to release, plant thousands of trees on the banks of the creek each year, and spend countless hours before, during, and after school passionately working on a project they truly love.[24]

Each year, for more than twenty-five years, the students have planted an average of 1,200 trees along the banks of what was once little more than a dry ditch, turning the creek into a vibrant riparian corridor once again. In the mid-1990s, they succeeded in getting the City of Petaluma to remove all of the diversion structures in the creek, allowing the stream once

again to flow freely from its headwaters to its confluence with the Petaluma River. Over time, the students have hauled more than 25 tons of tires and other debris from the creek bottom. In 1993, the dedicated students raised money to build a state-of-the-art fish hatchery on their campus. Their outstanding efforts were recognized by the U.S. Federal Government in 1994, and they were granted a permit to raise an endangered species of Chinook salmon from the nearby Sacramento River. Only two other institutions in the country have such a permit, and both are professional organizations.

The group's hard work has paid off handsomely. By 2000, the United Anglers had successfully hatched over 30,000

Chinook salmon and released them into San Francisco Bay. (Figure 4.29) Since 1995 they have recorded several hundred returning Chinook in the Petaluma River watershed each year. They have also had impressive results improving the native steelhead trout population in Adobe Creek.[25] Students are profoundly affected by their stewardship work on this project, and many have gone on to become professionals in related fields. (Figure 4.30)

🍃 Schoolyard Elements that Enhance Wildlife Viewing

Schoolyard wildlife sanctuaries are unique because they provide comfortable living environments for insects, birds, and other creatures, while also helping students develop scientific knowledge and their sense of wonder for the natural world.

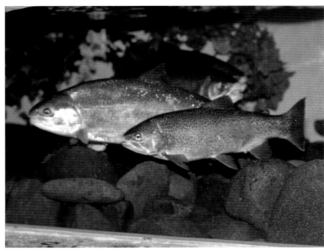

FIGURE 4.30 *Fish raised in the onsite fish hatchery at Case Grande High School.*

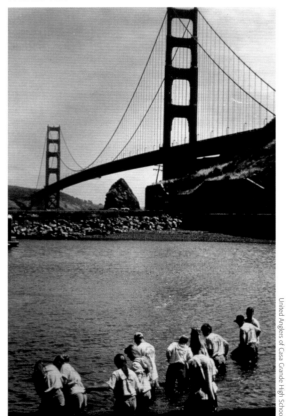

FIGURE 4.29

United Anglers of Casa Grande High School

To achieve these multifaceted goals, schoolyard wildlife areas often include educational and interpretive features, such as wildlife viewing platforms and signage, to make them more accessible to teachers, students, and visitors.

Bird blinds

Bird blinds allow students to spend time observing wildlife in close proximity without scaring the creatures away. They are most effective if built near locations that wildlife *already* frequent, such as a pond, a deep habitat patch or other quiet location.

St. Paulinus Church of England Primary School near London, England, built a bird blind using living willow plants in the midst of a meadow. Students crawl into the igloo-shaped structure and are concealed inside while they observe birds and other creatures that come to visit the colorful wildflowers and nearby pond and forest. This structure connects the science curriculum to the outdoor environment and is also a fun place for children to play.[26] (Figure 4.31)

Wildlife viewing platforms and observation areas

Sometimes, students can get the best view of local wildlife from observation platforms that permit them to stand in places that would normally be inaccessible or inadvisable. These wildlife

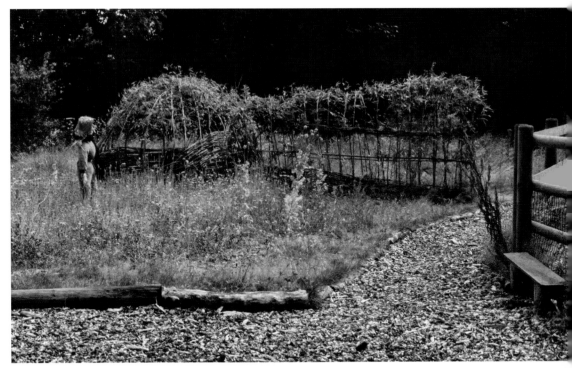

FIGURE 4.31 *The cozy bird blind at St. Paulinus Church of England School is proportioned for children, with an entrance tunnel only four feet tall.*

FIGURE 4.32 *A rustic log bird blind, built deep within the "Look and See" wildlife area at Cowick First School in England, allows students to hide inside and observe birds without changing their behavior.*

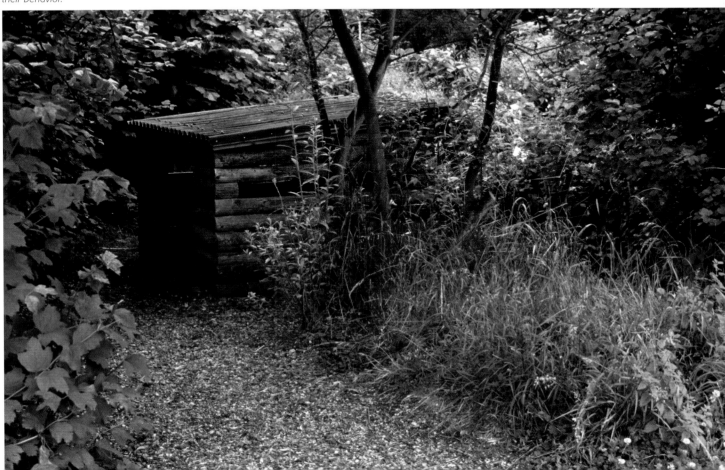

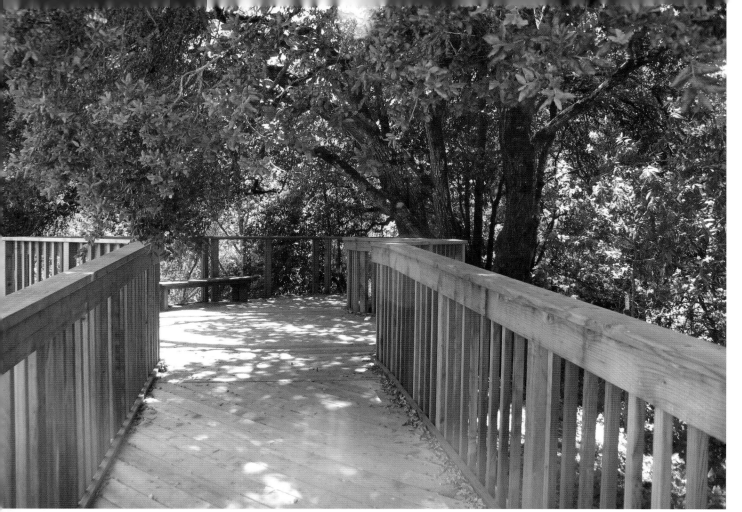

FIGURE 4.33 *A dramatic wildlife viewing platform at Salmon Creek School in Occidental, California, is suspended over a creek in a steep ravine. This carefully engineered, cantilevered deck allows students to watch the salmon jump up the creek's waterfalls as they swim upriver to spawn.*[27]

observation structures are as varied as the animals that are being observed. (Figures 4.33–4.35)

Interpretive signage

Interpretive signs enhance wildlife viewing and habitat appreciation on school grounds by providing educational information about local wildlife, and by alerting visitors to the presence of particular creatures so they can better observe them—or avoid stepping on them! Signs can also help children to remember the names and habits of each creature, and thus identify with them more closely. (Figure 4.36)

Interpretive signs should be used in all schoolyard wildlife gardens to inform the school community of the project's purpose and to help them appreciate the plant and animal lifecycles that are occurring in these special places. For example, seasonally dry plants or those with seed heads left for the birds, may appear "dead and uncared for" if not properly explained. Without explanatory signs, dead branches or brush piles that serve as wildlife nesting or foraging sites may be misinterpreted as sloppy maintenance work.

🍃 Habitat-Themed Installations that Enhance Educational or Play Value

In addition to onsite amenities that help wildlife thrive, some schools and children's venues extend wildlife themes throughout

FIGURE 4.34 *At the Living Class-rooms of the National Capital Region in Glen Echo, Maryland, children can climb an elevated observation deck to get a view of the treetops where they observe wildlife that live in the leafy canopy.*

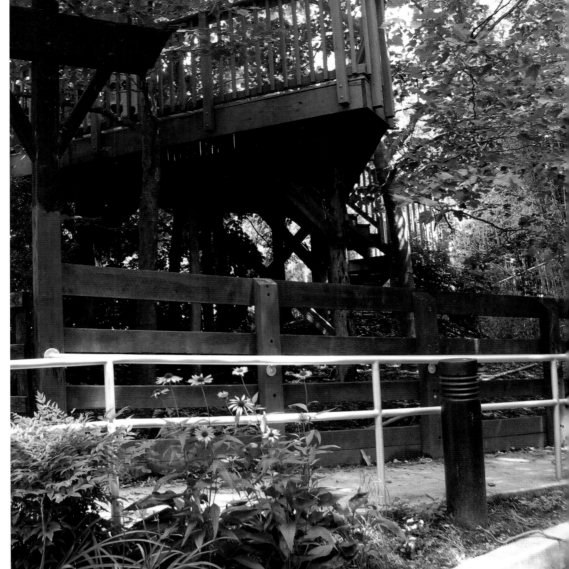

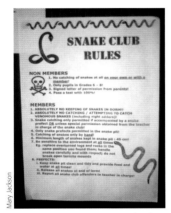

FIGURE 4.35 *Treverton School, outside Durban, South Africa, has an onsite snake viewing pit that is used to temporarily house snakes while students study them from a safe vantage point. Children in the snake club collect non-poisonous snakes and bring them to the pit for observation by their classmates. The snakes are returned to the wild after the children have finished observing them. The school's Snake Club has a list of posted rules to keep children, and snakes, safe.*[28]

FIGURE 4.36 *The sign at Lagunitas School in San Geronimo, California, raises visitors' awareness of the rare salmon that swim in Larsen Creek onsite.*

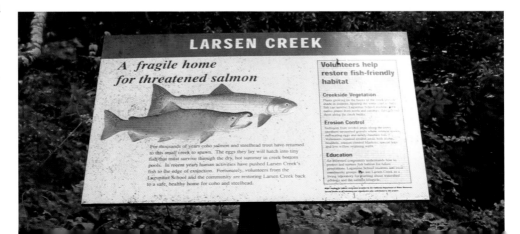

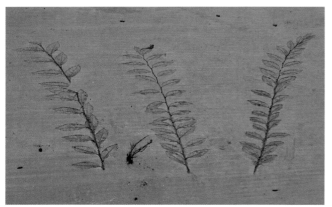

FIGURE 4.37 *Parents at Sherman School in San Francisco, California, pressed real leaves and branches into their new concrete path while it was still wet to create interesting plant patterns.*

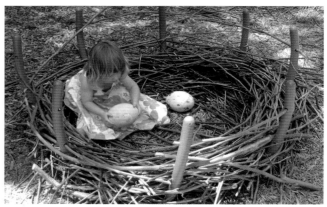

FIGURE 4.39 *Young children visiting the Bay Area Discovery Museum build "nests" big enough to sit in, using loose sticks supplied onsite.*

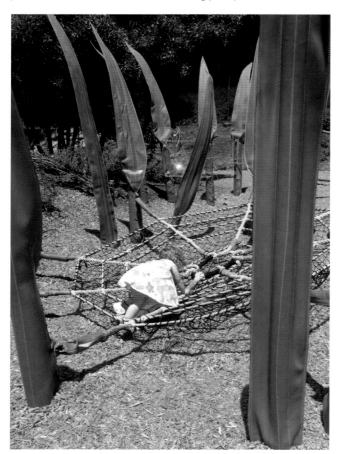

FIGURE 4.38 *The Lookout Cove exhibition's outdoor playground at the Bay Area Discovery Museum in Sausalito, California, includes a child-sized "spider web" climbing structure that rests among tall blades of "grass."*

their learning and play spaces. Paved pathways, for example, can be imprinted with leaves, wildlife "tracks," or other creative ornamentation. Some schoolyards and children's centers also use wildlife themes to encourage imaginative play. (Figures 4.37–4.39)

🍃 Wild Schoolyards

Wildlife habitats on school grounds are a reflection of their local context and are as varied as the schools that create them. Small demonstration-sized plantings can teach students about native plants and visiting wildlife, while providing food for neighborhood birds and pollinators. Larger installations go further to create environments that immerse students in the plantings and patterns that are unique to their geographic region—while simultaneously improving the living conditions for creatures large and small. They help to shape a school's sense of place and connect it to indigenous natural communities in the region.

All of these projects on school grounds have valuable educational and social components that contribute to making each schoolyard unique and memorable. Wildlife sanctuaries on school grounds allow children a closer and more personal view of native plant communities and living creatures in a way that helps them include the natural world as part of their developing self-identity. Animated by seasonal changes and individual creatures that come and go, wildlife zones pique children's curiosity and capture their hearts.

5 *Schoolyard Water Systems*

🍃 *Water Stewardship as a Teaching Resource*

Most of our communities' water systems are underground, hidden from view, and unnoticed by urban and suburban residents, young and old alike. Where does our water come from? Where does it go? How does it get there?[1] Are we managing our water systems in ways that are ecologically sound and sustainable?

Clean, fresh water is a precious resource. It comes to our schools and communities through municipal plumbing systems and natural waterways and in the form of rainfall. It leaves school grounds through man-made stormdrains,sewer networks, and by running over the landscape and percolating into the soil. In most cases, water from these sources is relatively clean when it arrives on school grounds and dirtier when it leaves.

School communities have the power to improve their local water systems and to use them as educational resources at the same time. Water is a dynamic teaching tool that can be harnessed to enrich the curriculum across disciplines and grade levels. Many schools around the world are teaching their students to act as watershed stewards and to use water responsibly. Some schools are taking control of stormwater flows across their landscapes, others are reducing the amount of water they consume, and a few are purifying some of the wastewater and runoff they produce.

The case studies that follow focus on schools with water projects that range from watershed education to water purification and conservation. They teach lessons about the water cycle and other fundamental processes that everyone should understand in order to be ecologically literate and to be able to steer our communities toward a more ecologically sound future.

🍃 *Site-specific Design for Water Conservation and Purification*

The design of schoolyard water systems varies with the climate and precipitation levels of each region, the school's location in its watershed, the shape of surrounding topography, and the size of the school building and grounds—but this is a topic that all schools can address in some way, because water is present and consumed at every school.

Schools in wet regions of the country, or in heavily paved neighborhoods, are frequently interested in finding ways to prevent flooding and slow down water movement so it percolates into the ground instead of overflowing the stormwater system. Some Los Angeles schools participating in the Cool Schools program, for example, found that they could reduce flooding by removing asphalt on their playgrounds and by planting "thirsty" trees where water pooled.[2] Schools in other areas are using living roofs to absorb part of their stormwater and slow its release to stormdrains.

By contrast, schools in dry regions frequently desire a system that conserves the precious water they have and makes good use of every drop. Designers of water systems for these schools frequently adopt dry gardening principles, selecting native plants that are adapted to local rainfall patterns and avoiding plant species that are "water hogs." These schools sometimes use rain barrels or cisterns to capture and store rainfall and water-conserving drip irrigation methods to efficiently water vegetation that requires supplemental moisture.

Schoolyard water systems in any geographic location are complemented by water conservation measures implemented *within* school buildings, such as low-flow faucets and toilets or simple, but effective, programs that instruct the school community to turn off water when it is not in use. These conservation programs often result in long-term financial savings by reducing water bills.

In most climates, schools can also cleanse stormwater and wastewater flows onsite. Stormwater purification systems that use low-tech, plant-based water purification techniques such as swales (vegetated "ditches") and wetlands can improve water quality. They are particularly important in urban, suburban, and agricultural areas where stormwater runoff is likely to be polluted—and are an engaging way to get students involved in improving the water quality of local streams and lakes. Wastewater treatment systems process water from sinks and, sometimes, toilets, purifying them onsite using constructed wetlands and treatment systems, and then reusing the water for irrigation and other purposes. These purification systems are often practical, as well as environmentally responsible and educational.

Schoolyard water resources, created for ecological and academic purposes, can be beautiful assets that contribute to curb appeal and school pride. For example, planted swales used for stormwater purification add ribbons of attractive greenery to the landscape when artfully designed. Stormwater detention ponds, usually an unappealing, utilitarian feature of many communities, can be reinterpreted as living wetland ecosystems or stepped plazas that double as seating areas in the dry season. Often a detention pond or a wetland, planted with native aquatic species, will also attract wildlife and be suitable for use by science, math, art, or other classes.

The best schoolyard water systems are sensitive to local water cycles and climate. They incorporate plant-based stormwater and/or greywater purification methods to reduce the school's contribution to local water pollution and to conserve water. Schoolyard water systems should favor onsite rainwater retention and groundwater recharge instead of sending stormwater into municipal drainage systems. Water conservation measures, such as dry gardens and low-flow water systems, can significantly reduce a school's annual water bills and its impact on the local environment. Building schoolyard water systems with student involvement, maintaining them with student assistance, and connecting them to the existing curricula maximizes their educational value as exceptional scientific resources.

❧ Watershed Education

Every school is located within a watershed and has access to rainfall during wet seasons—yet the educational potential of these resources remains untapped in most places. From an early age, children can be entrusted with reducing their school's environmental impact by taking charge of the water they use, conserving it where possible, and helping to ensure that rainwater is clean when it leaves the schoolyard to flow into nearby waterways. By tapping into this local educational resource in a manner that captures students' imaginations, schools help their students become good stewards of their community's ecological infrastructure.

Most students study the water cycle in an abstract way in elementary and middle school, following arrows on a simple diagram in a book. Connecting this type of water cycle curricula with the landscape at your own school brings these central concepts to life, and makes them relevant to students who ask, "Why is this important to me?"

Teachers might begin their investigation of water systems with a basic discussion about the school's own watershed, followed by a model-building project that illustrates how rainwater moves through their own local topography. Students can step outside to consider how rainwater moves across their schoolyard and ask questions about where the water flows when it leaves the grounds. Some schools also extend these lessons to incorporate related discussions about mapping techniques, climate patterns, geography, hydrology, and geology, depending on the students' grade levels.

Make the most of rainfall. Take children out into the drizzle and let them watch it as it flows down hills, across the pavement, through their garden, and into the stormdrain. Ask them

❧ What Is a Watershed?

A watershed is a stormwater drainage basin—an area of land that shares a natural drainage network of creeks and rivers. Its boundaries are the high points in the landscape—the tops of gentle hills or tall mountains—that cause rainwater to "shed" (flow downhill) toward the center of the basin where it forms creeks and rivers. Rainwater that falls in a single watershed drains to the same receiving water body—such as a river, pond, lake, or ocean—at the end of its downhill journey.

where it comes from, where it goes, and what it might pick up on its journey through the schoolyard (and the city!). Use maps, models, and field trips to help them find their school's place in the watershed and bring these lessons to life. Plant rainwater gardens to clean water flows onsite and create ponds to observe aquatic creatures. Teach students responsible irrigation practices, remove some asphalt from your schoolyard to let water soak into the ground, and experiment with the properties of this fascinating liquid.[3]

Schoolyard watershed models

Some schools use hands-on projects to enliven watershed studies for their students and to illustrate how stormwater travels through the neighborhood. Students at Monarch Grove Elementary School in Los Osos, California, for example, worked with the local San Luis Obispo 4-H chapter to build a large-scale model of the entire 48,000-acre Morro Bay watershed on their schoolyard. To create the model, children and their parents used foam insulation boards covered with layers of cement and colored cement stucco. Approximately 12 feet square at the base with the highest peaks in the watershed almost 3 feet tall, the model reflects the 2,400-foot topography, rendered with a vertical exaggeration of 3x in order to make it easier to use. The model is used to teach the school community about water quality and how to keep local waterways and estuary clean. Some classes also use the model as a resource for teaching about the water cycle, local geology, and Native American history.[4] (Figure 5.1)

Lockwood Elementary School in Oakland, California, is surrounded by busy streets and a mostly flat, paved urban environment. It is only a mile from San Francisco Bay, but the water can't be seen from the school. From the playground, the most prominent and visible natural features are the Oakland hills, about three miles inland.

In 2001 the school had the opportunity to redesign its schoolyard and bring awareness of natural systems onto the grounds. The playground design that I helped to create in collaboration with the Trust for Public Land includes a "watershed" model painted on the asphalt, oriented along the approximate path that rainwater follows across the playground. My original design concept called for this pathway to be a functioning swale network or stormwater runnel, but it wasn't feasible to have flowing surface water present on this school site.[5] (Figure 5.2)

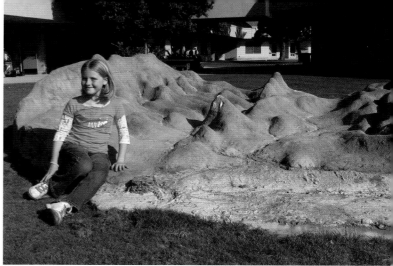

Judy Neuhauser

FIGURE 5.1 *The model at Monarch Grove Elementary is durable enough to walk on. Classes can spray it with a garden hose to simulate rainfall and erosion processes.*

Make stormwater flows visible on school grounds[6]

The built environment in urban and suburban landscapes often obscures the underlying natural systems that predate them. Typically, urban creeks are channeled into pipes that run under our streets, houses, and schools. Though hidden from view, they continue to receive rainfall through our stormdrains. In some places, creeks are left above ground but are forced into narrow, steep-sided, engineered channels that make the water flow faster, deeper, and straighter than nature intended. Urban development often pushes up against these channelized creeks,

FIGURE 5.2 *The painted creek at Lockwood Elementary "flows" downstream from the hills (and kindergarten building), east toward the bay.*

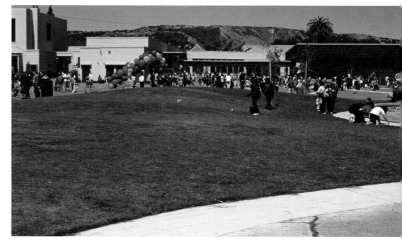

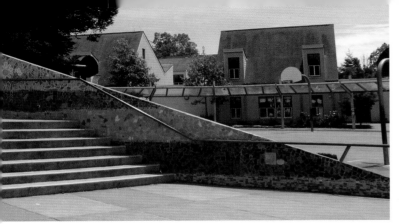

FIGURE 5.3 *This tile mosaic mural at Rosa Parks School depicts the natural world, including a soil profile with an artistic representation of the buried creek, shown in the lowest layers of the mural.*[7]

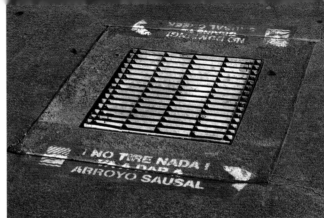

FIGURE 5.4 *The painted markings next to this schoolyard stormdrain in Oakland, California, help students to recognize buried Sausal Creek as an asset the school should help to protect.*

so they are frequently locked behind tall fences and treated as hazards, rather than revered as vital life-giving systems.

Visit your local historical society or map library to find old maps of your school's neighborhood. Ask students to look for any historical creeks that run close to the school. If a creek once flowed in your neighborhood, can you locate it now?

If you find a hidden waterway in your midst, try to bring it back into the school community's consciousness in some way and make it easier for everyone to see. In urban areas with creeks buried underground in pipes, schools can mark the ground surface in a way that traces the water's flow, or paint signs near the stormdrains that lead to these underground waterways. If there is a channelized creek near your school-yard, it might be possible to provide students with safe visual and/or physical access to the water.

Channeling rainfall from school rooftops into onsite water features, such as ponds, wetlands and swales, is another way to make part of the watershed visible and improve water quality at the same time. These man-made additions to the schoolyard can be artfully designed to celebrate the beauty and educational value of rainwater.

Mark the location of buried waterways onsite. In 2006 I worked with Rosa Parks School in Berkeley, California, to create a green schoolyard master plan that now guides the gradual transformation of the school grounds. (See chapter 2, Figure 2.3) Urban development placed a small historical waterway in pipes under the schoolyard, making it physically inaccessible to the students. As the schoolyard design is implemented, we

plan to raise awareness of the buried creek using schoolyard artwork above the buried waterway and elsewhere onsite. In spring 2009, students worked with local artists to create a tile mosaic that incorporates this theme. In the future, we also hope

FIGURE 5.5 *Sometimes it is possible to seek access to a hidden or blocked water flow onsite. A fifteen-foot fence separates this school from a nearby creek, which runs along the edge of its playground. The students engaged in a green schoolyard design process that investigated the possibility of creating visual or physical access to the waterway. In the meantime, to raise students' awareness of the hidden stream, the school painted a creek mural on the asphalt in front of the fence.*

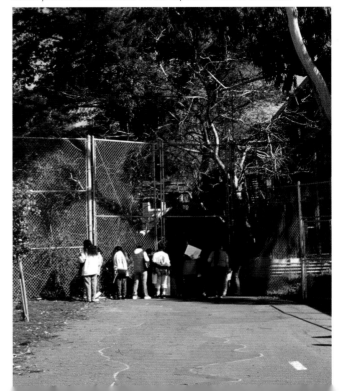

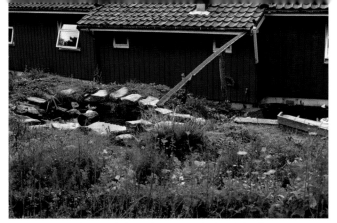

FIGURE 5.6 *Rainwater-fed pond at Bergen Steiner School.*

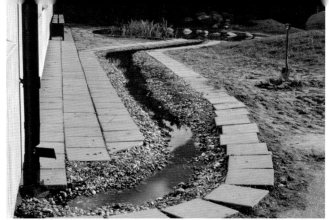

FIGURE 5.7 *Mårten School in southern Sweden has a small pond fed by runoff from the school's roof. The stormwater flows across the roof, down the building's downspout, and through a long winding channel at ground level before filling the pond.[9]*

to develop a "listening station" near the stormdrains to allow auditory access to the underground creek. (Figures 5.3–5.5)

Connect downspouts to schoolyard water features. At most schools, students do not follow rain patterns closely enough to be able to tell if a given year is a wet year or a dry year. At Bergen Steiner School in Norway, however, rainfall patterns are directly connected to a schoolyard pond. When it rains, roof runoff flows across a rain gutter, directly into the pond. When the pond is full, the excess water spills into the adjacent garden and is absorbed by the ground. When the weather has been dry for a while, the students monitor that pattern

through direct observation of the pond's water level, and re-fill the pond with water from a hose. This system not only emphasizes the importance of rainfall to natural systems, but also focuses the students' attention on how much rainfall they receive.[8] (Figures 5.6 and 5.7)

Use stormwater flow in an artful manner. Parents at Bergen Steiner School built a simple, playful stormwater art piece onsite. When it rains, water drains from a stairway into an adjacent channel and cascades downhill in a series of small waterfalls. This feature keeps the stairs from flooding and provides an interesting, attractive play element for the children.[10] (Figures 5.8 and 5.9)

FIGURE 5.8 *Playful drainage system at Bergen Steiner School.*

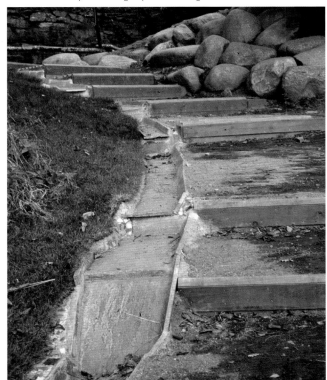

FIGURE 5.9 *The cobblestone runnel at Svendstuen School in Oslo, Norway, directs stormwater as it flows downhill and keeps the stairs free of puddles.*

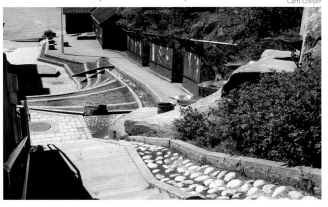

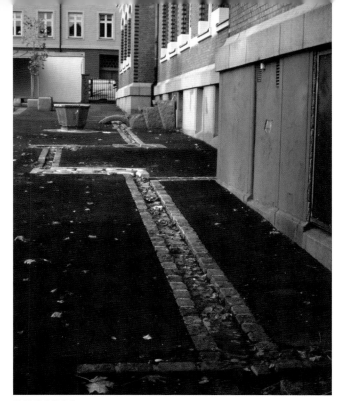

FIGURE 5.10

FIGURE 5.11 *Argyle Primary School in London, England, channels a portion of its stormwater across the paved schoolyard in a meandering, colorful, mosaic-covered runnel, decorated with water-themed artwork. At the end of the channel, children may observe the water disappearing underground through a round stormdrain.*[12]

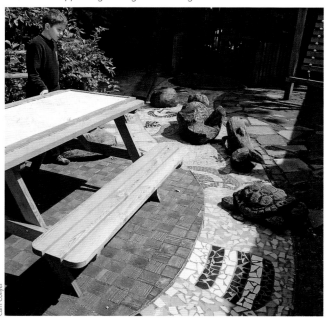

Grünerløkka School in central Oslo, Norway, includes artful stormwater features that double as enticing play elements. Water from the downspouts and an outdoor drinking fountain is directed into an intricate network of surface-flow channels that guide it under small bridges, through swirling pathways, and ultimately into the stormdrain. (Figure 5.10) This complex arrangement must be cleaned regularly to prevent clogging.[11]

🍃 *Teaching Water System Ecology through the Design of the Schoolyard Landscape*

After students understand watershed and water cycle processes, they can begin to use their own schoolyard to mitigate the effects of urban development on local water systems. The first step in this process is to analyze the school grounds to see where water is flowing from, where it is going to, and what it might be picking up on its journey. Next, school communities should consider how they can (1) modify water flows to increase rainwater infiltration; (2) slow and filter stormwater to make it cleaner and less likely to flood the stormdrain network; and (3) conserve as much municipal tap water as possible. Achieving these goals often requires some physical modifications to the school site, but as the examples in this section illustrate, these are worthwhile and achievable tasks.

Many of the following projects incorporate multiple water conservation and purification strategies in an integrated manner. I have highlighted particular characteristics of these systems to bring them to your attention.

SITE DESIGN GOAL #1: *Reduce stormwater runoff by increasing infiltration on school grounds.*

Asphalt and concrete are two of the most commonly used materials in our playgrounds. Unfortunately, they are not healthy choices for our watersheds. Rainwater that falls on these impermeable surfaces runs off quickly before it can soak into the ground to recharge the water table, disrupting stormwater flow patterns and causing erosion due to the water's high speed. Rainwater flowing over asphalt or concrete also picks up pollutants such as oil that drips from cars, pollution that settles out of the air and accumulates on the ground, and other materials that are spilled on the ground. Pollutants are washed off the pavement and into the stormdrains when it

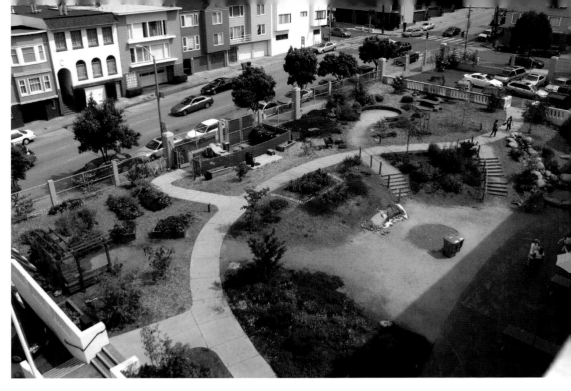

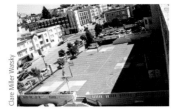

FIGURE 5.12 *Sherman School's playground, September 2006, before construction began.*

FIGURE 5.13 *Sherman School's green schoolyard, April 2009, after plants have grown for one year.*

rains, eventually ending up in our rivers, lakes, and oceans where they harm sensitive aquatic environments. Sometimes stormwater pollution also threatens the quality of our drinking water, as well.

To alleviate these problems, some schools are removing asphalt and concrete to increase the amount of permeable (water-absorbing) surfaces onsite. Permeable pavement may be used for pathways and other areas that need to remain accessible for wheelchairs or vehicles. Permeable pavement options include decomposed granite (similar to firmly-packed course sand), and bricks or flagstones set on sand. Hard surfaces may also be replaced with soft, child-friendly ground coverings that are conducive to play, such as planted areas, wood chips, or sand. "Rain garden" wetlands that allow water to soak into the ground can also be used to achieve stormwater infiltration goals. Larger, more technical water infiltration projects, with underground pipe systems, can be employed to alleviate flooding.

Rain gardens and stormwater wetlands. Rain gardens are wetlands or ponds that are connected to a building's downspout or drainage swale that receives stormwater runoff when it rains. They are generally placed on permeable surfaces to encourage rainwater to soak into the ground. Small-scale stormwater ponds are useful for processing small quantities of rainwater in a manner that is attractive and educational. (See Figures 5.6 and 5.7)

Schoolyard asphalt removal. Sherman School in San Francisco, California, is a dramatic example of the power of schoolyard asphalt removal to change the character of a schoolyard landscape. As part of a large green schoolyard renovation project, the school removed 68 percent of the impermeable surfaces on one of their playgrounds.[13] The renovation replaced approximately 9,500 square feet of flat asphalt with a rolling hillside filled with plants, mulch, and permeable decomposed granite pathways that allow rainwater to soak into the ground. The new design also features a wheelchair accessible concrete pathway that meanders through the yard and a curved asphalt patio along the school building, totaling approximately 4,500 square feet.[14] (Figures 5.12 and 5.13)

SITE DESIGN GOAL #2: *Slow and filter schoolyard stormwater flows*

Stormwater moves through urban environments with greater speed than nature intended, running off rooftops, streets, sidewalks, and ground surfaces that resist water absorption. During

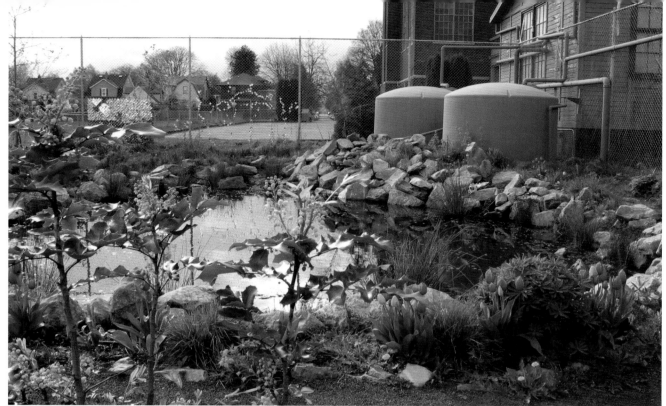

FIGURE 5.14 *Surface water in the garden at da Vinci Arts Middle School provides habitat for beneficial insects and supports a great variety of plants and wildlife.*

Rosey Jencks

large rainstorms or in places where a high percentage of the land is paved, the resulting water surges can overwhelm the stormdrain network and pollute the receiving water bodies.

These problems can be addressed by providing areas where stormwater can soak into the ground and by reducing the water's speed. Densely planted areas slow stormwater runoff because leaves and branches partially block the water's path. As the water slows, particulates drop out of the water column and settle to the bottom of the planted zone. Plants also collect nutrients from the water, and they can be used to filter or remove other water impurities, if the proper species are selected and placed appropriately. Water that does not soak into the ground during its slow passage through vegetation is often released from the end of a swale or wetland with improved quality, and at a speed that stormdrains can manage.

Schools can help repair their watersheds and protect their local streams, lakes, and oceans by designing their landscapes to (1) slow down stormwater, so it can soak into the soil, (2) filter stormwater by using planted swales and wetlands, and (3) create living roofs on their buildings to help moderate peak flows.

Stormwater gardens filter and capture rainwater to improve local water quality. The da Vinci Living Water Garden project, founded in 2001, is a collaboration between da Vinci Arts Middle School in Portland, Oregon, and Urban Water Works, a local nonprofit organization.[15] The goal of the project is to educate students and citizens about stormwater runoff and water quality, while celebrating the beauty of rainwater.

The project reroutes stormwater runoff from the school's roofs and parking lots into a 7,200 square-foot water garden that includes cisterns, a pond, a constructed wetland, and a bioremediation swale. Located on the site of an abandoned tennis court, the project was designed and built by the school's students, teachers, and parents. It now cleans and absorbs 100 percent of the water it captures, reducing runoff to the Willamette River, providing recreational and educational opportunities for the school and surrounding communities, and creating a model for stormwater diversion that can also be implemented on residential and commercial sites.

The rainwater harvesting system consists of two tanks capable of holding a total of 5,000 gallons of water, supplied by gravity-fed runoff from a 2,840-square-foot roof. In a region that gets over 30 inches of rain a year, just 3 inches of rain can fill the tanks. Overflow from the tanks is directed into the pond. The cisterns supply a gravity-fed garden irrigation system, which is used during dry summer months.

The garden also captures stormwater runoff from nearby parking lots and filters it though a bioremediation swale before it enters the pond. Plants in the swale slow the flowing water, allowing pollutants and sediment to settle out. Some of the water percolates into the ground during this journey, helping to recharge the water table. This system keeps the water garden clean, and removes some of the pollutants that would have otherwise entered the local watershed.

The da Vinci Living Water Garden is an attractive, clear demonstration of sustainable rainwater harvesting techniques and an important asset for the school. It provides a living laboratory, educational and recreational opportunities, and green space for relaxation. Students who participate in this project have a greater understanding of stormwater management methods and are empowered by the experience of transforming their immediate environment in a lasting, beneficial way. (Figure 5.14)

Living roofs on school buildings moderate stormwater flows.
"Living roofs" are building rooftops, covered with waterproof drainage membranes, a thin layer of lightweight soil, and hardy, drought tolerant plants. Living roofs act as sponges when it rains, holding some of the water on the rooftop for a short time, before releasing it to the gutter and downspout systems below. This moderation of stormwater flows helps to protect stormdrains from sudden surges of water during rainstorms, which can help to keep them from overflowing.

Living roofs are also useful for insulating buildings, resulting in lower energy needs for winter heating and summer cooling. Rooftop plants also keep the surrounding outdoor environment cooler by reducing the "urban heat island" effect that is usually produced by traditional, dark roofing materials like asphalt shingles. Additionally, living roofs sometimes provide habitat for birds, butterflies, and other beneficial wildlife. They are visually attractive and help a building to blend in with other vegetation onsite. Large living roofs have more pronounced environmental benefits than smaller ones, but even tiny projects can be used as successful demonstration projects. (Figures 5.15–5.17)

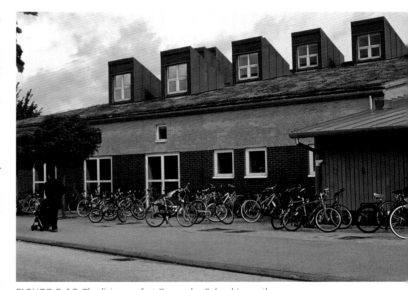

FIGURE 5.16 *The living roof at Gunnesbo School in southern Sweden is planted with drought tolerant, waxy-coated sedums that are well-suited to hot, dry roof conditions.*

FIGURE 5.15 *The barn at St. Hansgården in southern Sweden is part of an after-school permaculture center for the local school district. The building and its living, grassy rooftop were constructed by local middle school students, with the help of an architect.[16] (See Chapter 8.)*

FIGURE 5.17 *This small, red tool shed included in our 2008 "Sustainable Schoolyard" exhibit at the United States Botanic Garden in Washington, DC, was built with a living roof and planted with sedums.[17]*

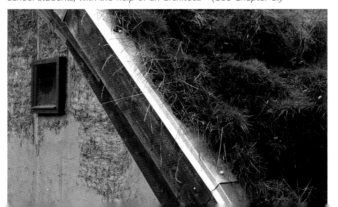

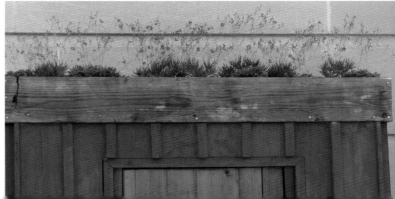

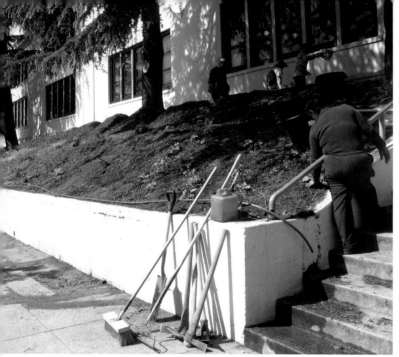

FIGURE 5.18 *Volunteers from Sequoia School in Oakland, California, planted a large hillside garden along their perimeter sidewalk, shown here during installation. The native plants will be watered using a drip irrigation system until they are established. The soil is covered with a layer of mulch to preserve moisture.*[18]

FIGURE 5.19 *Cowick First School in southwest England teaches its young students that water is a precious resource. This concept is noted on schoolyard signs and reinforced at the school with the use of low-flow bathroom sinks and toilets. A rain barrel also collects stormwater runoff from the school's roof for watering the garden.*[19]

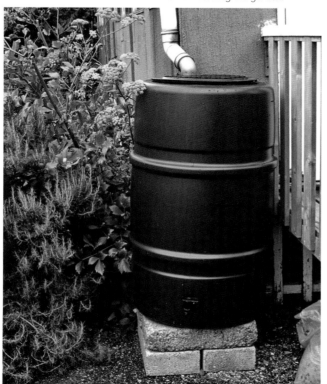

SITE DESIGN GOAL #3: *Use as little potable water as possible*

Many of us take it for granted that purified water flows from our taps and "dirty" water goes "away," down the drain to be treated elsewhere. However, fresh water is in short supply in many places and a lot of energy is expended to make water clean enough for us to drink and use in our schools and homes.

Schools can choose to reduce the amount of fresh, clean water they import to their site from municipal water systems by instituting water conservation programs. They might also choose to capture and temporarily store rainwater in rain barrels or cisterns to supplement irrigation supplies or to flush toilets onsite. Schools can also recycle used water by filtering it in wetland gardens.

Improve water conservation with drought tolerant plants, drip irrigation and mulch. To conserve potable water, schools can initiate water conservation programs that include good landscape design choices, such as native and drought tolerant plants that are adapted to local rainfall patterns. Native plants benefit from irrigation in their first year after planting, but usually require very little supplemental moisture after they are established. Efficient drip irrigation systems coupled with water-retaining mulch on the soil's surface, to slow evaporation, often effectively reduces further water usage. (Figure 5.18)

Capture rainwater for use onsite. Stormwater can be captured and stored for later use inside school buildings or for landscape irrigation. The most common types of rainwater storage devices are rain barrels, which have a relatively small capacity, and cisterns, which tend to be larger. Each of these storage devices can be connected to a clean source of water, such as runoff from a building's metal rooftop. Storing water in closed containers, such as rain barrels and cisterns, helps keep the water clean and prevents mosquitoes from breeding in it.

Rain barrels are most frequently installed outside schools at the base of a downspout, where they can be easily seen and used for educational purposes. Due to their relatively small storage capacity, rain barrels are most useful in places that receive intermittent rain year-round, so they will be refilled frequently. Cisterns can be buried under the playground, placed in school building basements, or installed in gardens, where the water is needed. They can be used for much larger irrigation tasks

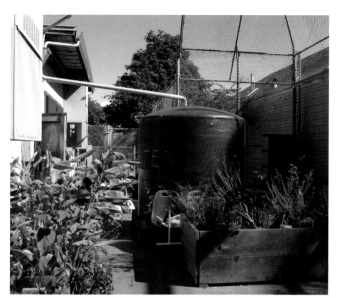

FIGURE 5.20 *In San Francisco, California, Alvarado Elementary School has a large metal cistern that collects rainwater from the adjacent classroom rooftop. The water is used to irrigate plants in the neighboring "secret garden," tucked into a corner of the schoolyard.*[20]

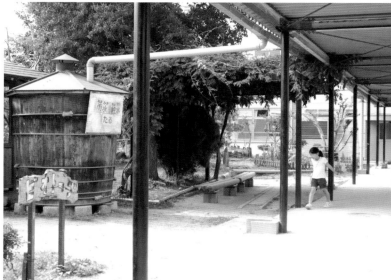

FIGURE 5.21

Sandra Koike

FIGURE 5.23

Sandra Koike

such as storing winter rains for summer irrigation, watering wide expanses of thirsty grass, or storing water for other school gardening or pond-related uses. (Figures 5.19 and 5.20)

Sagano Elementary School in Kyoto, Japan, employs several different methods to reduce its need for potable, municipal water. The school collects roof runoff in a 528-gallon (2,000 liter) wooden cistern, used to irrigate flowers in the schoolyard, and (Figure 5.21) the children leave empty buckets out in the rain to collect smaller amounts of water for hand-irrigation. (Figure 5.22) They also use a well in their culinary garden to water crops.[21] (Figure 5.23)

FIGURE 5.22

Sandra Koike

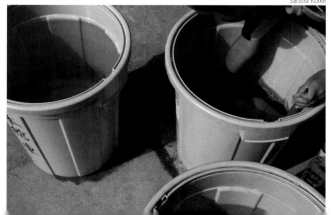

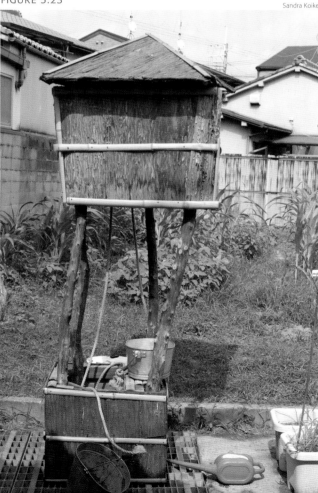

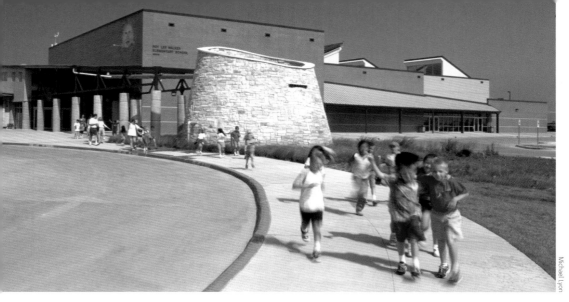

FIGURE 5.24

Michael Lyon

Roy Lee Walker Elementary School, in McKinney, Texas, has an impressive rainwater harvesting system that captures runoff from the school's entire roof area. Six large stone cisterns hold a total of 68,000 gallons of rainwater when they are full. (Figure 5.24) Students monitor the amount of stormwater held in the cisterns using a gauge in their main hallway. The collected stormwater irrigates buffalo grass plantings and other native vegetation. A 30-foot-tall windmill in front of the school powers a filtration system for the collected stormwater and circulates it to the irrigation network. The school building also has an extensive solar panel array that meets most of their needs for hot water. Other ecology education features—sundials, a pond, and a weather station—help students tune into the natural cycles around them.[22]

The grounds at Open Charter Elementary, near Los Angeles, were renovated to convert acres of impermeable asphalt into an asset for the school community and the local watershed. In 1999, the school created vegetated swales (planted depressions)

Melinda Kelley, TreePeople

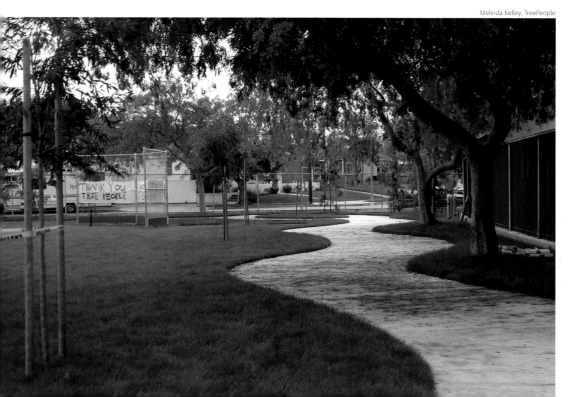

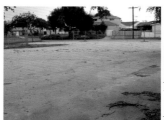

Rebecca Drayse, TreePeople

FIGURE 5.25–5.27 *Open Charter Elementary shown before and after schoolyard renovation. Underground cistern during construction (below).*

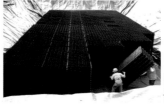

TreePeople

to absorb part of the site's stormwater and planted 88 trees to absorb water and provide shade. In 2002, the school installed a substantial 110,000-gallon underground cistern, and an accompanying stormwater treatment device, that removes oil residues and other pollutants from the stormwater before storage. The water collected in the cistern irrigates the school's ball field and other vegetation during Los Angeles's long, hot, dry season.[23]

The cistern, water treatment filter, and plantings at Open Charter Elementary work together to provide a comprehensive approach that accomplishes the project's stormwater management goals. "All stormwater on the site is either percolated in the tree wells and swales; collected, treated in a sedimentation basin and stored in an underground cistern for later use; or treated and released to the stormdrain system if the cistern is full."[24] Students at the school also benefit from the beautiful shady, green learning and play space. (Figures 5.25–5.27)

Conserve water by recycling it onsite. Most of our communities and schools are *designed* to waste water—using it only once before sending it down the drain to be cleaned in energy-intensive treatment plants far away. Some of the water that currently runs down our drains can be reclaimed by savvy school communities and put to additional uses onsite, conserving water and energy in the process.

The water that flows down our bathroom and classroom sinks, usually only lightly "dirty" from hand washing, is called "greywater." Greywater may be reclaimed relatively easily for landscape irrigation if simple protocols are followed to maintain hygiene. The water flushed in our toilets usually has a more complex load of contaminants and is referred to as "blackwater." Blackwater can also be reclaimed using thorough, but manageable, water purification processes. Schools can illustrate these treatment processes for their students by installing wetland-based treatment systems on their grounds.

When Östratorn School in southern Sweden expanded to accommodate more students in 1997, they chose to create a building addition that showcases green practices. Among its wide array of exemplary features—from recycled materials to renewable energy—is an innovative system that combines rainwater collection and onsite blackwater treatment to reduce use of potable municipal water. (Figure 5.28)

At Östratorn School, rainwater is collected from the building's roof and channeled into its basement where it is stored in

two large cisterns that hold a total of 18,000 liters (4,755 gallons) of water, used to flush bathroom toilets. The toilets are a two-chambered variety that separate urine and feces, and use *very* little water for each flush. A mere two deciliters (6.8 fluid ounces) of water is used to flush urine and four deciliters (13.5 fluid ounces) to flush feces—a dramatic savings over standard toilet models that use up to six liters (202.8 fluid ounces or 1.6 gallons) of fresh water for each flush.

When flushed, the urine is sent to two underground storage tanks that are emptied periodically by a local farmer who uses this nitrogen-rich material as fertilizer for his off-site fields. Feces and its flush water are sent down a different set of pipes. The feces solids are collected in a basement composting unit where they are processed for use as fertilizer for the same farm. The feces flush water, called blackwater, is separated from the solids and is treated onsite in a constructed wetland built specifically for this purpose. (Figure 5.29 on the next page)

The blackwater is pumped from the toilet system into a lined, constructed wetland filled with gravel and planted with tall reeds in front of the school. The plants' roots slowly filter the nutrients out of the water and the water is gradually released

FIGURE 5.28

White Arkitekter AB

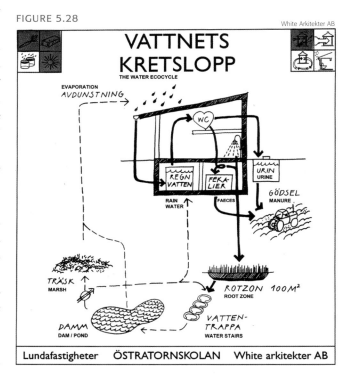

from the wetland. (Figure 5.30) This area of the wetland is fenced off from the schoolyard to prevent children from digging in it—but there is no surface water visible above the gravel, and I did not detect any odors from it when I walked nearby.

After the water is released from this subsurface wetland, it flows downhill in an attractive, waterfall-like series of "flow form stairs," which aerate it. Next, the water crosses through the root zone of an adjacent shrubby area and into a beautiful, small pond in front of the school. Water then evaporates from the pond, and perhaps falls again as rain on the school's rooftop. The water in the pond is clean enough to use again in the toilet flushing system, if desired.[25]

FIGURE 5.29

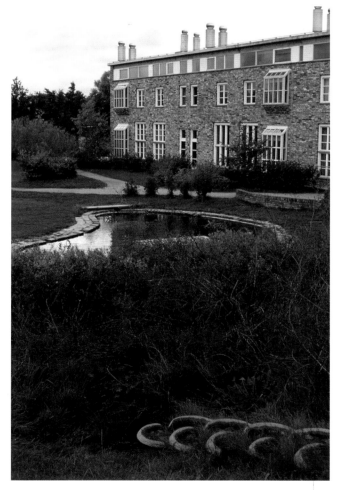

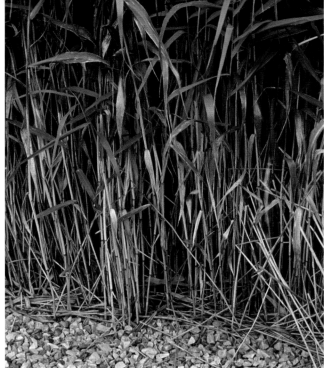

FIGURE 5.30

Comprehensive Model

In 2006 Sidwell Friends Middle School in Washington, DC, completed a major building expansion that resulted in a large new addition and a substantial renovation of existing school buildings. Following the environmental stewardship philosophy and Quaker values of the school, the new construction and renovation were designed to be as green as possible; they achieved an impressive "Platinum" rating from the LEED® Green Building Rating System—the first K-12 school in the United States to achieve this distinguished status.

Green building systems are thoroughly incorporated into every facet of the building, but the design's close attention to water systems is truly exceptional because it includes onsite blackwater treatment and addresses water systems in three other ways as well.[26]

The most unusual water-related feature onsite is the substantial blackwater treatment system that cleans and processes wastewater from the building's toilets, sinks, floor drains and janitor basins so that it can be later reused in urinals, toilets and the building's cooling tower. This saves a substantial amount of water and energy in comparison to standard offsite treatment systems.

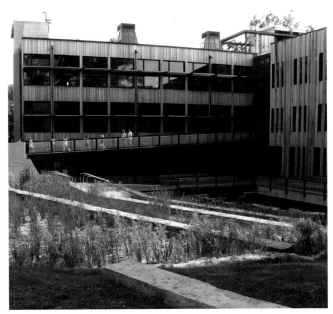

FIGURE 5.31

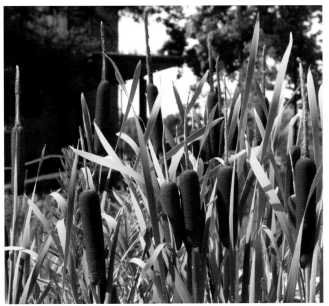

FIGURE 5.32

FIGURE 5.33

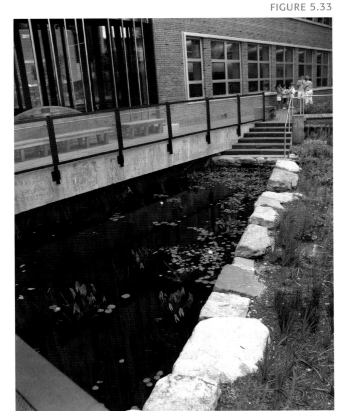

After the water runs down the building's drains, it enters an underground settlement tank where liquids and solids are separated. The liquids proceed to an attractive wastewater treatment wetland garden just outside the building. (Figure 5.31) The wastewater circulates through the garden repeatedly, passing through three tiers of subsurface flow wetlands where cattails (*Typha* spp.) (Figure 5.32), bullrushes (*Scirpus* spp.), and other plants rooted in deep, odorless gravel beds remove nutrients from the water. As it circulates through this system, the water also cycles through a trickling filter that aerates it and removes excess ammonia. The purified water passes through a sand filter on its way to the building's basement, where it is further treated using three filters and a UV disinfectant system. The resulting water is clean enough to meet municipal wastewater treatment standards, but its use is restricted by health codes; it is only used in the building's cooling tower and the toilet flush system, where it then repeats the cycle.

The school grounds also include a separate stormwater harvesting system that captures roof runoff to create a beautiful pond and rain garden. (Figure 5.33) When it rains, water flows from the roof through downspouts and chutes to the pond below. The pond is filled with fish and aquatic plants that are dynamic teaching tools for the science classes. To help the

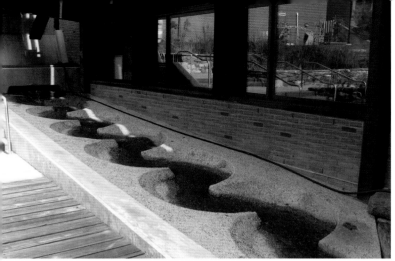

FIGURE 5.34

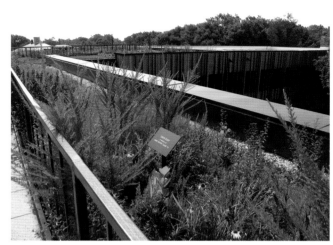

FIGURE 5.36

fish thrive, the pond includes a 4-foot deep section, protected by an underwater metal grate designed to allow fish to successfully over-winter. The pond water is continuously circulated using an attractive, swirling aeration system that deters mosquitoes. (Figure 5.34) After large rainstorms, the pond water spills into the adjacent rain garden's floodplain, where it percolates into the ground to recharge the water table. (Figure 5.35) Excess water from very large storms is channeled into the municipal stormdrain network. During dry periods, the pond can be refilled using an additional 3,000-gallon cistern nearby that is also fed by rooftop stormwater runoff.

FIGURE 5.35

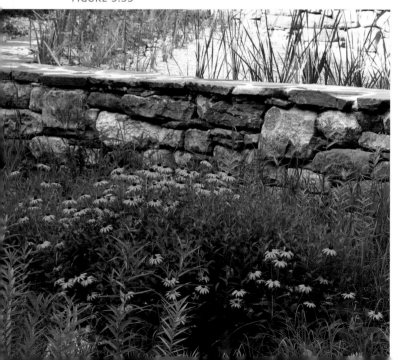

The school building's innovative design includes a living roof that helps to filter stormwater and slow it down on its journey to the pond below. Composed of a 5-inch layer of lightweight soil, planted with drought-tolerant species, the living roof insulates the building and protects the waterproofing membranes and roofing materials from the sun, prolonging their durability. (Figure 5.36) The new building's rooftop also includes a raised-bed organic garden where students grow edible crops and other plants. Other portions of the roof, over the older building, hold solar panels and a weather station. Finally, the school's landscape design strongly emphasizes native plants, which are naturally adapted to local rainfall patterns and, therefore, need little irrigation. The school grounds also include an artificial turf field so students may play games on a soft surface without the high maintenance levels and large irrigation needs typically associated with a live lawn.

According to the school's estimates, their wastewater treatment wetland and the water efficient landscaping features reduce their use of municipal water by 93 percent, as compared to similar schools with conventional water treatment and usage.[27] Their stormwater pond and living roof improve the health of the local watershed in ways that are harder to quantify, but are equally important.

At this writing in 2010, it is fairly unusual to have all of these systems in place on a single school campus, but I hope that more schools will follow Sidwell Friends School's example in the future and take greater responsibility as stewards of their own water systems.

generate may help offset their monthly electric bills or may simply serve as a hands-on educational demonstration.

If schools wish to teach their students using onsite renewable energy systems, they have many choices open to them. To begin, the school community must first determine the goal and scale of their desired project. Energy systems of any size, from small demonstration projects to large installations, will be of educational value and can be connected to the school's curriculum. Large scale projects, aimed at improving the school's energy footprint in a significant way, may also be enticing from financial and ecological perspectives.

The following sections include renewable energy examples from schools around the world. Some of these systems are tied to the electrical grid, while others are smaller stand-alone features that power an individual demonstration or schoolyard feature. Solar power, in the form of photovoltaic (electric) panels and solar thermal panels, seems to be the most common type of renewable energy used at schools, but wind, geothermal, and biomass energy generation methods are also used in an increasing number of places. When selecting a renewable energy

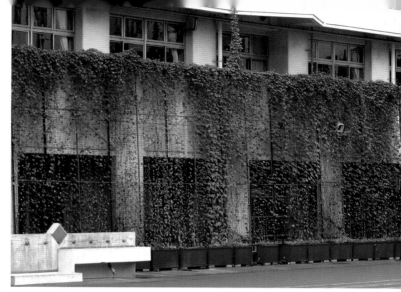

FIGURE 6.6 *The green curtain at this school in Tokyo, Japan, rests on a strong, lightweight metal framework that supports a sturdy wire mesh. In this design, the vines grow up the wire trellis from small planter boxes on the playground, and also grow down from additional planters located on the first floor balcony.*

FIGURE 6.7 *The green curtain at Miyako Ecology Center in Kyoto, Japan, softens the light inside the building and makes a beautiful backdrop for this room. It also provides some visual separation from the adjacent outdoor parking lot, reduces heat gain for the building, and reinforces the Center's environmental education philosophy.*

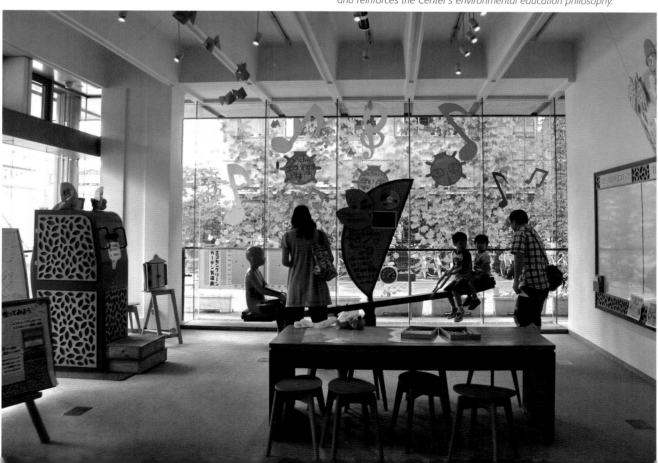

system, consider the school's location, its regulatory and policy context, local climate, physical constraints of the site, and budget. Every school community should be able to find an energy system that suits their needs from the wide range of options.

Solar power

The sun is the ultimate source of most of the energy for our planet. Over millions of years, solar energy has helped to produce oil, natural gas, and coal by fostering plant growth that was eventually transformed into fossil fuels with the addition of tremendous heat, pressure, and time. Because these fuels took so long to form, they are considered "non-renewable," at least in a time frame that is meaningful for human lifespans.

Other types of solar energy are renewable in a much shorter amount of time. For example, the sun heats and lights our atmosphere on a daily basis, providing "free energy" we usually take for granted. It is also the driving force behind continued plant growth, from which we gather "biomass energy" when we burn plant materials such as wood.

We also harness solar energy "passively" by designing buildings to soak up or reflect the sun's rays, and can use natural daylight to illuminate their interiors, as described earlier in this chapter. Solar energy can be captured "actively" with high-tech equipment, to warm a building's water supply or produce electricity. Schools around the world are incorporating these techniques to turn their buildings into solar teaching resources while also reducing their environmental footprint.

Solar thermal systems. Solar thermal systems use the sun's rays to heat a liquid circulating in a closed loop system on a building's rooftop. Once warmed by the sun, the fluid flows through sealed pipes into the building to transfer its heat to a separate, clean water supply inside a heat exchange unit. It takes very little additional energy to then heat the pre-warmed water to the desired temperature for use in school sinks, showers, or radiant heating systems. Most solar thermal systems are installed on top of existing roofing materials, but some may also be integrated into the roof's structure, if desired.

Östratorn School in Sweden uses a custom-made solar thermal system embedded in its roof to preheat water for the school's sinks. "Solar heat is collected by water pipes cast in about a third of the total surface of the concrete roof. [The building's architects felt that in Sweden's climate, this was] a

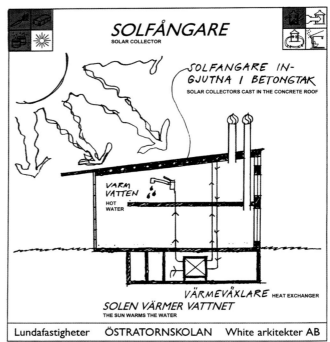

FIGURE 6.8

more reliable solution than resting the collectors on the surface, subject to weather, wind, and other external influences."[31] The liquid that circulates in this closed system travels to a heat exchanger in the basement where it transfers its heat to water that ultimately comes out of the taps. (Figure 6.8)

Oliver McCracken Middle School in Skokie, Illinois, uses rooftop solar thermal panels (Figure 6.9) to preheat all of the school's hot water for 70 percent of the year, significantly reducing the use of its natural gas-powered water heater. The solar

FIGURE 6.9

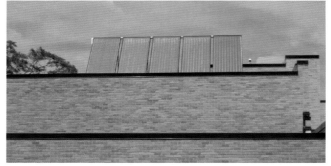

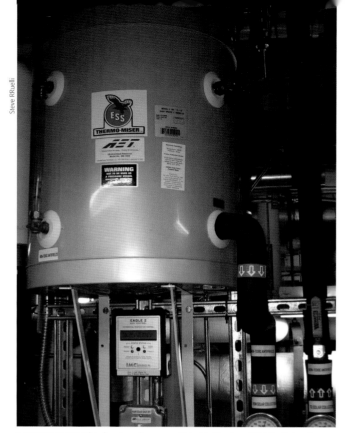

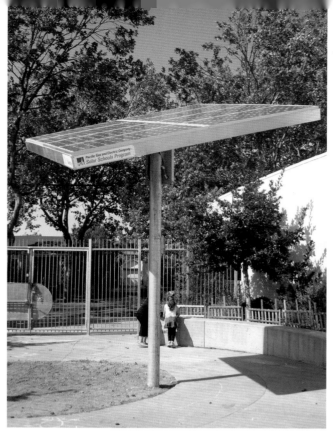

FIGURE 6.10 *This heat exchange unit in McCracken Middle School's utility room transfers warmth—gathered by the liquid circulating in the solar thermal panels—to the building's separate potable water supply.*

FIGURE 6.11 *The PG&E Solar Schools Program installed identical pole-mounted solar arrays in prominent locations in over 100 schoolyards in California.*

thermal panels, and a 1-kilowatt solar electric (PV) system, are also used as teaching tools for science classes.[32] (Figure 6.10)

Solar electric systems. Photovoltaic (PV) systems, commonly referred to as "solar panels," harness the sun's energy to create electrical power for use in the school building or grounds. This electricity may also be sent to the electrical grid to offset the school's annual energy bills. Photovoltaic panels are commonly mounted on school rooftops, or somewhere close to the building, to simplify the wiring process and protect what is usually a large financial investment. Some schools also install elaborate monitoring devices so their students can track energy production in real-time.

Pacific Gas and Electric Company (PG&E), a major California energy utility, started a shareholder-funded Solar Schools Program in 2004.[33] By 2008, the program had awarded 100 grid-tied photovoltaic arrays to schools in its service area to help teach students about renewable energy production, and

to inspire their communities to produce their own energy. The output from these 1-kilowatt PV systems varies somewhat with their geographic location, but generally each produces approximately 2,000 kilowatt hours of electricity each year. The school is credited for this energy, saving them each a few hundred dollars annually.[34] The energy output from each solar installation is recorded on a website set up for the school, so science classes can track it and compare results to those of other schools in the system. PG&E also offers teacher-training sessions about renewable energy.[35] (Figure 6.11)

At Argonne Child Development Center in San Francisco, California, a 1.8 kW photovoltaic system was incorporated into the design of the school building to demonstrate renewable energy generation. South-facing skylights include photovoltaic modules sandwiched between two layers of skylight glass. These polycrystalline silicon PV cells help soften the sunlight coming into the spaces below, and provide approximately 10 percent of the electricity the school uses each year. Completed

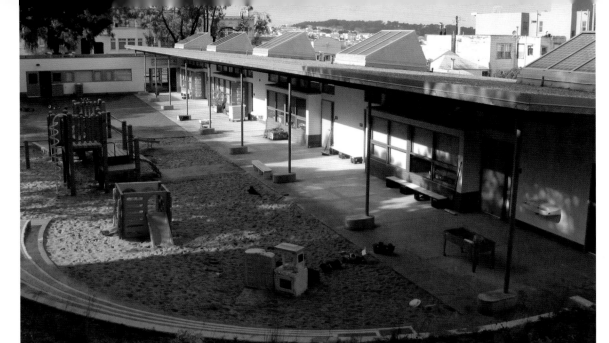

FIGURE 6.12

in 2002, the system has generated a total of 58,000 kilowatt hours over its first seven years.[36] (Figure 6.12)

Wind power

Wind power is a clean, renewable energy production method within reach for many schools. Wind turbines come in a variety of shapes and sizes—from small educational models that demonstrate energy generation and power freestanding schoolyard features, to larger units connected to the electrical grid, which provide sizable quantities of electricity to power school buildings.

Unlike silent solar panels, most wind turbines make some noise as they spin, and they produce vibrations. They are best installed in locations with consistent breezes, away from trees and other potential obstructions, and where their noise and vibrations will not be troublesome. Large or particularly noisy turbines should be placed away from neighbors and classrooms. Wind turbines should also be sited carefully to avoid interfering with bird populations, which can be harmed by spinning blades of many models. Some newer wind turbine designs reduce the risk to birds by using alternate blade configurations.[38] (Figure 6.14)

Royston High School in central England created a watershed model in one of the building's courtyards to demonstrate renewable energy systems, riparian ecosystems, and geology concepts. A recirculating artificial river now flows from its "headwaters" to the "sea," passing flora that is typically encountered along a river's path and rocks that represent the appropriate geology—from boulders to sand.

The school uses two sources of renewable energy to power the water pump for this educational "watershed": a nine-meter (29.5-foot) tall wind turbine (Figure 6.15) and two solar panels mounted on the roof. This dual system ensures that the watershed model functions properly on cloudy or windless days. Electricity produced by the wind turbine and solar panels is also stored onsite in two 24-volt truck batteries for later use.[40] The wind turbine is quiet enough to operate in close proximity to the classrooms surrounding the courtyard.

Cassop Primary School in northern England is a small rural school with a large wind turbine and big goals for renewable energy production and education. In 1999, the local energy utility, Northern Electric, worked with the school and the Durham County Council to install a 50-kilowatt grid-tied wind turbine on their grounds, making Cassop Primary the first wind-powered school in England.[41] (Figure 6.16)

The 60-foot (18 meters) tall turbine produces approximately 50 megawatt hours of electricity per year—more electricity than the school uses. This renewable energy system is a key part of the school's environmental science and technology curricula, and is enhanced by an electronic interpretive panel

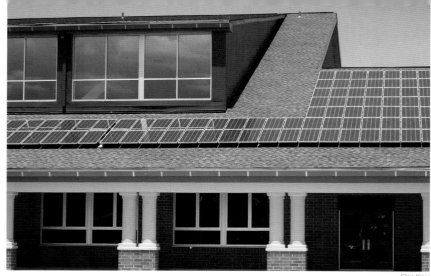

Glen Kizer

FIGURE 6.13 *This 24-kilowatt rooftop PV system at Twenhofel Middle School in Independence, Kentucky, provides about 30 percent of the energy the school uses each year.*[37]

FIGURE 6.14 *The wind turbine at Sagano Elementary School in Kyoto, Japan, is paired with a solar panel to power a decorative schoolyard clock.*[39]

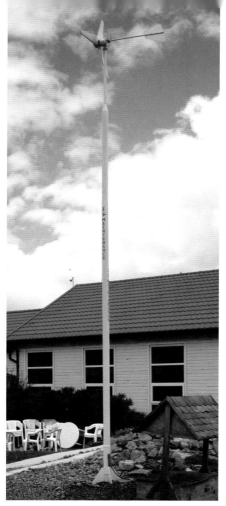

FIGURE 6.15

FIGURE 6.16 *The turbine at Cassop Primary School sits at the far edge of a large field onsite; the noise it makes as it spins is not disruptive to classes.*

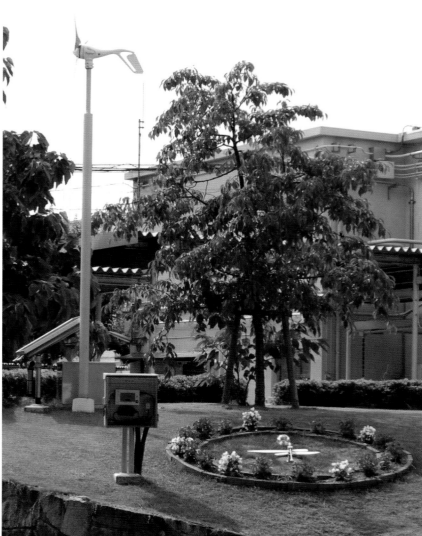

Sandra Koike

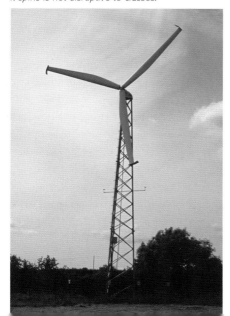

FIGURE 6.17

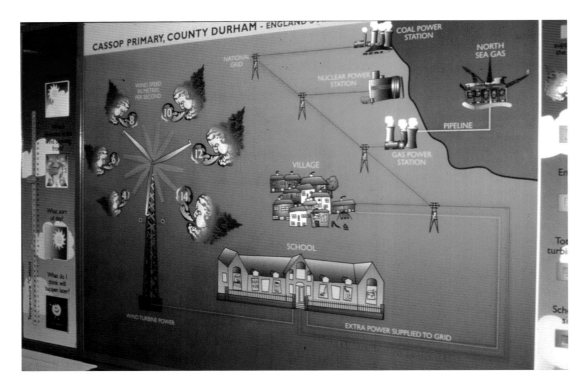

in the front hall. (Figure 6.17) The panel includes real-time energy production and consumption data, and records the total amount of energy the turbine has produced to date. It also illustrates how the turbine's energy benefits the school and contributes to the electrical grid. The panel includes a weather forecasting station so students can make connections between the weather and the amount of energy produced each day.

The school also produces renewable energy in other forms. Since 2003 Cassop's heat has been generated with an onsite boiler that runs on locally produced biomass—recycled wood pellets from the community and wood grown onsite. In addition, the school's hot water is produced by solar thermal panels. In 2005, Cassop School installed a small array of grid-tied photovoltaic panels on the south-facing portion of their roof to add to their electrical generation capacity. They also conserve energy onsite using efficient light bulbs and appliances, increased insulation in the walls, and detailed energy audits. All of these renewable energy systems are fully integrated into the school's curricula and are understood even by very young pupils.[42]

Geothermal energy

Some school buildings are designed to take advantage of geothermal energy. The temperature of the earth, deep in the ground, remains fairly constant throughout the year even when the air temperature experiences wide fluctuations from winter to summer. This constant ground temperature varies by latitude but is generally between 45°F–75°F at a depth of six feet.[43] Geothermal heating and cooling systems are designed to take advantage of this thermal constant by pumping air or water into the ground to be heated or cooled to the earth's stable temperature. Once the ground warms or cools the circulating air or water, it takes very little extra energy to bring it to the desired temperature for a comfortable building. The conditioned air or water may then be used in radiant heating or cooling systems embedded in the building's floors, or as part of the building's HVAC (climate control) systems. Geothermal climate control systems make buildings more comfortable and may save their schools a substantial amount of energy as compared to conventional heating and cooling options. These systems have reasonably short payback periods, generally take up less room in the

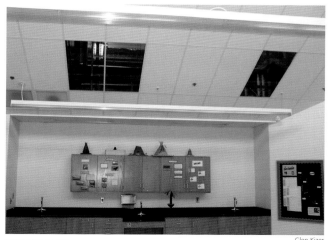

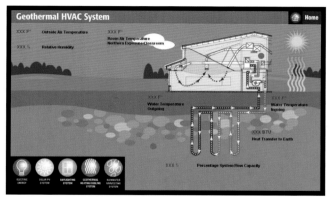

FIGURE 6.19 *This diagram from Twenhofel School's Vital Signs Monitoring System website illustrates how outside air travels through the geothermal heating and cooling system and into the classrooms.*[45]

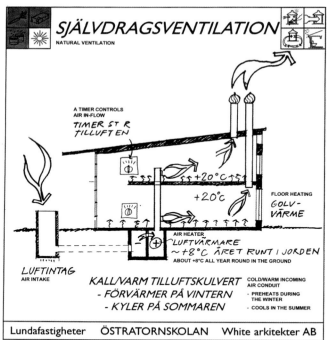

FIGURE 6.20

school than conventional heating and cooling equipment, and run quietly.[44]

Twenhofel Middle School in Independence, Kentucky, has a geothermal heating and cooling system that uses only half the energy of a typical climate control system. Each classroom can adjust its own temperature independently to maximize comfort. The building includes a "truth window" in the science lab's ceiling so students can see the climate control system's ducts and other utilities.[46] (Figures 6.18 and 6.19)

In 1997, the architecture firm, White Arkitekter, helped Östratorn School in Sweden to create a large school building

addition that includes many innovative green building techniques. The overall building design incorporates passive solar features including numerous surfaces made from concrete and brick, which absorb heat and help to moderate the temperature inside. Awnings are placed strategically on the east and west sides to reduce indoor temperatures in the spring and summer. The building relies heavily on daylight as a primary lighting source, so it avoids much of the typical heat gain that results from standard lighting fixtures. (See Figure 6.3.) It also has a radiant heating and cooling system.

One of the most innovative features of the building's design is its energy efficient, geothermal ventilation system that heats and cools the classrooms. The building's ventilation system takes in outside air and channels it into conduits underground where the temperature is always a moderate 46°F (8°C). This ground temperature either cools or preheats the air, depending on the season, and the conditioned air is circulated through the building's ventilation and radiant flooring system.(Figure 6.20)

During the summer, warm outside air is drawn through the underground conduit to cool and then is released into the classrooms. The cool air cools the concrete floors which, in turn, keeps the rooms cool even after the conditioned air has left the space.

In the winter, the moderate-temperature underground preheats the freezing outside air before it enters the building's heating system. At that point, it takes very little additional energy to actively heat the air to a comfortable temperature for the building's occupants. Again, the warm air is circulated through pipes in the floors before being released into classrooms, warming the thermal mass of the floors so that they continue to radiate heat after the warm air in the ventilation system has left the room. Each of the classrooms has a set of controls to increase or decrease the airflow in the room and operable windows that do not interfere with the ventilation system.[47] (Figure 6.21)

Interpretive displays and interactive energy demonstrations

All school renewable energy systems will be more useful if they are well explained to students through the use of interpretive displays and hands-on science lessons that connect energy curricula to the physical site. The most successful interpretive energy displays have features that change, such as readouts of electricity produced onsite, which draw students back to the display time and time again.

The interpretive panel at Cassop Primary School (See Figure 6.17) and the truth window in the ceiling of Twenhofel Middle School's science lab, (See Figure 6.18) along with its interpretive display online (See Figure 6.19), are examples of

FIGURE 6.21 *Turban-topped towers on the roof at Östratorn School rotate in the wind, creating low pressure in the building's ducts that draws air through the building.*

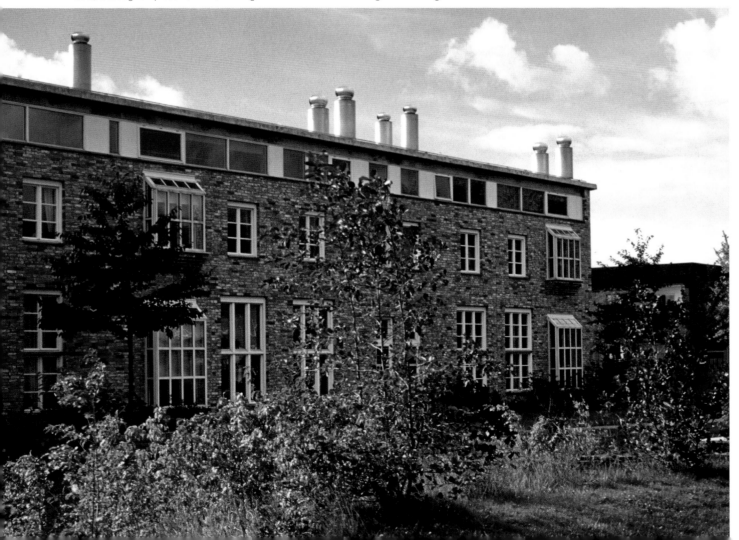

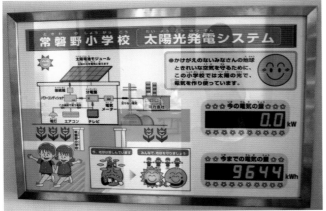

FIGURE 6.22

Sandra Koike

playful and effective educational displays. Tokiwano Elementary School in Kyoto, Japan, also developed an exemplary interpretive display for its PV system that includes a real-time read-out of the energy the school produces. The interpretive panel uses cartoons to explain that the energy generated on the roof is used onsite and that this is beneficial for the environment.[48] (Figure 6.22)

In northern California, the Rahus Institute's Solar Schoolhouse program playfully engages students in their renewable energy projects. Many of their solar powered fountains (they assist with installation) have pivoting mounts so students can turn the panels away from the sun to watch the water stop or turn them toward the sun to watch it go. The solar panels can also be placed within students' reach so that they may shade

them with their hands to get the same "stop and go" effect. These interactive features make the simple solar panels continuously fascinating for children. (See chapter 4, Figure 4.10)

🍃 Bringing Energy Issues Home

As this chapter illustrates, there are many ways to teach about energy conservation, renewable energy production, and how to live well while using less energy. Some of these ideas relate to the school buildings and grounds, and others relate to our behavior and the daily choices we make. It is important to make these issues personally relevant to students and to illustrate how the relatively simple actions of each child can help to improve the environment of their school and community.

One way schools can personalize energy issues and empower their students is to encourage them to commute to school under their own power, if possible, rather than riding in cars. Some schools combine their physical fitness goals with fossil fuel reduction targets by encouraging students to walk or ride their bikes to school. Successful programs provide bicycle racks and organize "bike to school" days to increase participation. Similarly, some schools organize walking days or "walking bus" routes, where parents chaperone groups of children as they walk to school, creating an effective, non-motorized carpool alternative.

Reducing climate change is an enormous task that will require creative thinking on many levels, from large projects to small ones, around the world. It will be an easier task, however, if we all contribute in our own way, starting with the youngest students at our schools. (Figure 6.23 and 6.24)

FIGURE 6.23 *Communities can encourage students to walk to school by creating special "walk to school" events and publicizing them well.*

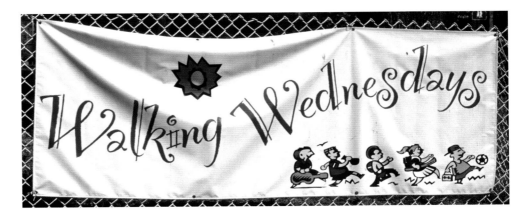

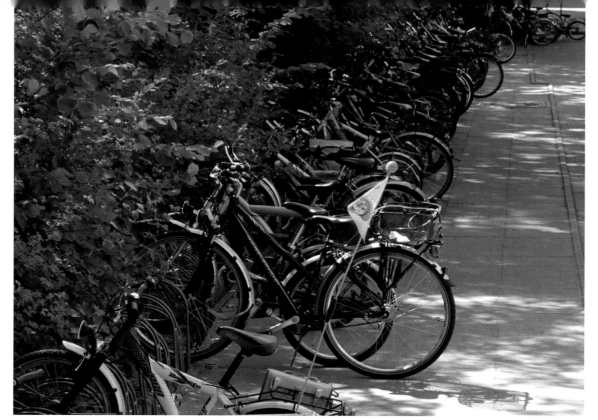

FIGURE 6.24
*Biking to school
saves fossil fuel
and promotes
physical fitness.*

🌼 Creative Curricula

Renewable energy concepts can be taught in an interactive, hands-on manner that is not connected to the school building's function. At Rosa Parks School in Berkeley, California, for example, the school's creative science teacher collaborated with the Rahus Institute's Solar Schoolhouse to hold a school-wide solar festival that brought renewable energy curricula to children in grades K-5. In preparation for the festival, young

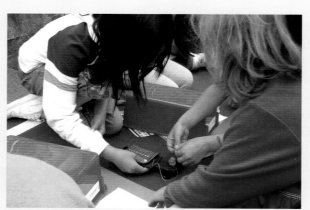

FIGURE 6.26

Hal Aronson

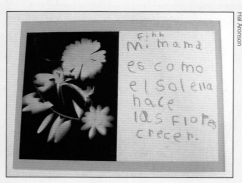

FIGURE 6.25

Hal Aronson

students explored the power of the sun through plant growth and light sensitive materials (Figure 6.25), while older students made model solar powered homes and cars (Figure 6.26).[49] Projects like these are valuable learning experiences that help teachers initiate discussions with their students about many types of energy-related topics.

7 *Schoolyard Agriculture*

🍃 *Why Garden at School?*

In our increasingly urban society, people of all ages have become disconnected from the natural and agricultural environments that sustain us. The effect is most profound for children growing up in our cities, but touches the rest of our population as well. Starting a school garden is one way to reconnect students and school communities with local agricultural and ecological systems, and at the same time create new, vibrant learning environments that can be used in countless ways.[1]

School gardens take many forms and contain a wide array of different physical and programmatic elements. They are found across North America, and all over the world, in public and private schools at the elementary, middle, and high school levels.

For **students**, school gardens engage all of the senses, allowing them to taste the sweetness of ripe fruit and crunch on freshly harvested carrots, smell fragrant flowers and moist earth, listen to bird calls and buzzing bees, touch smooth stones, fuzzy leaves, and rough tree bark, and see plants grow and change with the seasons. They are places to feel the breeze, take in fresh air, and stretch one's legs after a long morning at a desk. Many children who have trouble sitting still in the classroom turn into leaders in the garden, gaining new confidence and respect from their peers. Gardens are places where even the youngest students can be helpful and responsible for nurturing living things. Culinary gardens give students insight into where their food comes from, what it takes to produce it, and the art of bringing it to the table in an enjoyable manner.

For **teachers**, school gardens are cost-effective, hands-on learning laboratories for natural science curricula, commonly used to teach lessons about soil, weather, plant growth, insect lifecycles, and decomposition processes. Culinary gardens may be springboards for lessons about social studies, world cultures, and history that bring these subjects to life. They are also engaging environments for teaching arithmetic and geometry, health and nutrition, art and music, reading and foreign languages. Ongoing lessons may be taught in school gardens over the course of an entire school year, rather than reduced to short sound bites between class bells. Students might follow a plant from seed to seed, watch it grow through the semester, harvest and eat its bounty, then compost the leftover biomass to use as rich compost on the following year's crops, produced from seeds they saved themselves. Lessons like this give students a deep understanding of agriculture and the intricate ecological dances performed by insects and other creatures that coexist among the plants.

Gardens are natural gathering places for the **school community** and they foster a culture of stewardship at the school. They are spaces for parents to relax after dropping off their children and comfortable locations to read a book on the weekend. Gardens bring school communities together around the common goal of improving the school grounds, allowing parents to bond with shovels in hand at monthly work parties, or relax together at school-wide barbeques and festivals.

Culinary gardens and related cooking classes may open discussions about students' health and nutrition. Schools with food gardens often grow fruits, herbs, and vegetables for the cafeteria and cooking classes, and some encourage students to "nibble" produce when they visit the garden. The garden's bounty may also be shared with people outside the school: students may raise vegetables and fruits as part of a social service program or turn their garden into a school-based business.

Many school gardens are started with donated materials, such as child-sized hand tools, rich garden compost, inexpensive seeds, and rustic seating circles made from logs or straw bales. PTA funds or grants often pay for larger items like tool sheds, outdoor kitchens, garden furniture, and drip irrigation. Many schools find they have talented parents who are capable gardeners, woodworkers, stonemasons, and designers. Others who have never gardened are often happy to lend a hand to those who are more skilled in these areas.

Search your own school community to find people who can help you from within. Build a network that will support you in harnessing their talents. If you are successful, any funds you raise to purchase building and planting materials will stretch further if you have willing hands to help assemble and maintain the garden.

The physical form of school gardens is usually determined by the following combination of factors: the shape and size of available land, the garden's intended uses, the project's budget, the types of inexpensive building materials that are available locally, and the range of skills that participating students, teachers, and community members contribute. Some schools in spacious rural or suburban settings have the freedom to grow large gardens or even create demonstration "mini-farms" onsite. In most cases, gardens are located at schools with much less available land, tucked into tight spaces between school buildings and the sidewalk, hidden in previously underutilized corners, nestled in quiet interior courtyards, or even placed on sturdy rooftops.

The best gardens emerge slowly and grow over time as they are nurtured by students and others in the school community. School gardens should never be "finished." To remain relevant through the years, they need to continually shift to reflect the school's changing population and interests. Each year, students have the opportunity to contribute something long-lasting—a

"On any given day, 35 percent of elementary school kids eat no fruit, 20 percent don't touch a vegetable, and many of those who do come no closer than French fries. A shocking 90 percent consume fat above the U.S. Department of Agriculture's recommended level, and 27 percent of children between the ages of 6 and 11 are obese. Many schools have abandoned school lunch programs altogether, turning them over to fast-food chains."[2]

special pathway, a raised garden bed in a unique shape, a whimsical bench, a set of hand painted tiles, a dramatic entryway, or welcoming informational signs. Taken together, these contributions create a profound "sense of place" that connects the school community to the garden in personal, meaningful ways.

Growing Food: Edible Crops and Agricultural Systems on School Grounds

Many schools now have culinary gardens to introduce students to nutrition concepts and the delicious flavors of freshly harvested produce. Even the pickiest eaters, if given the opportunity to grow and pick fresh produce, frequently find vegetables an enjoyable snack.[3]

Many places around the world have productive food gardens at their schools, but California has made these gardens a state-wide priority. In 1994, chef Alice Waters collaborated with the principal and community members at ML King, Jr. Middle School in Berkeley to begin a project called the Edible Schoolyard, which sought to change the urban students' relationship with food by helping them to grow organic produce and learn to cook it themselves. In 1995, under the guidance of Delaine Easton, then Superintendent of Public Instruction for the State of California, the state initiated guidelines to create a "garden in every school." These two related programs became national models that have "borne fruit" throughout the United States, inspiring schools to grow organic produce and healthy children.

Renewed interest in local self-reliance, organic foods, and the Slow Food movement, as well as concern about the alarming prevalence of childhood obesity, have helped to increase the popularity of school gardens around the world over the last 20 years. From England to New Zealand, schools are planting culinary crops ranging from herbs and vegetables to berries, fruits, nuts, grain, culinary mushrooms, and agricultural products like honey, milk, and eggs. The crops each school grows typically reflect their local culture and regional agricultural methods.

Many schools keep maintenance manageable and maximize food production by planting a large percentage of permanent and perennial crops, such as fruit trees and berry bushes, that are reliable food producers with relatively low maintenance needs. They supplement these crops with more labor-intensive plants—lettuce, beans, carrots, and tomatoes—that are sown

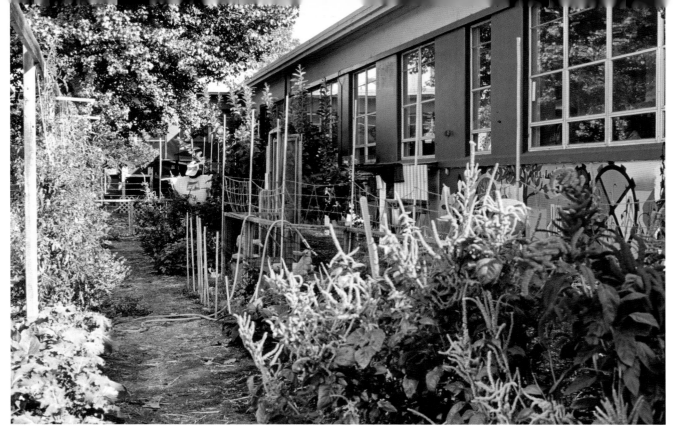

FIGURE 7.1 *At LeConte Elementary School, students coax twelve-foot-tall sunflowers from the soil and harvest tomatoes until December in Berkeley's moderate climate.*

seasonally and can be easily changed from year to year. Into this mix may be added a variety of herbs, to compliment their cooking programs, and flowers to brighten the garden and attract beneficial insects. Crops that grow on vines, such as kiwi fruits, grapes, and passion fruit, may also be used to layer the garden vertically, giving it added visual interest while making use of all available growing spaces.

Many excellent books about school gardens include techniques and tips for starting new projects, working with groups of children, and maximizing food production. (See Resources, chapter 18) Rather than duplicating these efforts, this chapter highlights a variety of innovative school gardens with strong programs and unique features.

Schoolyard culinary gardens

When students at LeConte Elementary School step from the hallway into their school's courtyard, they are transported from urban Berkeley, California, into a mini-farm filled with lush, colorful, and seasonal vegetables, herbs, fruits, and flowers.

Founded in 1982, the Farm and Garden program at LeConte is one of the oldest continuously tended school gardens in California. It connects Berkeley's urban children to the land by giving them a taste of what it is like to grow some of their own food and care for small farm animals. The courtyard is currently home to two free-range chickens and several rabbits. Over the years, it has also housed goats and ducks. The program seeks to improve the children's nutrition and to teach them about natural systems such as plant growth cycles and composting processes. A garden instructor manages the program, assisted by AmeriCorps participants.[4] (Figure 7.1)

The long, narrow courtyard is oriented along an east-west axis. Its microclimate is 15–20 degrees warmer than the neighborhood, extending the growing season by several weeks. The concrete walls of the surrounding two-story building are painted a light color, reflecting additional light into the partly shaded courtyard, further improving plant growth.

The courtyard's garden is managed organically to protect the children and the animals, so no chemical pesticides,

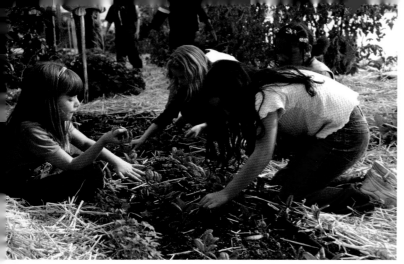

FIGURE 7.2 *LeConte students participate in hands-on garden work such as planting seeds, weeding, composting, and harvesting.*

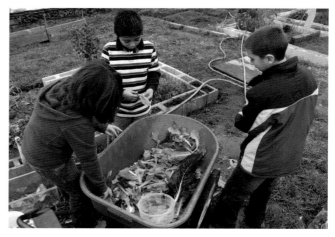

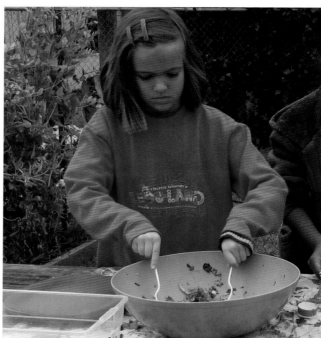

FIGURES 7.3 and 7.4 *Students at Green Acres Elementary School are experts at making salads from their garden. They harvest and wash the greensand mix salads for themselves—and sometimes lucky garden visitors.*

herbicides, or fertilizers are used. Crops are rotated on an informal basis. Winter cover crops and loads of compost—produced in the garden—enrich the soil. Several compost piles and worm compost bins process garden plant waste, vegetable scraps from cooking classes, and rich droppings from the chickens and rabbits. Two chickens patrol the courtyard, devouring the slugs, snails, and insects they find.

In 2006 the school added a second garden on their playground. The spacious new plot has an outdoor seating area, raised beds, and pathways that are wheelchair accessible. The garden beds throughout the school grounds are not subdivided by classroom, so students work in both spaces and think of the entire garden as "theirs." In cooler weather, the gardens include multiple varieties of lettuce and crops such as garlic, onions, beets, and turnips. Students sometimes harvest the lettuce and prepare it for their lunchroom salad bar. Some garden produce is also used by cooking classes. Tomatoes, always popular among the students, are enjoyed in early fall and include heirloom varieties such as green zebra and Russian Black Krim. When school is closed for the summer and holidays, the garden instructor maintains the garden and helps to care for the animals with assistance from other teachers, students, and parents.

Students visit the Farm and Garden once every two weeks for an hour-long class in groups of 10 to 14. The garden instructor connects his lessons to their classroom curriculum and to nutrition education goals established by the California Nutrition Network, one of their funders. A portion of each lesson includes a "tasting" of fresh fruits or vegetables, grown onsite or purchased from an organic farm, that encourages the children to try a wider variety of foods.[5] (Figure 7.2)

Green Acres Elementary School in Santa Cruz, California, has had a culinary garden since 1978. Classes come to the garden regularly to grow crops and participate in lessons—but

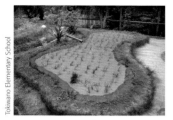

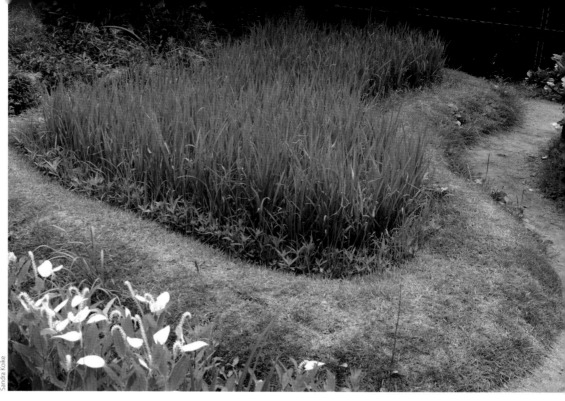

FIGURES 7.5 and 7.6 *The schoolyard rice paddy at Tokiwano Elementary, shown newly planted and mid-season.*

the space is also used during students' free time. Interested third, fourth, and fifth graders may eat their lunch in the garden and can sign up to have their own garden bed, or to share that responsibility with their friends. Self-directed students tend their own plot and plant, water, maintain, and harvest crops they grow themselves.[6] (Figures 7.3 and 7.4)

Around the world in Kyoto, Japan, the school community at Tokiwano Elementary School transformed their school grounds into a microcosm of what the region looked like before it was heavily urbanized. Referred to as a "biotope" (nature study area) in Japan, the students study the schoolyard's rich ecological features and investigate the insects, aquatic creatures, and birds onsite, learning from and playing in a beautiful landscape.

The culinary portions of the space include terraced "fields" with grassy sides, intended to recall the look of traditional agricultural areas. The school grows common garden crops, such as lettuce, and an eye-catching rice paddy planted in a traditional manner. To keep the water level high in their earth-bermed rice bed, the plot was lined with a plastic sheet, hidden in the soil. The students plant the rice in the spring, watch it grow, and then harvest and collect the rice in the fall. After processing the rice by hand, students cook a meal to share with each other.[7] (Figures 7.5 and 7.6)

Fruit and nut orchards

Some schools have orchards that produce delicious fruit and nuts in great abundance, which are very useful for cooking classes, and handy for schoolyard snacks. As with all edible crops on school grounds, orchards should be managed organically for the safety of the children and pollinators, and trees should be selected for their suitability to the schoolyard microclimate.

In Berkeley, California, the Edible Schoolyard at ML King, Jr. Middle School grows a great variety of fruiting trees including citrus crops, figs, hazelnuts, loquats, mulberries, olives, pears, persimmons, plums, and quince. Fruiting vines and brambles, such as blackberries, cape gooseberries, chayote, currants, grapes, kiwis, and raspberries, also thrive onsite. Espaliered apple trees, pruned and trained into a flat form, are planted along a supportive trellis on one side of the garden.[8] Espaliered fruit trees take longer to establish and produce less

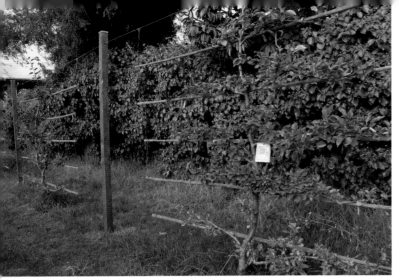

FIGURE 7.7 *Espaliered fruit trees, pruned flat against a fence, at King Middle School.*

fruit than standard trees, but they are very space efficient, beautiful, and easier for students to harvest. (Figures 7.7 and 7.8)

Farther south, in Los Angeles, California, Multnomah Street Elementary School planted an extensive fruit and nut tree orchard as part of a larger effort to shade the schoolyard.

The fruit trees are concentrated around the playground's outdoor eating areas and the perimeter of the school. The schoolyard orchard includes apples, apricots, cherimoyas, gingkoes, kumquats, persimmons, plums, pomegranates, macadamia nuts, olives, and white sapotes. The trees are watered with drip irrigation and the ground is covered with a thick layer of mulch to conserve water in this hot, dry climate.[9] (Figure 7.9)

Schoolyard animal husbandry

Most urban and suburban students have not spent much time in close proximity to farm animals. Including them on school grounds helps to teach animal husbandry, while also fostering responsibility and imparting nutrition concepts that apply to both the animals' and students' health. Some farm animals, such as chickens, are also assets to garden ecology as they happily eat weed seeds and insect pests, while recycling garden nutrients.

Farm animals, including chickens, ducks, rabbits, goats, and sheep can be raised in rural, suburban, and urban schoolyards. The space needed for each animal varies with its species and size. It is important to check your city's ordinances before

FIGURE 7.8 *The Edible Schoolyard at King Middle School, Berkeley, California.*

Cam Collyer

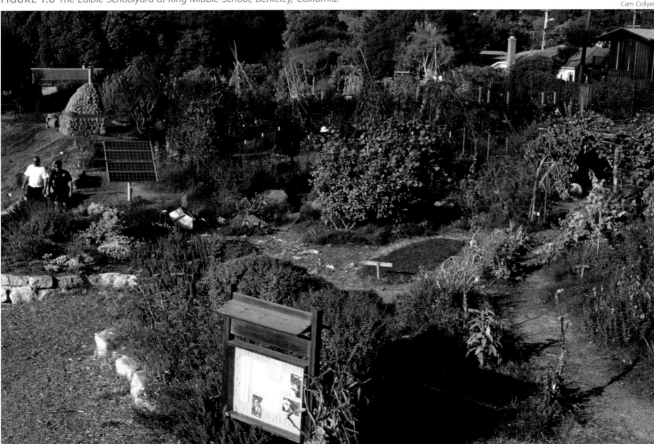

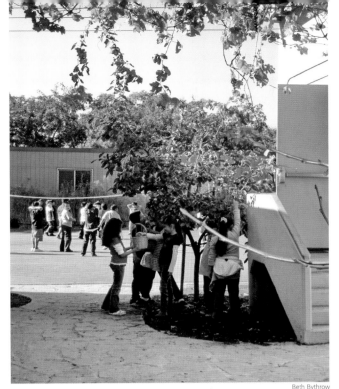
Beth Bythrow

FIGURE 7.9 *The trees at Multnomah Street Elementary were selected to provide the school with tasty snacks year-round.*

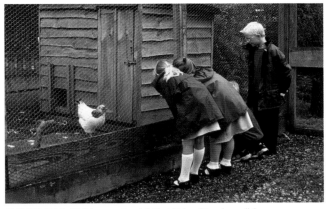

FIGURE 7.10 *Children at Cowick First School tend small farm animals onsite and delight in watching them in their free time.*

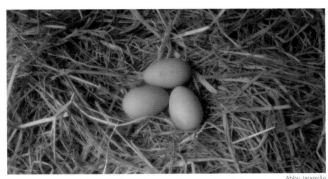

Abby Jaramillo

FIGURE 7.11 *High school students at June Jordan School for Equity in San Francisco, California, are raising three chickens and a rooster. The garden coordinator reports that students' observations of the rooster's behavior, coupled with the appearance of eggs, provides a graceful introduction into age-appropriate conversations about puberty and reproduction.*[11]

bringing farm animals into a schoolyard as some municipalities restrict the types of animals allowed within their boundaries.

Chickens, guinea pigs, and rabbits live on school grounds at Cowick First School in downtown Exeter, England. The five- and six-year-old students are responsible for daily care of the animals year-round, in all types of weather. The school allows some of the youngest students to care for and nurture these creatures to help instill a sense of pride and responsibility in each child. The eggs produced by the hens are sometimes used for school cooking projects and are also occasionally sold at fundraisers.[10] (Figure 7.10)

FIGURE 7.12 *During my site visit in 1999, Children's Day School in San Francisco, California ran a mini-farm that was home to a large Corriedale sheep, two Alpine goats, and five chickens. The animals have a spacious corral with a sheltering roof, a small barn for the sheep and goats, a chicken coop, places to store hay and animal food, and compost bins for processing used straw bedding. The children help to grow row crops nearby that supplement the animals' diets. Students who help with the morning chores are often rewarded with a freshly laid egg to take home with them at the end of the day.*[12]

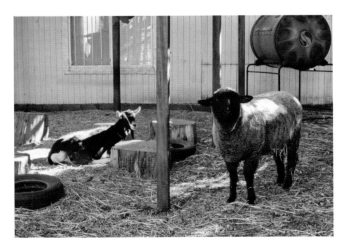

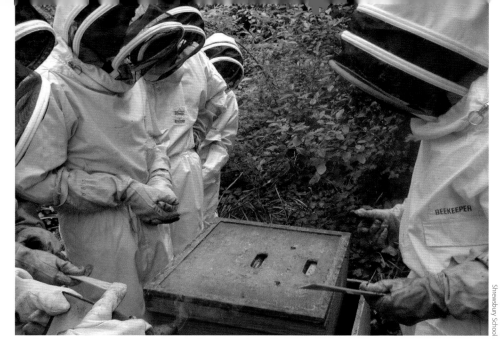

FIGURE 7.13 *Students at Shrewsbury School harvest their own honey. They report that the "flavour of the honey is excellent, with the principal nectar source being the many lime trees on the school site and in the Quarry park nearby."* [14]

Shrewsbury School

Beekeeping

Some schools have ventured into the exciting and rewarding world of beekeeping, harvesting honey onsite and benefiting from the bees' pollination services. Some beekeeping schools sell their honey to raise money for school activities or to make donations to charities, while others use the honey in student cooking classes or for home consumption.

Most schools with honeybees work with a trained beekeeper to keep the hives well maintained. Students and teachers wear proper beekeeping clothing when tending the hives to minimize the risk of bee stings. It is also wise to survey the school's students, teachers, and administrators about bee sting allergies to avoid serious medical complications that can result if an allergic person is stung.

Bergen Steiner School, in western Norway, has been keeping bees for many years. Students tend ten hives at school from late fall through late spring. In the summer, the bees are moved to nearby islands off Bergen's coast to feast on abundant heath flowers. The fall harvest alone usually produces approximately 50 kilograms (110 pounds) of honey per hive. Students enjoy some of the harvest at school, but most of the honey is sold to raise money for future school projects.[13]

At Shrewsbury School in central England students have had a Beekeeping Society for over 30 years. The beekeeping program includes a total of ten hives. Seven hives are each managed by an individual student who may sell the honey that

he produces, or keep it for his own use. The remaining three hives are jointly managed, and the honey they produce is sold at the school's store to raise money for charity. The students in the Beekeeping Society receive hands-on training and attend lectures to learn about honeybee management and crop production. They are required to pass a proficiency test before working with their own hive. (Figure 7.13)

Bees can also be kept on school grounds using a type of hive that is valued for its educational and pollination value, rather than honey production. These small observation hives are generally installed inside school buildings or nature centers, near a window or exterior wall where their entrance tube can be extended outside. The bees come and go from the hive as they please, while the students safely watch them through glass walls. (Figure 7.14)

Garden infrastructure

School gardens run more efficiently with effective garden infrastructure. Access to a reliable and convenient water supply is one of the most important prerequisites for a schoolyard garden. Small gardens may be hand-watered, but many schools prefer to use drip irrigation systems, which conserve water by delivering it slowly and precisely to the soil's surface.

Tool sheds are very helpful for keeping school gardens well organized, and they provide secure and convenient places

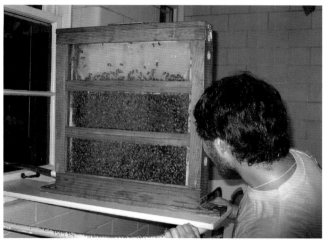

FIGURE 7.14 *Bees can be observed through glass panels in this educational hive.*

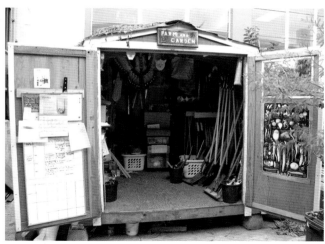

FIGURE 7.15 *LeConte Elementary School in Berkeley, California, has a classic garden tool shed.*

to store equipment. In addition to shovels, clippers, boots, and gloves, many garden teachers also keep educational gear in their tool sheds—class-sized collections of small magnifying lenses, clipboards, pencils, bug collecting boxes, and watercolor paints. (See chapters 8 and 14 for additional tool shed and garden infrastructure examples.) (Figure 7.15)

Greenhouses and cold frames nurture young plant starts and extend the growing season. This is particularly important in climates with snowy winters, where they can make school gardens more productive between September and June. Even schools in moderate climates can use these protective structures to improve seed germination rates and to provide insect protection, increased moisture, and a little extra warmth in the spring.

Both greenhouses and cold frames allow sunlight into an enclosed space through glass or plastic windows, trapping the

FIGURE 7.16 *The garden at Bergen Steiner School in Norway includes a small greenhouse (pictured) and an extensive set of cold frames that help to extend the growing season.*

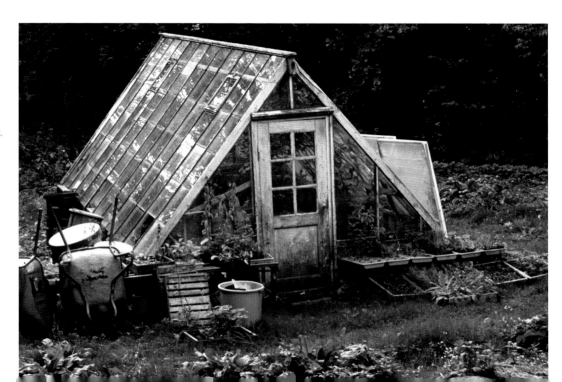

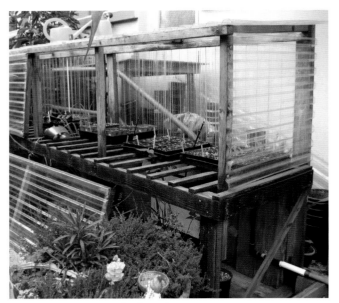

FIGURE 7.17 *LeConte School in California uses an elevated cold frame to give seedlings an added boost.*

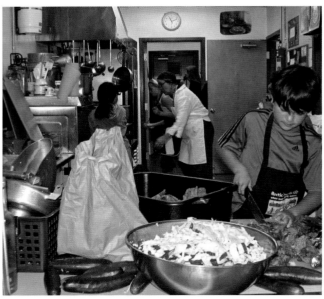

FIGURE 7.18 *The student-cooked lunch menu at Pacific School includes organic, seasonal ingredients—whole grains, leafy greens, fresh vegetables—from local farms, and sometimes herbs and produce from the school garden.*

warm air inside. On warm days, most structures open to allow excess heat to escape so the plants don't cook. Greenhouses are generally large enough to walk into, while cold frames are smaller and are usually accessed from the outside. Each comes in many shapes and sizes. (Figure 7.17)

🍃 Cooking on School Grounds

Many schools with active edible garden programs also cook with their students inside school kitchens and outside on their grounds to capture students' interest in fresh, healthy foods and to increase their cooking expertise. The lunchroom, in the form of salad bars or more extensive meals, may be the focus for garden produce and cooking lessons. Indoor kitchen classrooms may be elaborate spaces, with multiple built-in ovens, sinks, and burners for students to use in small groups, or they may be simple electric plates brought into a regular classroom when it is time to cook. Students may eat at their desks or at communal tables. Outside, schoolyard cooking spaces range in complexity from fire circles and barbeques to full outdoor kitchens with designated food preparation and picnic areas.

Student-driven lunch cooking program

Pacific Elementary School in Davenport, California, has had a phenomenal hands-on lunch program since 1984. As part of the school's Food Lab curriculum (affiliated with the national Life Lab garden program), fifth and sixth grade students take turns in the school's kitchen to prepare lunch for the whole school—almost 100 people per day! Students work with nutrition coordinator Stephanie Raugust—who founded the program 25 years ago—to plan the menu based on nutritional requirements and food preferences. They practice their math skills as they scale recipes up to the right size, calculate the amount of food they will need, and check their budget. When it is their turn to cook menus they have chosen, several students work with Raugust—assuming the roles of kitchen manager, baker, prep chef, or cook—to prepare and serve the meal. The menu features healthy, delicious, seasonally and globally-inspired cuisine, and is warmly received by both students and staff.[15] Students learn valuable culinary skills, confidence, and healthy living practices as they participate in this program. (Figures 7.18 and 7.19)

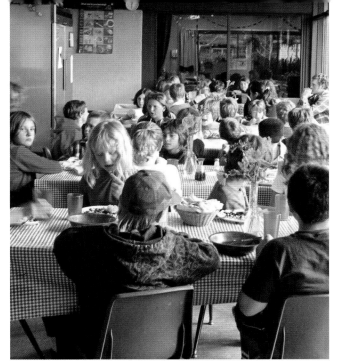

FIGURE 7.19 *Tasty meals prepared daily by students at Pacific School are served to their peers on checked table cloths, with flower bouquets on each table.*

Outdoor cooking over open fires

Some schools use portable camp stoves or temporary barbeques to enhance outdoor cooking lessons. When I visited Malcolm X School in Berkeley, California, one day, they were using a portable gas camping stove, a griddle, and a hand tortilla press to make traditional tortillas outside on the school garden's picnic table. On another visit, the garden teacher used the same stove and a pot to boil a very large, fresh beet that had just been harvested from the garden. Everyone tried a slice of the beet, hot from the pot. (Figure 7.20) The garden coordinator at Willard Middle School, also in Berkeley, California, sometimes uses a larger portable gas grill to cook corn from the farmers' market during recess. The middle school students smell the corn and come over to nibble on an ear as it comes off the grill.[16]

For many years, the after-school and preschool programs at the Jewish Community Center of the East Bay in Berkeley, California have celebrated the Passover holiday by making matzoh (unleavened bread) with the children in a temporary outdoor cooking area, over a period of several days. The cooking fire is built on bare earth inside a circle of concrete cinderblocks.

FIGURE 7.20

Students at Malcolm X School in Berkeley, California, often harvest produce from their garden and eat it with their class.

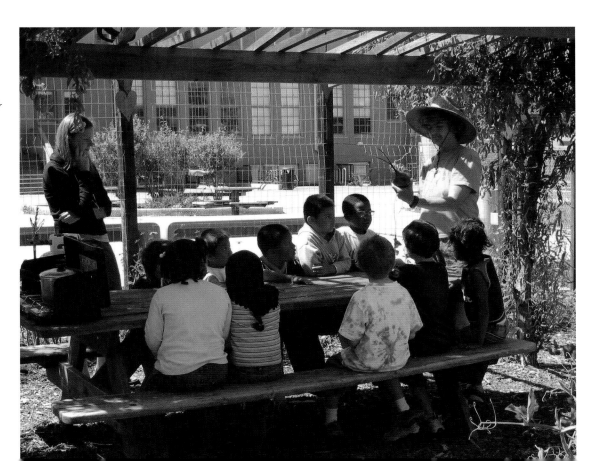

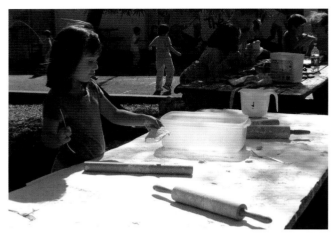

FIGURES 7.21 and 7.22 *The playground at the Jewish Community Center in Berkeley, California, becomes a temporary outdoor kitchen for their Passover holiday celebration.*

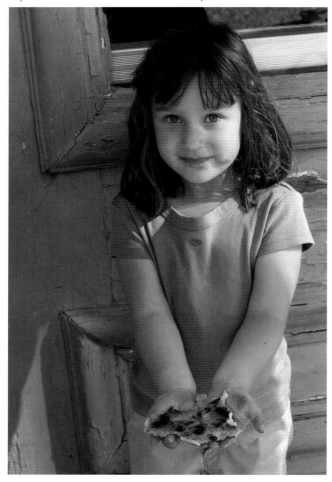

The cooking surface is composed of two restaurant-sized cookie sheets that are placed over the fire, upside down, to become temporary griddles. The children make the matzoh dough from scratch, then each one rolls out his or her ball of dough into a wide, flat circle. (Figure 7.21) The teachers place the children's dough on one of the hot cookie sheets to bake briefly on each side. When the matzoh is fully cooked, the happy children eat their fresh treat while it is still piping hot. (Figure 7.22)[17]

Outdoor, fire-based cooking methods may also include traditional campground-style fire circles and fire pits of many shapes and sizes. Fire circles are simple to install, and can be used at well-supervised class times, lunch hours, and school festivals. Cooking over an open fire permits culinary techniques including grilling, baking, roasting, frying, and boiling—offering a wide range of cooking options with very simple equipment.

In Hawai'i, more elaborate *imu* pit ovens, dug into the ground, are a type of traditional outdoor cooking fire that produces juicy, tender meat and roasted vegetables after hours of slow cooking with hot stones and steam from banana stalks and leaves. Schoolyard *imus* in Hawai'i are used to mark annual events, celebrate local Hawaiian culture, and raise funds for school projects.

Kailua High School in Kailua, Hawai'i, has a large *imu* that it uses to cook foods for the school and community members. Initiated in 1996, the pit oven at Kailua High is fired up quarterly as a fundraiser. The school's *imu* holds enough for 500 food trays. Each family pays a modest fee to have their tray of prepared foods cooked in the underground oven overnight. The *imu* is run by the high school students who collect donated banana leaves and stems used in the cooking process (Figure 7.23), assemble the rocks, tend the fire throughout the night, and ensure that the food doesn't burn as it cooks. In 2005, with the help of local businesses and community members, the school erected two open, roofed structures over their *imu* and the food distribution area to enable cooking, rain or shine.[18] (Figure 7.24)

Outdoor ovens

For schools that are serious about outdoor cooking, and want to cook for a crowd, large earthen and stone ovens, run on firewood, are an appealing choice. Some ovens can be built by a group of novices with the help of a single expert. They are

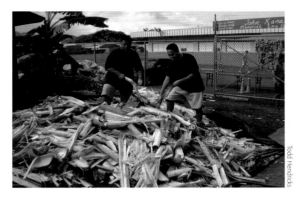

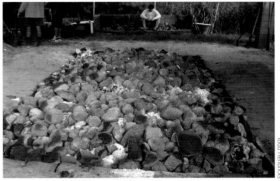

FIGURE 7.23 and 7.24 *Meat and vegetables that cook overnight in the* **imu** *at Kailua High School are tender and delicious, infused with fragrant banana-leaf steam in the traditional Hawaiian style.*

generally as safe or safer than other outdoor cooking devices, if used properly by adults. They can also take many physical forms, making them appealing centerpieces and "place making" features in a schoolyard, even when they are not in use.

Most earthen and stone ovens have high thermal mass: they are made from heavy materials that absorb heat from the fire and then radiate it back onto the food during the cooking process. In an earth oven, the inner sand- and clay-based heat absorbing layer is often surrounded by an insulating layer, made from clay and straw, on the outside of the oven; when the inside is amazingly hot, the outside is still only gently warm to the touch. Many earthen ovens are designed with the door as the only place that heat can escape, while other configurations may also have a chimney on top.

Some ovens have one chamber for the fire and another for the food. Most, however, are single chamber devices that first hold the fire, to preheat the oven, and then hold the food, which cooks in the residual heat after the wood ashes have been swept away. To run the oven, the chef/teacher lights a fire in the chamber and feeds it a large quantity of wood over the course of several hours. The inside of the oven can easily reach temperatures in the 500°–600° F range when the oven has been adequately heated.

This initial temperature will bake pizzas and other types of bread in a matter of minutes—a good way to feed a large group of students or a whole community at a school festival. As the temperature starts to fall, additional wood may be added again to bring it back up, or the falling temperature can be used as an asset, to bake different dishes that require lower and lower temperatures as time passes. For example, following a pizza party, the oven could be used over the course of another six hours to bake potatoes at 400° F, and then cakes at 350°, slow cook stews at 200°–300°, and then used as a food dehydrator to preserve the school garden's bounty when the oven drops under 150° F.[19]

Earthen ovens can be built by a group of 10–15 adults over the course of an intensive weekend or two, or by a class of middle school students over the course of a semester. The primary materials are simple: clay, straw, and sand are used in different combinations to make the layers needed for the domed cooking chamber, bricks are generally used for the oven's cooking floor, and stone or recycled concrete chunks may be used for the base. The construction process requires some precision, so it is wise to hire someone with experience building earth ovens to lead a team of novice volunteers. There are excellent books available that explain step by step earth oven construction. (See Resources, Appendix II)

Install earthen ovens under a non-flammable canopy to protect them from the elements. Locate them in a convenient place for cooking, near a water source for food preparation and clean-up. Build them far enough from the school building's walls to avoid creating a fire hazard or staining the wall with smoke.

Three hundred students at Willard Middle School in Berkeley, California, collaborated to build a well-crafted earthen oven over a two-month period in 2007, aided by their garden teachers and several earth oven experts. The exterior of the traditional, dome-shaped oven is decorated with a sculpted phoenix design, the school's mascot, rendered in two colors of

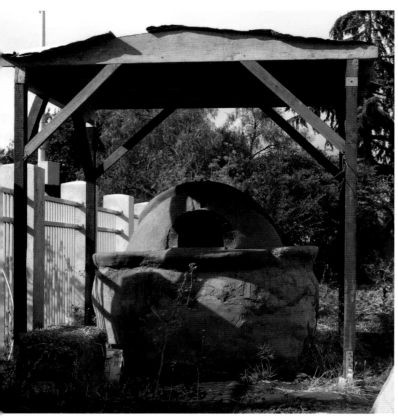

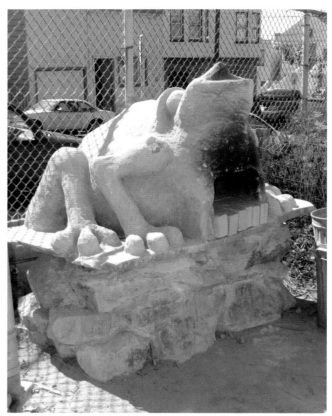

FIGURE 7.25 *The garden and cooking teachers at Willard School use their earthen oven to bake pizza and make other snacks for the students.*

FIGURE 7.26 *When the oven at San Francisco Community School is lit, the smoke comes out the frog's upturned mouth, which acts as a chimney.*

natural clay plaster. It sits in the school garden on a tall platform made from stuccoed, earth-filled sandbags surrounding a core of broken concrete and rocks. The oven is protected by a wooden canopy that keeps the winter rain from eroding the clay surface. It is now an important part of the school's nutrition education program.[20] (Figure 7.25)

In 2002, students in grades 4–8 at San Francisco Community School in San Francisco, California, built a frog-shaped earthen oven, with the assistance of their garden teacher and others at the school. The oven was made from clay, straw, and sand with a fire brick cooking surface. It sits on a base made from rough stone blocks, cemented securely together.[21] (Figure 7.26)

Stone ovens are more complex undertakings than their earthen counterparts. Their construction usually requires the expertise of stone masons and other craftsmen, and the heavy materials and cement used during construction prevent young children from participating. Once built, however, they are wonderful, permanent additions to a schoolyard landscape.

The Edible Schoolyard in Berkeley, California, has a tall, graceful stone pizza oven that can be seen from almost anywhere in the garden. It is set on a cement-block base that provides storage for the wood used to heat the oven. After the oven is preheated by a log fire and the ashes have been removed, bread, pizza, or other foods are baked inside.[22] (Figure 7.27)

Outdoor cooking with solar energy

The sun is a powerful and effective tool for schoolyard cooking, when channeled into solar ovens. In their most basic forms, solar ovens are boxes lined with reflective surfaces that focus the sun's energy on dark, heat-absorbing materials. The devices are typically enclosed by a glass pane or heat-resistant plastic that works like a greenhouse to let the sunlight in and keep it there to cook food. Most solar ovens are portable devices that are used outdoors, but are stored inside when cooking is finished.

Students can make a simple solar box cooker in a single afternoon using a cardboard box, tin foil, and a sheet of glass or plastic. These ovens are useful, safe demonstration tools that work by cooking food at a low temperature for a long time. They are used to bake cookies, dehydrate garden produce, cook

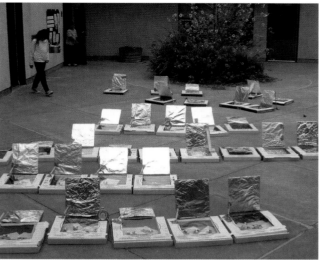

Hal Aronson

FIGURE 7.28 *Solar box cookers in use at Rosa Parks School in Berkeley, California.*

FIGURE 7.27 *A stone pizza oven at the Edible Schoolyard in Berkeley, California.*

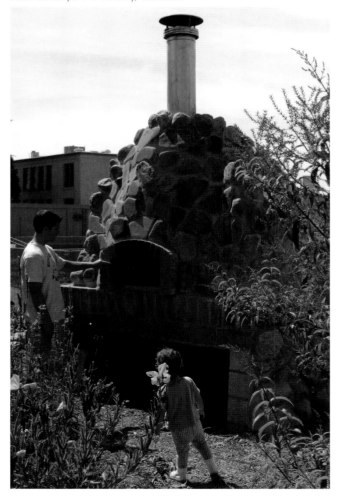

an egg, melt cheese for *quesadillas* or other similar low temperature baking and roasting projects.

A solar energy festival at Rosa Parks School in Berkeley, California, included a solar box cooker demonstration. The third grade students built their cookers out of pizza boxes, fitted with black paper to absorb heat and aluminum foil to reflect the sunlight into the box. (Figure 7.28) A portion of each box top was replaced by a plastic panel to let the light in and trap heat. The school's science teacher connected this project to the students' physical science curriculum, illustrating how renewable energy can be harnessed to achieve important daily tasks.[23]

More elaborate, commercially produced solar ovens, built from durable materials, incorporate advanced features such as insulated sides and powerful reflectors to capture heat more efficiently. Some ovens can reach temperatures of approximately 400° F or more—hot enough to cook a meal or pasteurize water. Ovens like this may be used to cook more elaborate classroom meals, such as simmering stews or roasting vegetables at higher temperatures. These reusable ovens are also very beneficial in many parts of the world where firewood and clean water are not available to everyone. Inexpensive, heat-sensitive water pasteurization indicators may be used with these ovens to ensure reliable water pasteurization results and to demonstrate this technique to students.[24]

Food Preparation/Clean-Up Areas and Outdoor Seating

After growing their own food in a school garden, and cooking it onsite, students need a welcoming place to sit down together to share their meal. Eating areas need not be fancy—a simple group of picnic tables will do. However, many schools find that the addition of a table cloth, or a vase of flowers from the garden, makes the meal feel special and creates a stronger sense of "family" and "community" around the table. Eating in this way also helps busy students and teachers relax and enjoy each other's company.[25] (See chapter 13 for seating examples.) For schools that do a lot of cooking, it is also quite helpful to have places set aside for food preparation and clean-up, with sinks and counter space. (Figure 7.29)

FIGURE 7.29 *Lessons about cooking and nutrition occur in Grattan School's garden in San Francisco, California, aided by a sink and countertop at the center of the teaching space.*

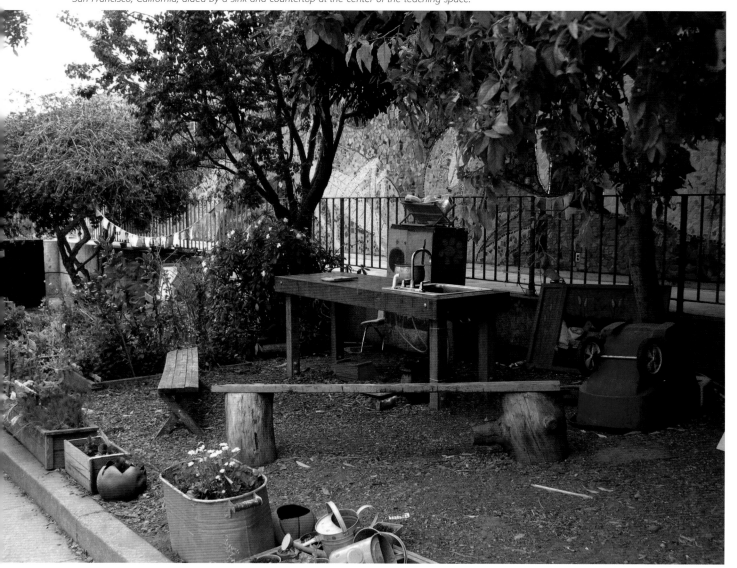

❧ Garden Configuration

Some school grounds have wide open, unstructured fields or large expanses of asphalt that can be turned into gardens. Others have smaller sites or are constrained by competing needs from other activities that occur on their grounds. These physical factors help determine whether the garden should be planted directly in the ground, in raised beds, or in containers. There are pros and cons for each type of configuration, but all of these design choices can be equally successful. Gardens, of any configuration, located close to the school building are easier to observe closely and maintain regularly.

FIGURE 7.30 *Students at Malcolm X School in Berkeley, California, collaborate to tend in-ground beds filled with herbs, vegetables, and brightly colored flowers.*

In-ground plantings

In-ground planting beds are almost always my first choice when I help a school design an ecological schoolyard. In-ground beds can be any size or shape and the configuration can change each year as the garden matures and its needs shift. Plants that are placed directly in the ground are usually more drought tolerant and hardier because their roots can search for water and nutrients over a wide area. Larger, more effective root systems help plants grow more easily to their full size and reach their full potential. It is important for school gardens with in-ground plantings to mark the edges of the beds in some way to avoid accidental trampling. Garden beds can be clearly marked using small rocks, artwork, attractive fencing, or creative garden edging.

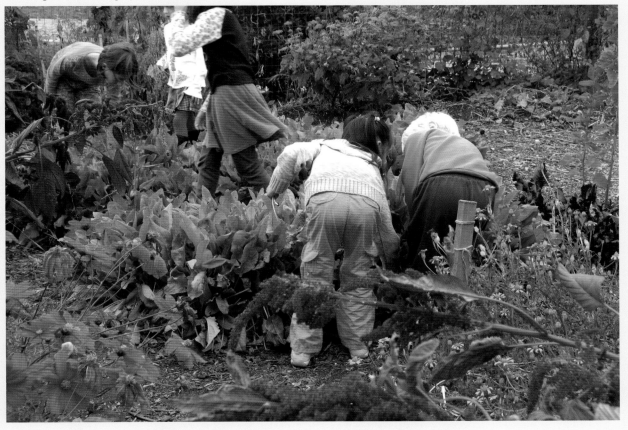

Before starting a new schoolyard culinary garden, test the soil to determine its pH and nutrient balance and to look for possible lead contamination or other soil pollutants. Lead is most likely to be found next to building walls (where old paint chips may have fallen) and near busy roadways (where car exhaust may have settled when gasoline contained lead). Other soil contaminants may be present near areas previously used for industrial purposes, or around places where cleaning chemicals, fuel, or landscape poisons have been stored in the past.

Raised beds

Raised beds are garden plots that are built upward from the natural ground level, supported by a durable perimeter material. This garden format can be very useful for school gardens that need clearly defined garden beds, that have drainage problems, or that contain garden mulch materials within the boundaries of each bed. Raised beds are also useful for terracing hillsides to make level garden spaces, raising the soil level to accommodate students in wheelchairs, and for providing seating along their perimeter.

It is helpful to arrange raised beds so that a class can gather around them on all sides for discussions. They are easiest for the children to use and maintain if they are narrow enough for the younger students to reach into the middle of the bed (generally less than three feet wide for elementary school gardens), and if they are placed at a height that is comfortable for the age group that will be using them.

Raised beds may be built from a wide range of materials including: untreated wood that is naturally long lasting, such as cedar or redwood, untreated logs, recycled plastic "lumber" (without wood fiber), stone or bricks, chunks of broken concrete, and concrete pipes (placed vertically, partially buried). The recycled materials and logs on this list are generally low cost, and may even be free. Other materials, such as thick redwood boards and attractive stone, can be quite expensive if purchased.

It is very important to avoid using poisonous materials in all gardens on school grounds. Do not use pressure treated lumber, railroad ties, telephone poles, tires, or other materials that have been chemically treated or have come into contact

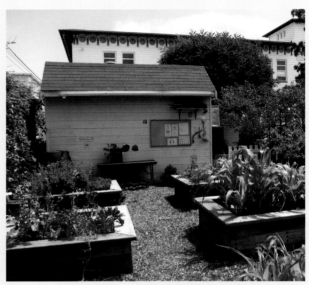

FIGURE 7.31 *The wooden raised beds at Tule Elk Park Child Development Center in San Francisco, California, help keep preschool children from accidentally trampling delicate plants.*

with poisons, heavy metals, or other contaminates. These chemicals may rub off on children's hands or leach into the soil where they could contaminate edible crops. Also avoid using plywood or other engineered wood products that may contain poisonous binding materials and preservatives such as formaldehyde. Many of the new "plastic lumber" brands also include pressure treated lumber fiber in their formulas, so inquiries are advised before purchasing these materials for use in children's gardens. If reusing old painted wood or metal, be sure to test it for lead. (See chapter 8 for more information about materials.)

Container gardens

At some schools, in-ground beds are not possible due to paved surfaces, or not desirable due to soil contamination or drainage problems. Other schools prefer temporary or portable garden spaces to accommodate changing needs. Schools in these situations may start a garden using containers, placed on the pavement or raised off the ground above contaminated soil.

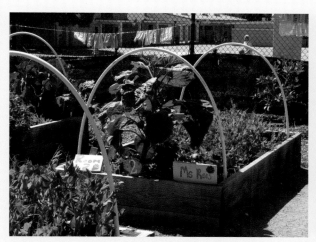

FIGURE 7.32 *Edna Maguire School in Mill Valley, California, encourages interested teachers to sign up for their own garden bed and plant it with crops they select.*

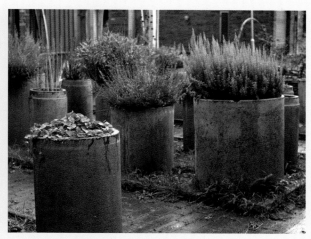

FIGURE 7.33 *Klostergård School in Sweden features raised beds made of concrete water pipes of varying widths and lengths. Each pipe, partially buried for stability, is filled with potting soil and planted with herbs or flowers.*

FIGURE 7.34 *As part of the science curriculum at St. Kentigerns School in Auckland, New Zealand, each student is responsible for maintaining his or her own plot of vegetables and flowers.*[26]

Judy Walsby

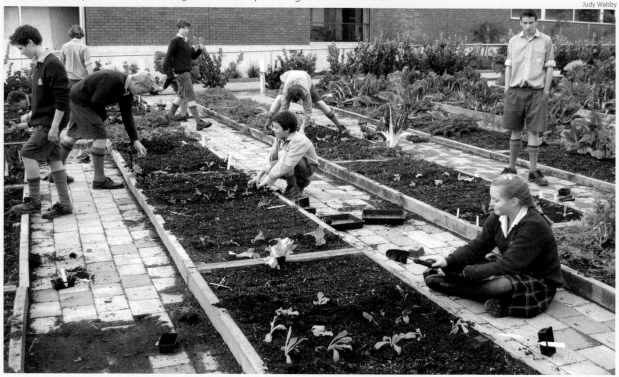

FIGURE 7.35 *Alice Fong Yu School's terraced, hillside garden in San Francisco, California, was created with flexible, wood-free, recycled plastic boards. The plastic boards were secured to metal pipes that were hammered into the sandy soil. These garden beds have held up well for almost ten years.*[27]

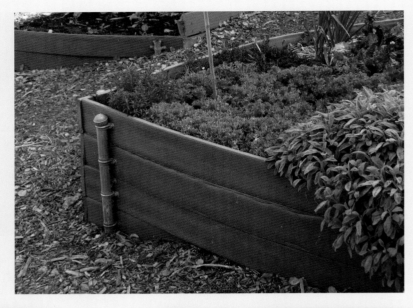

FIGURE 7.36 *Ossington/Old Orchard Junior Public School in Toronto, Ontario, Canada, terraced a hillside adjacent to the playground to create dramatic garden beds. The long, wooden planting beds alternate with walkways so the students can easily tend them.*[28]

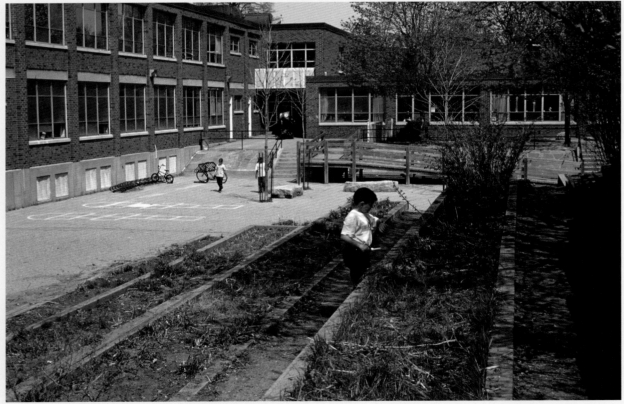

trees and large shrubs in small containers as their growth will be stunted.

Many California schools use wine barrels, a by-product of the local wine industry, as garden planters (with drainage holes drilled in the bottom). They are inexpensive, attractive, and have about a five-year life span in a school garden context. Their porous sides, however, allow moisture to escape so they require extra watering. To improve water retention, some schools line the barrels' vertical sides with plastic sheeting or paint the inside walls with a non-toxic wood sealant. (Figure 7.37)

Rooftop gardens

Sometimes schools cannot spare any space at ground level and turn to their rooftops to create outdoor classrooms and gardens, complete with planter boxes, seating, chalkboards, and other teaching amenities. They are particularly useful for schools with strong, flat roofs that have limited playground space or need protection from neighborhood vandalism. Rooftop gardens may also provide wonderful views of the surrounding neighborhood, which can be enjoyed by both children and adults.[29]

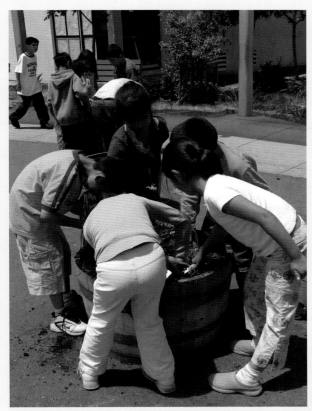

FIGURE 7.37 *Wooden wine barrels make nice garden planters.*

Some schools reuse porcelain or metal fixtures such as bathtubs (with lead-free finishes), livestock water troughs, and other water basins. Wooden wine barrels and other large containers previously used for food storage are also good choices. Large plastic and clay pots (with lead-free glazes) are also available for purchase at most garden stores.

By their nature, container gardens have limited soil volume, which restricts plants' root space and constrains their growth. Container plants are completely dependent on their gardeners for regular watering and nutrient replenishment. They also generally require more water than in-ground plantings; some of the water applied to containers runs out the bottom or evaporates through the sides of porous wood or clay surfaces. Small plants, including many herbs, flowers, and strawberries, often do quite well in containers. Avoid planting

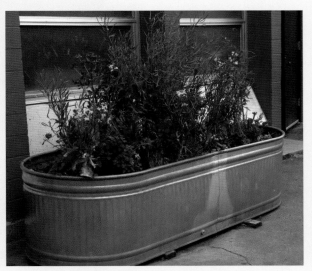

FIGURE 7.38 *Grattan School in San Francisco uses metal horse troughs as attractive, distinctive planters. Metal troughs are long-lasting, durable, non-toxic, and affordable.*

Rooftop gardens are not as simple to construct as ground level plantings. They require careful planning and consideration of the building's engineering specifications and the children's safety. Before embarking on this type of project, talk to your school district and get professional advice from an engineer to ensure that the roof will be able to hold the weight of a garden and its visitors. Also follow school district advice about perimeter safety fences and other precautions. Check to make sure the roof's surface is waterproof and durable enough for foot traffic, garden construction, and maintenance. Plants on the roof will be subjected to hotter, windier microclimates than ground level gardens, so select plants that thrive in these conditions and water carefully so they don't dry out.

Tenderloin Community School near downtown San Francisco, California, has outdoor space on two different rooftop levels. The playground on the second floor includes a play structure, painted game striping, seating, and perimeter planting beds. Lush garden plantings in deep wooden raised beds are on the third floor with picnic tables and other outdoor classroom amenities. It also has a spectacular view of the city, including San Francisco's City Hall. (Figure 7.39)

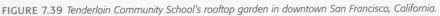

FIGURE 7.39 *Tenderloin Community School's rooftop garden in downtown San Francisco, California.*

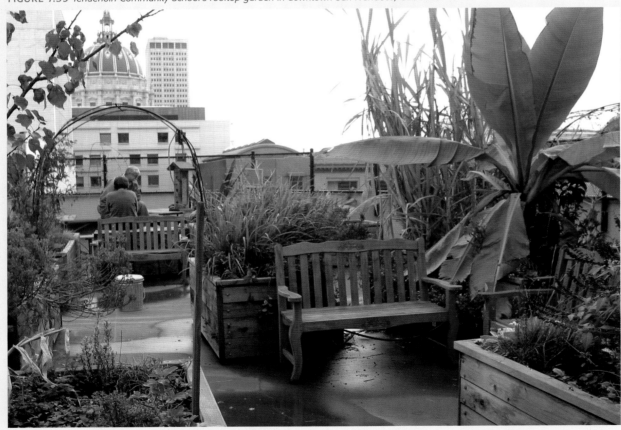

8 *Ecologically Sensitive Materials for Schoolyard Landscapes*

🍃 *Material Choices Matter*

Everything a school chooses to add to its environment says something about what it values.[1] Over the last decade or so, as the green building movement has taken hold around the world, a growing number of schools have started to question the playground materials—asphalt, concrete, stainless steal, plastic and rubber—that have been widely used for decades.

These materials didn't appear in schoolyards by accident. They are fairly durable, low maintenance, relatively inexpensive, and can be mass produced—all qualities that make them appealing to school districts with low budgets, few maintenance staff members, and heavily used playgrounds. If these are the only criteria against which the materials are measured, they fulfill these specific needs and do their jobs fairly well. But is that all there is to it? These materials require extensive energy investments to produce, transport, and install—and also contain ingredients or byproducts that are harmful to the environment. Many are also from non-renewable sources.

As school communities envision a greener, more environmentally friendly schoolyard, and come together to collaborate as schoolyard stewards, many more options unfold. They have a palette of high quality, natural, and renewable materials available to them. For example, they can substitute sustainably harvested, non-toxic wood for plastic when it is time to purchase new play structures, build tool sheds and benches from straw bales and earth, and choose local stone over concrete where new paved pathways are needed. Some schools also salvage previously used building materials—putting "waste" to use as a resource on school grounds.[2] Metal salvaged from local sources may be reinvented as garden artwork, broken ceramic tiles transformed into colorful schoolyard mosaics, or garden walls created from pieces of broken sidewalk.[3]

Choosing to include natural and reclaimed materials on school grounds shows students and visitors that the school cares about its ecological footprint[4] and is committed to minimizing its environmental impact on the surrounding landscape. Natural materials are teaching tools for lessons on environmental stewardship and on time-tested construction techniques that are still relevant today.

Natural and reclaimed building materials also lend themselves well to artistic expression; they add a variety of interesting textures and tactile experiences that enrich the environment for students more familiar with metal and plastics in their daily play routine. Reclaimed materials generally show age-related patinas or patterning that suggests their earlier uses. Wooden elements can be polished to show unique wood grain patterns or growth rings, or they can be left rough and rustic. Earthen structures radiate warmth on sunny days and have an appealing irregular texture. All of these characteristics add depth, variety, history, and intrigue to their new forms in the schoolyard. For children going to school in urban areas, this—in and of itself—can be a revelation.

> Green building is the practice of creating structures and using processes that are environmentally responsible and resource-efficient throughout a building's life-cycle from siting to design, construction, operation, maintenance, renovation, and deconstruction. This practice expands and complements the classical building design concerns of economy, utility, durability, and comfort.[5]
>
> —U.S. Environmental Protection Agency

What should schools look for when selecting natural and reclaimed building materials for their school grounds? There are many factors that contribute to making a material "green," and sometimes the pros and cons of each substance should be considered on a case by case basis. Environmentally responsible building and landscape professionals typically look for materials that are:

- **From renewable sources**—materials that are sustainably harvested and are quick to replenish.

- **From reclaimed sources**—materials that have outlived their usefulness in their original context and may be reused in another place.

- **From local sources**—materials that do not require a lot of energy to transport to the project site. Using local materials also reinforces the unique character of each location, which contributes to its "sense of place."

- **Nontoxic**—materials that do not pose health risks to the site's users or those who process the material.

- **Non-damaging to the environment**—materials that do not cause pollution at any point in their lifecycle, including extraction/harvest of raw materials, processing, manufacturing, during use, and after their useful lifespans.

- **Recyclable/reusable**—materials that are easily recycled or composted at the end of their useful lifespans.

🍃 *Natural Building Materials on School Grounds*

Natural building is the oldest form of construction on our planet. Plant materials, such as wood, straw, and bamboo, may be nailed, woven, stacked, or tied to create durable schoolyard site furniture, structural elements, and garden artwork. Materials found in the ground, such as clay, sand, and stone, may be mixed, sculpted, stacked, or baked to build monumental forms that are durable and enchanting. Ephemeral natural materials, such as snow, can also be used to create temporary schoolyard landforms to be enjoyed in the winter, when the weather is right.

Using natural materials in a schoolyard landscape requires a paradigm shift in the ways that schools and their maintenance staff relate to their grounds. Natural building materials are part of a living landscape and frequently have shorter lifespans than their manufactured counterparts. They change over time as they respond to the weather and active use, often requiring annual care, such as a new coating of linseed oil or paint, and replacement every five to ten years. This process of ongoing alterations and renewal mimics social processes that occur in school communities: students grow up and graduate each year, shifting the composition of the PTA and staff cycle through the school as their careers progress. From a social perspective, the cycle of schoolyard construction, decomposi-

tion, and rebuilding is a way to keep the continuously changing school community actively engaged in schoolyard stewardship. In some ways, the relatively short lifespan of natural materials is ideal because it allows this changing community to add something to the grounds each year to make it their own. This keeps the community far more engaged with the schoolyard, and each other, from what typically occurs in an environment with permanent pavement and industrial materials.

Wood

Wood is one of the most versatile, natural building materials for schoolyards. It can be incorporated in its roughest forms—as stumps, logs, branches, twigs, and mulch, and in its more refined form—as milled lumber. Some green schoolyards include entire trees, downed in a storm or felled by disease, as ornamental play elements. Others use portions of tree trunks, large branches, and sturdy twigs, obtained from local arborists or cut onsite, in their outdoor seating areas, stairways, and pathways.

Standard milled lumber and unprocessed logs can be purchased from many places. Look for local, sustainably harvested lumber, if possible. In my area, for example, reasonably priced, sustainably harvested dimensional lumber can be purchased from an urban mill that specializes in creating lumber from trees that local arborists remove from our region.[6] Local arborists are also good sources for logs, branches, mulch or other wood products; often they would rather donate these materials to schools than pay a fee to dump them at a landfill.

When purchasing lumber from hardware stores and other conventional sources, do *not* buy pressure treated wood for use in a schoolyard—particularly for areas in or near edible gardens. Some types of treated wood contain highly poisonous substances that are intended to kill fungi and insects and resist rot—but they are also very hazardous for children. Some of the chemicals used to treat wood leach out over time and permanently contaminate the surrounding soil. Children may come into contact with these poisons by touching the wood or by inadvertently consuming the contaminated soil when they get it on their hands.[7] Some types of pressure treated wood commonly sold in home improvement stores are banned from playground uses, but are not clearly marked as such in the store. Similarly, it is important to avoid the use of railroad ties, which usually contain poisonous creosote, treated telephone poles, "marine grade wood," and other chemically treated wood products. Many types of plywood are also poor choices for the schoolyard – and edible garden beds in particular—since they often contain formaldehyde and other chemical binders. Because it is often difficult to tell exactly which chemicals the wood has been treated with, and how poisonous they are, I recommend avoiding treated wood entirely in a schoolyard context. Some school districts, such as the San Francisco Unified School District, adopt a similar approach district-wide and request that their schools avoid using treated wood in their schoolyards, if possible.[8]

Naturally rot-resistant woods such as redwood or cedar are good choices for schoolyards, if they come from sustainably harvested local sources. If these are not available, choose other hardwoods or softwoods that have shorter lifespans in the outdoor environment, and protect them with a natural finish or nontoxic stain or paint. Another good source of untreated wood is reclaimed lumber from material reuse centers or from buildings that have been carefully deconstructed.[9] Timber from these older sources may be of a higher grade than what is currently available; old growth timber frequently has tighter grain than younger wood. Be sure to avoid wood painted with lead-based paints, however.

Over the last four years, I have worked with Rosa Parks School in Berkeley, California, to green their school grounds.

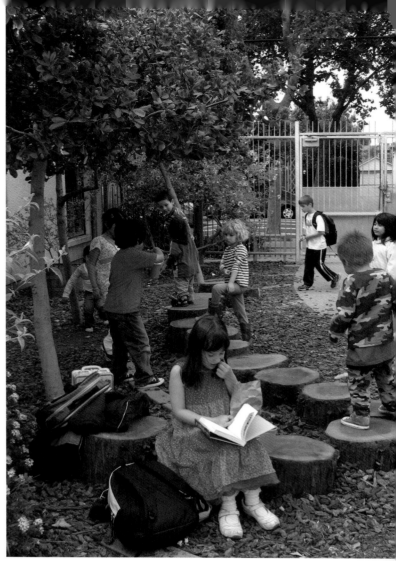

FIGURE 8.1

Many of the schoolyard improvements, installed or handcrafted by the school community, are made of wood. For example, we used redwood logs, donated by an arborist parent, to create a sturdy and sinuous bench. The log segments, each 1.5 to 2 feet long, were installed by parents and volunteers who dug a narrow, curving trench and buried half of each log firmly in the ground. The finished project, surrounded by a soft bed of woodchips, is enjoyed by the entire school community. (Figure 8.1) Leftover logs, placed in small clusters around the schoolyard, act as informal benches. We also placed a few 3-foot diameter eucalyptus tree slices, retrieved from another neighborhood tree removal project, under several bushes along the

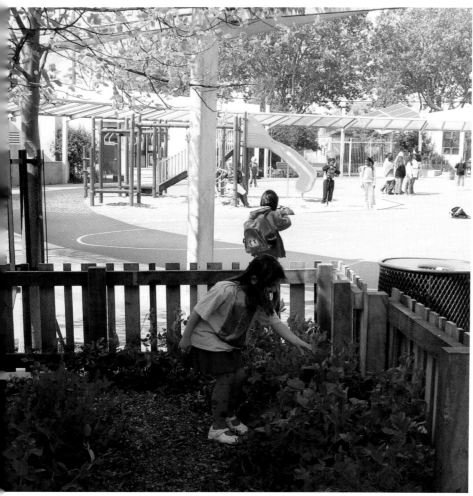

FIGURE 8.2 *Sustainably harvested wood was used to build fences for Rosa Parks School's "nibbling garden" in Berkeley, California.*

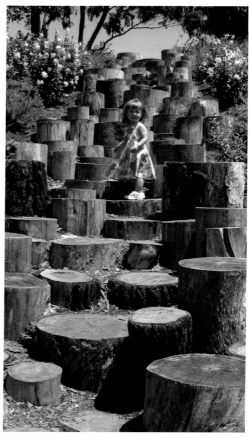

FIGURE 8.3 *This multileveled log "stairway" in the outdoor play area at the Lookout Cove exhibition at the Bay Area Discovery Museum in Sausalito, California, beckons children to climb.*

playground's perimeter to create comfortable seats nestled in the leaves. (See chapter 11, Figure 11.3)

I worked with parents and teachers at the school to build several small garden fences adjacent to the playground, using local, sustainably harvested dimensional lumber. The Monterey cypress and redwood we selected are naturally rot resistant, but we also added a soy-based wood sealer to further extend the wood's longevity. The new edible gardens are filled with raspberries and other crops for the children to freely "nibble" at recess. The fences define the edges of the new gardens and keep (most of!) the balls out of the plantings. (Figure 8.2)

Bamboo

Bamboo is a fast-growing plant in the grass family that is well adapted to climates ranging from tropical locations to places with snowy winters. The strong stalks, called "culms," are hollow cylinders, subdivided into individual chambers by nodes along the stalk. Some species of bamboo form dense clumps, while others spread prolifically by sprouting from underground rhizomes. Bamboo is used in countless ways around the world to construct everything from buildings, bridges, construction scaffolding, flooring, furniture, baskets, chopsticks, and paper. Its young rhizomes are also a delicious edible food crop.[12]

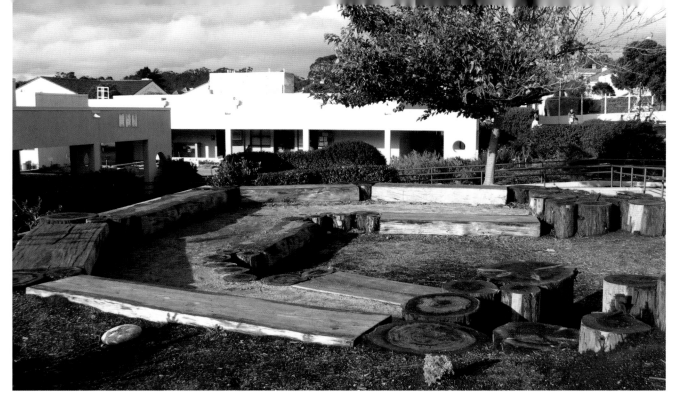

FIGURE 8.4 *Commodore Sloat Elementary School in San Francisco, California, used large eucalyptus logs, downed in a storm, to create wide outdoor classroom seating tiers. Smaller redwood rounds complete the amphitheater.*[10]

FIGURE 8.5 *The Edible Schoolyard at ML King, Jr. Middle School, in Berkeley, California, includes a tool shed, expertly crafted by a local designer and King students from a single, naturally fallen redwood tree.*[11]

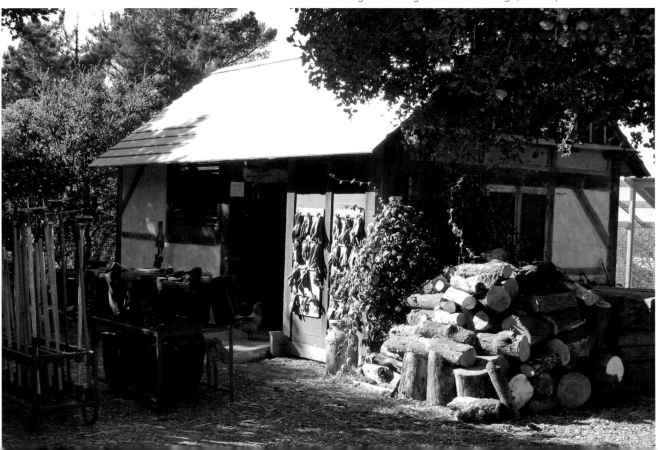

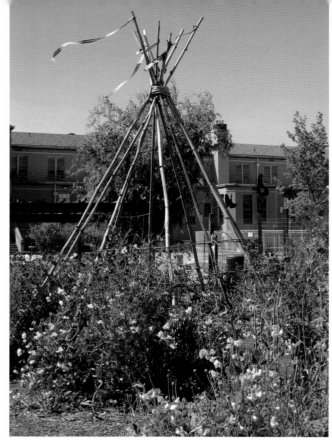

FIGURE 8.6 *This whimsical, teepee at Malcolm X School in Berkeley, California, was built using sturdy 12-foot long bamboo poles, two inches in diameter.*[13]

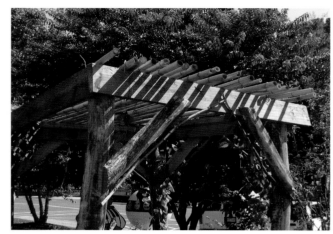

FIGURE 8.7 *Horizontal bamboo rods on the roof of this outdoor classroom shade the seating area below.*[14]

Bamboo has an appealing linear aesthetic with subtle color variations and a smooth surface. Many types of bamboo are green when they are alive, then dry to a golden yellow that fades to a weathered grey over time. In a school garden, use dried bamboo stalks to build fences, trellises, bean teepees, irrigation channels, and rain gutters. (Figures 8.6 and 8.7)

Straw bale

Straw bales are blocks of tightly packed, fibrous stalks from wheat or rice plants that remain after the grain has been harvested. Straw is used in an agricultural context as animal bedding or mulch. It is also a key component of many natural building techniques, either in bale form, or mixed with varying amounts of clay and sand to create materials called "wattle and daub," "light clay," and "cob."

Stacked like bricks and reinforced with metal rebar or bamboo, straw bales become durable garden walls, benches, and building walls. Straw bale structures require "dry feet" and a "dry hat" to prevent damage from moisture, so they are usually placed on a slightly elevated foundation and, generally, have a roofline with deep overhanging edges to protect the bale walls from precipitation. Straw bale structures are commonly finished with earth-based or cement stucco, or lime-based plaster, to further protect the walls. If built properly, straw bale structures are very resistant to fire, earthquakes, and vermin.[15] Because the walls are thick and built from naturally insulating materials, the interiors of these buildings are very quiet, comfortable, and protected from wide temperature fluctuations.[16] (Figures 8.8–8.10)

FIGURE 8.8 *Simple straw bale garden seating at Prospect Sierra School in El Cerrito, California. After bales like these outlive their use as seating, they may be disassembled and used as mulch.*

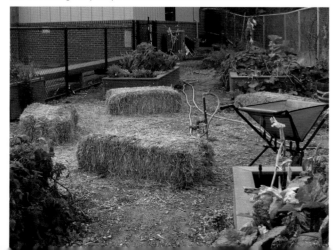

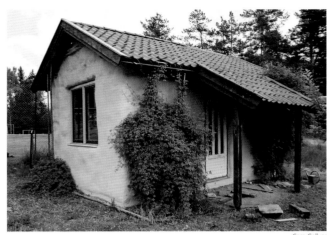

FIGURE 8.9 *Maridalen School in Norway has a charming straw bale tool shed, built by school staff members with help from the students' parents.*[17]

Cam Collyer

Light clay

Light clay is a building material made from loose straw that is coated with mud, then forcefully packed between the joists of wood framed structures. It is a relatively fast building technique used to create well-insulated, lightweight, sturdy walls. Light clay building methods are simple enough that untrained volunteers, assisting a natural builder, can create long lasting structures.

Sankt Hansgården in Sweden is an after-school recreation center with an agricultural and ecological theme. It is also a superb example of natural and green building techniques. The center serves 90 local children between the ages of 9–12 on a daily basis, and is open to the public. Over time, the students

FIGURE 8.10 *Salmon Creek School in Occidental, California, built a stunning, straw bale "garden classroom" in the midst of the school's bountiful culinary garden.*

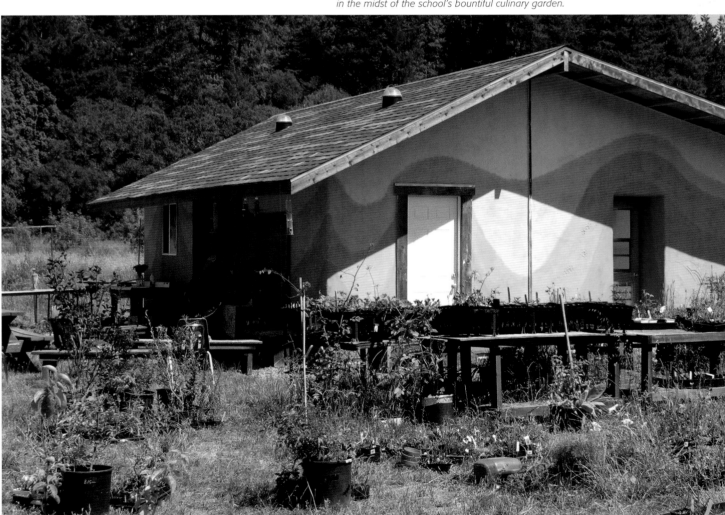

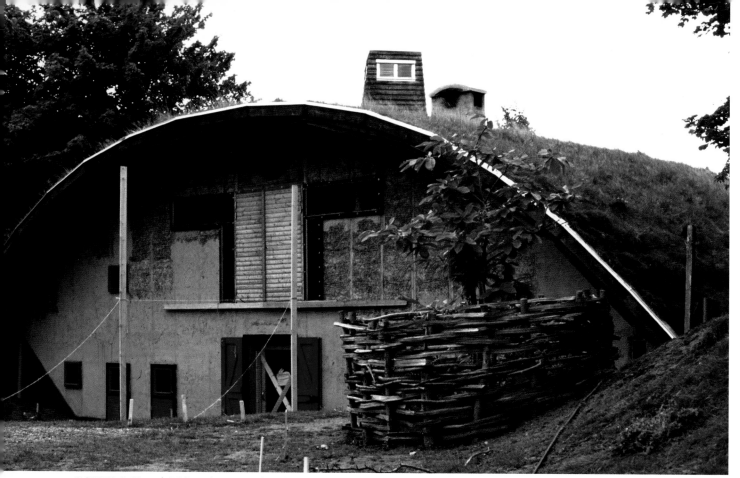

FIGURES 8.11 and 8.12 *Sankt Hansgården after-school center in Lund, Sweden, uses light clay as one of its primary building materials.*

helped a professional builder construct an elaborate barn to house chickens, goats, sheep and rabbits, and provide the center with added meeting space. (Figure 8.11)

Every aspect of the barn was selected with ecological design principles in mind. The structure is formed from massive wooden beams that spent the last three hundred years in another building and were reclaimed for this use. Light clay techniques were used to fill the cavities between the wooden joists in the outer walls, and the exterior of the building was receiving its coating of clay and lime plaster when I visited the site in September 2001. (Figure 8.12) The barn uses the constant temperature of the ground to preheat and precool incoming air flowing through an underground duct. Heat is supplied by a radiant system under the floor bricks. Solar thermal panels warm the building's water. Solar electric panels and a wind turbine provide a portion of the electricity used

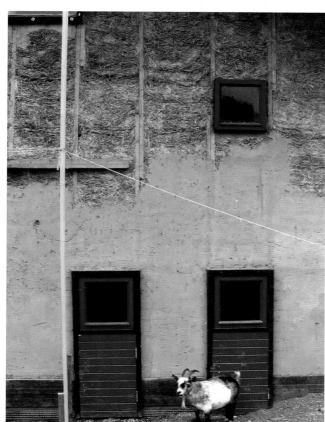

onsite. The barn is capped by a living roof planted with turf grasses.[18]

Wattle and daub

Wattle and daub is an ancient building technique used for thousands of years in Europe, Asia, North and South America, and Africa. It was commonly used to build homes in England until the 1700s and is currently growing in popularity again as part of the green building movement in Europe and North America.[19] In wattle and daub construction, a woven wooden lattice, used as the framework for a wall, is plastered with an earthen "daub" mixture that fills the lattice's holes to create a smooth surface. The daub usually contains clay soil, animal manure, and sand, but may also contain other fillers, binders, and fiber. (Figure 8.13)

Cob

Cob is also an ancient material, used in northern Africa and parts of Europe for hundreds of years. In modern times, it is strongly associated with traditional home building methods in places such as England's Devon and Cornwall counties. Like adobe, cob is a combination of clay, straw, and sand, but it is not formed into precise bricks or dried prior to construction. Instead, the sticky mixture is worked in a sculptural way to slowly build up heavy forms that have great strength. Workers add handfuls or bundles of wet cob to the structure they are building, and then use pointed sticks to weave the new material into previous layers. The haphazard network of interlaced straw that results reinforces the growing form and expands its ability to hold self-supporting sculptural shapes. Varying the proportions of clay, sand, and straw in the cob mixture results in different properties that are useful for building more complex projects, such as earthen ovens, or constructing large buildings. The more sand that is added to the mixture, the heavier the finished structure will be and the more thermal mass it will have. The more straw that is added, the better insulation value the resulting form will have, and the more interconnected the structure will be.

Cob, like straw bale, is sensitive to moisture. It is wise to build a cob structure on top of a raised foundation, and to build it in a place that will be protected from rain. Many natural builders apply an earth plaster coating to the exterior of their cob forms, made from finely screened clay, sand, lime,

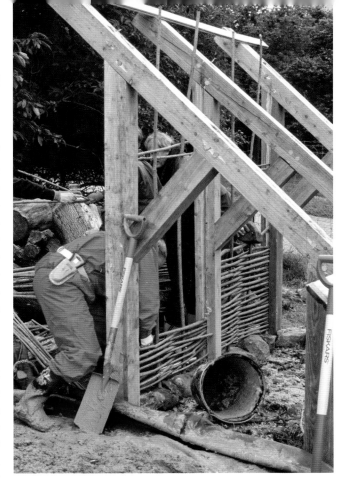

FIGURE 8.13 *This small wattle and daub pump station was under construction at Sankt Hansgården after-school center in Sweden during my September 2001 site visit.*[20]

and small fibers, to create a smooth finished surface. Next, they often seal their cob creations with linseed oil or other natural sealants to further protect it from moisture.[21] Despite this protection, most cob structures need to be touched up from time to time and their surface coatings refreshed, due to gradual erosion from weather and use.

In a schoolyard context, cob may be used to create fanciful benches (see chapter 13), curving seat walls, earthen ovens (see chapter 7), and other small structures. Though it is a labor intensive material that requires more time and effort than straw bale or light clay techniques, it can also be more forgiving, more creative, and more flexible. Sometimes, labor intensive materials are an asset if there are many hands willing to pitch in to work collaboratively. This can be an ideal material to use

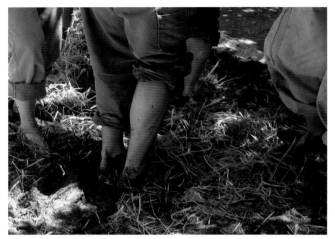

FIGURE 8.14

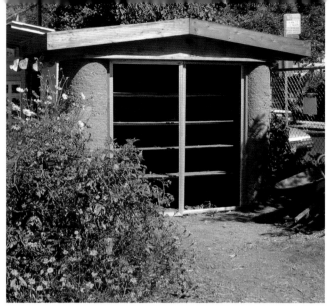

FIGURE 8.16 *This small cob greenhouse at Malcolm X School in Berkeley, California, was built by the school community and volunteers over a two-month period in 2001. Its walls are composed of clay, straw, and sand, and it has a living roof of wildflowers that blooms during the rainy season each winter. The thick walls (with high thermal mass) soak up the sun's heat during the day and then radiate that warmth to the plants at night.*[23]

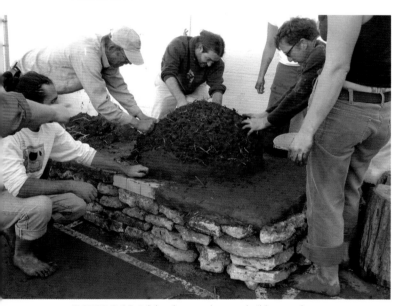

FIGURE 8.15 *Adult volunteers learn to build an earth oven at Harvey Milk Civil Rights Academy in San Francisco, California, during a green schoolyard conference workshop.*[22]

Rammed earth

Rammed earth is a technique that combines local soil or sand with small amounts of concrete to form a mixture that is "rammed" (tamped down with great force) into a mold to make a solid form. The resulting material looks and feels like stone; it is striated, somewhat like sedimentary rock, and is hard and smooth to the touch. Machines, run by professionals, are generally used to tamp the earth for large projects, but small structures and benches may be created with earth rammed by hand within wooden forms. I have not yet seen this material used in a schoolyard context, but it would be suitable for creating a greenhouse with high thermal mass, sturdy walls for a tool shed, or a seat wall.

As a graduate student at UC Berkeley in 2000, I participated in a hands-on green building class that constructed a tool shed for the Berkeley EcoHouse in Berkeley, California. The tool shed's walls are each made of a different natural building material (wood, straw bale, rammed earth, and light clay) to help educate visitors about natural building techniques. The rammed earth wall, created by hand-pounding a mixture of sand and cement into wooden forms, has beautiful striations in the finished surface.[24] (Figure 8.17)

with a class of middle or high school students, as it requires more strength than younger children generally have. "Playing in the mud" is also fun, and tactile activities like this have too often been removed from older children's experiences at school. Working with cob, and mixing clay, sand, and straw with one's bare feet, can be a refreshing change for students and their teachers. (Figure 8.14–8.16)

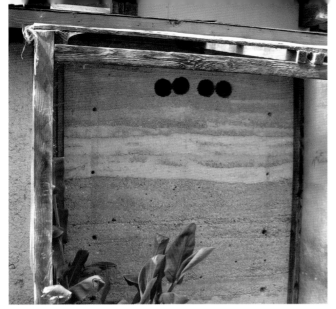

FIGURE 8.17

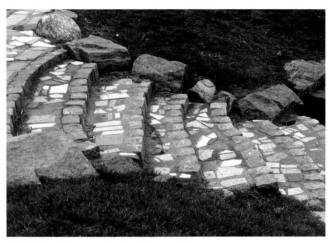

FIGURE 8.18 *The multicolored stone stairway at Maridalen School near Oslo, Norway.*

FIGURE 8.19

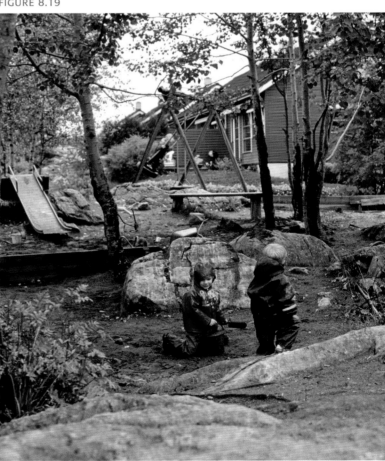

Stone

Stone is a good fit for school grounds because it is quite durable, visually interesting, and can be connected to the geology curriculum. Group stones and boulders for informal seating, arrange them along drainage channels or the edges of garden beds, or display them as prominent schoolyard landmarks. Rock can also be cut and carved to make paving materials, bricks, and sculptures. Use stone to create long lasting landscape features including benches, walkways, walls, and play areas. Significant amounts of fossil fuel are needed to transport stone as it is quite heavy. To conserve resources, it is best to use stone from a local source—which will add regional character to the schoolyard as well. (Figure 8.18)

Stone is an abundant building material in Norway, where it can be found on many schools sites and in the local fjords. In most of the Norwegian schools I visited, stone was used to create pathways, seat walls, climbing structures, and garden beds, but it was also an integral part of the school's natural landscape. It not only provided visual interest, but also served as play props for active and imaginative games. (See chapter 10, Manglerud School, Figures 10.16–10.18)

The kindergarten playground at Lørenskog Steiner School outside Oslo, for example, is built among naturally-occurring boulders, and children are allowed to play on the rocks as they please. (Figure 8.19) In 2000, the school also worked on a large project with architect Frode Svane to build a sinuous

FIGURE 8.20

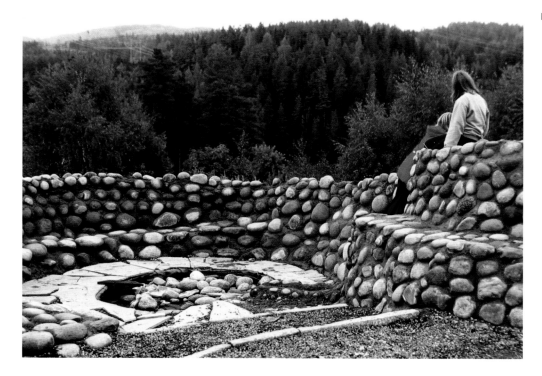

stone wall. (Figure 8.20) Students gathered stones at a local glacial moraine and then spent six weeks building the seat wall with the help of their parents and teachers. The top of the wall includes a water channel connected to a recirculating fountain system in the center of the seating area. On the day of my visit to the school, the middle school students were hard at work building another smaller mortared stone wall to create a garden bed near their classroom buildings.[25]

Earthbag

Sand or soil found on school grounds can be shaped into sinuous benches and seat walls using "earthbag" construction techniques. Sandbags are first filled with sand or soil from the site and then stacked in overlapping layers (like bricks) following the builder's design. The bags are pinned in place with metal rebar and wrapped tightly with a layer of chicken wire. A thin coating of concrete applied to the chicken wire creates a durable and weatherproof exterior surface that can be embellished with incised patterns, tile mosaics, or pigments. This building method is inexpensive, straightforward, and reason-

ably quick; a group of 10–15 adults can build a bench in a single day. (Figures 8.21–8.23)

Snow

In places like Canada, Scandinavia, and the northern United States, winter snow serves as an ephemeral natural building material. Snow encourages children to build dens and forts and brings sledding and skiing opportunities to school grounds, adding some seasonal variety. Snow can also be used to create temporary outdoor classroom spaces, seat walls, hills and other landscape features. (See chapter 11 for additional examples.)

Material Reuse in a Schoolyard Context

Many schools around the world are taking part in recycling programs for their used glass, paper, and metal waste products. Far fewer schools are reclaiming or reusing building materials—concrete, metal, tiles, wood—in their classroom buildings and playground environments. Using salvaged building materials on school grounds is valuable from an ecological perspective because it diverts bulky waste products from landfills and recaptures the remaining value of the materials for further use. It also reduces the need to mine, harvest, process, and transport virgin materials, which in turn, saves additional energy, fossil fuel, and effort, and preserves environments at the extraction source.

Finding new uses for materials is a creative endeavor that, if accomplished successfully, adds a sense of history and continuity to the new environments the materials are used to create. Both the history the materials bring with them, and the environmentally conscious design process they represent, are educational in a school context. The "stories" behind salvaged materials should be saved and repeated to each class of students to preserve this special aspect of their schoolyard's genesis.

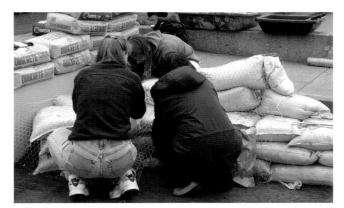

FIGURE 8.21 *Earthbag bench construction, in progress.*

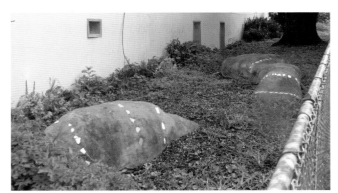

FIGURE 8.22 *This earthbag bench in the garden at John Muir School in San Francisco, California, is shaped like an earthworm, diving in and out of the ground.*

FIGURE 8.23 *This inviting, "couch-like" outdoor classroom at Willard Middle School in Berkeley, California, was built using "earthbag" construction techniques. The school also applied a tile mosaic design to the cement coating on the bench.[26]*

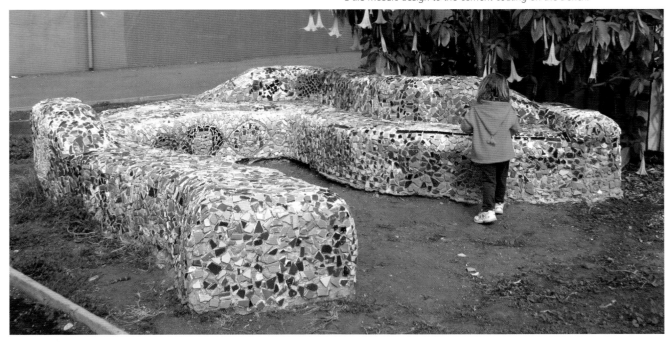

Concrete ("Urbanite")

Concrete is a material that has many uses; however, it is resource-intensive and environmentally unfriendly. Portland cement, a key ingredient, requires a great deal of energy to manufacture and emits large amounts of carbon dioxide into the atmosphere.[27] Because an enormous amount of concrete already exists and challenges landfills with its disposal, it is preferable to re-use it rather than create more, whenever possible. Stack pieces of broken concrete like bricks to form walls around garden beds, to create seating and foundations for straw bale and cob projects, and to terrace gentle hillsides. Sometimes mortar is used to make these walls more permanent, but it is not always required. Green builders often affectionately refer to these concrete chunks as "urbanite" ("ore" that is "mined" from urban locations). (Figures 8.24 and 8.25)

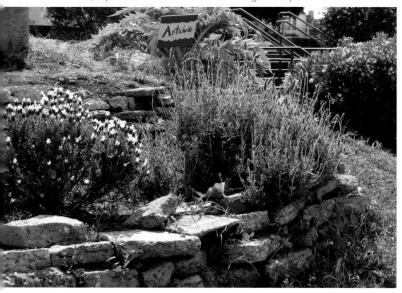

FIGURE 8.24 *Volunteers at Commodore Sloat School in San Francisco, California, terraced a shallow hillside using low, dry-stacked urbanite walls to create garden space.[28]*

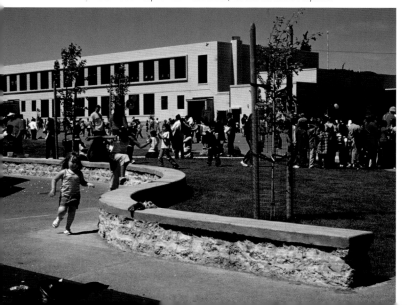

FIGURE 8.25 *Lockwood Elementary School in Oakland, California, used mortared urbanite to install a snaking seat wall. Professional stone masons built the wall and topped it with a smooth cap of new concrete, at the school's request.*

FIGURE 8.26

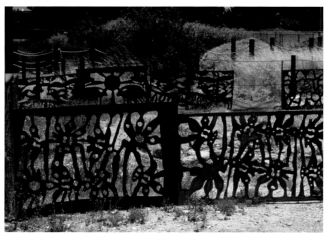

FIGURE 8.27 *A beautiful recycled metal gate graces Salmon Creek School's garden in northern California. A local artist welded retired metal tools together to create an entrance with a garden theme.[30]*

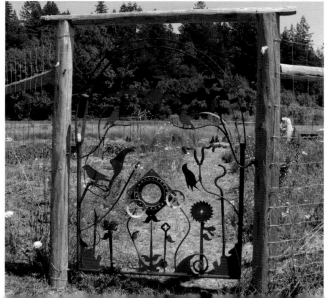

Metal

Used metal can be recut or reshaped to find new life as schoolyard fencing, gates, artwork, or other forms. At Montgomery High School in San Diego, California, for example, the school acquired metal bars and large metal sheets that were previously used as prison beds. They combined these materials, with their students' creativity and skills, to create attractive fences and signage for their extensive native plants garden. The school's art classes designed the wildlife-themed panels; other students in welding classes cut the metal and installed the fences.[29] (Figures 8.26 and 8.27)

Tile mosaics

Broken ceramic tiles, old dishware, and colorful glass can become decorative schoolyard mosaics. For example, Cowick First School in England commissioned a mosaic artist to make a stunning mural on a 60-foot long wall bordering the school's paved playground. The artist created the piece using old ceramic dishware students brought from home. The resulting exuberant scene, created in the mid-1980s, depicts children playing happily outside. More than twenty years later, the mosaic is still in excellent condition, illustrating that this type of art form can be a long lasting asset for a school.[31] (Figures 8.28 and 8.29)

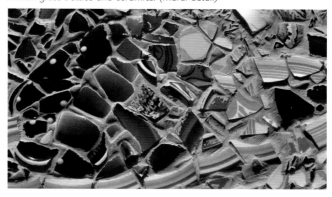

FIGURE 8.29 *This mosaic mural at a Brock Junior Public School in Toronto, Canada was created by students using broken glass bottles and ceramics. (mural detail)*

FIGURE 8.28 *An artist used recycled materials to create this tile mosaic mural at Cowick First School.*

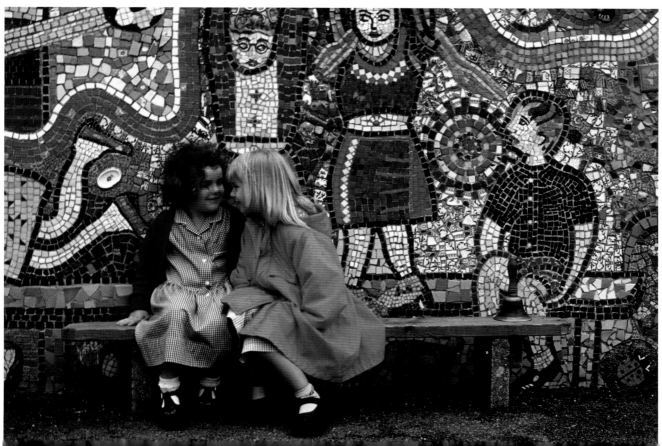

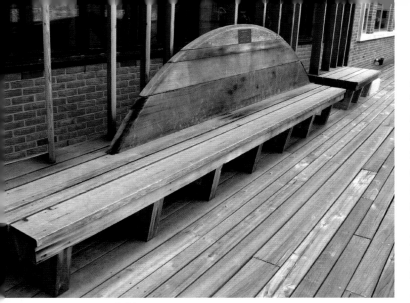

FIGURE 8.30

Salvaged wood

Wood is relatively easy to disassemble from previous configurations and to re-use in a new context. Once old nails, screws and other fasteners are removed, the salvaged wood can be refinished to clean and renew its surfaces. Some old, well preserved timber is actually superior to newly harvested wood since old growth trees frequently have tighter grain and greater strength than younger, newly harvested wood.

Eleven percent of the building materials used at Sidwell Friends Middle School in Washington, DC, came from recycled sources,[32] including some of the wood that is used in their classroom building and landscape. Greenheart wood from South America, salvaged from Baltimore Harbor's pilings, was used to make beautiful interior flooring at the school and a lovely deck located just outside the building (shown). The architects also used a very large wine cask, made from western red cedar, to create a unique bench that celebrates the wood's previous life by including a curved piece of the barrel top to make its source visible. The same wood was also used to make the building's exterior louvers, arranged vertically along the east- and west-facing windows to shade the interior at the hottest times of the day.[33] (Figures 8.30–8.32)

Composting

Schoolyard landscape clippings and plant wastes from the lunchroom (e.g. apple cores and banana peels) can be transformed into nutrient-rich compost and reused onsite in the school garden. Students learn about nutrient cycling and natural processes by observing decomposition processes onsite. Compost piles generally contain micro-ecosystems, rich with creatures such as earthworms, beetles, and pill bugs that fascinate children. The simple process of aerating a compost pile may turn into an entomology lesson or become a springboard for hands-on science studies.

Composting methods differ, but all have the same general principles. They start with raw, organic waste materials and

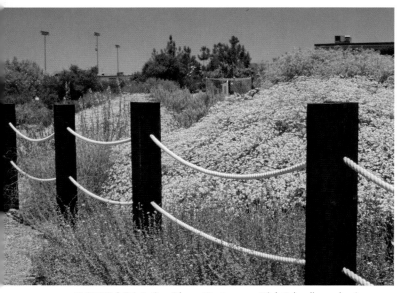

FIGURE 8.31 *In San Diego, Montgomery High School's garden includes fence posts made from recycled landscape timber and used nautical rope acquired from the nearby navy and shipping industries.*[34]

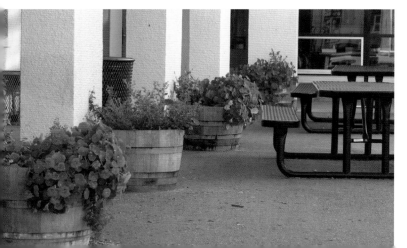

FIGURE 8.32 *The Rosa Parks School community in Berkeley, California installed twenty wine barrel planters and filled them with colorful flowers and culinary plants. These half-barrels, a byproduct of the local wine industry, last about five years as planters in their climate and schoolyard context.*

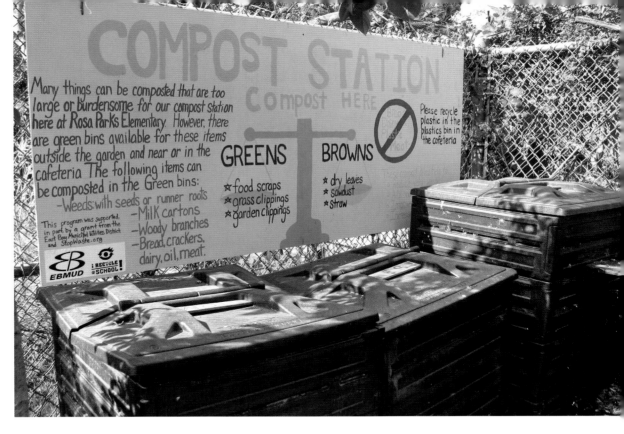

FIGURE 8.33 *Rosa Parks School in Berkeley uses three "biostack" compost bins to process garden clippings. The informative sign above the compost area helps students and garden volunteers to better understand the process.*[35]

end up with a rich soil amendment that works magic in the garden. Successful compost piles contain a balance of "green" materials—plants that were alive when they were picked such as garden clippings, vegetable and fruit peels and cores—and "brown" materials that were brown or dry when acquired, such as crunchy fall leaves, saw dust, or paper. To make compost, the green and brown items are chopped into small pieces, then mixed or layered in a pile. The pile is kept moist and turned occasionally to keep it well aerated, which speeds decomposition. Over time, microorganisms, fungi, insects, and earthworms turn the raw waste materials into a deep black, pleasant smelling soil amendment—similar to what many people purchase at garden stores.

If the volume of compost is large, and the mixture is just right, the compost pile will heat up as it decomposes, killing weed seeds and plant disease pathogens that may be present. Because it is difficult to ensure that a schoolyard compost pile will be hot enough to sterilize the mixture, try to avoid adding items you don't want to find later in your edible garden. For example, avoid adding yard clippings that include diseased plants, weed seeds, or runners from plants that spread prolifi-

cally. Also avoid adding animal wastes to the compost pile, as they can spread diseases. Milk, meat, and bread products will not harm the quality of the compost produced, but they have a strong rotten smell as they decompose, which makes the composting experience unpleasant for the school community and may also attract rats, raccoons, and other animals.

The choice of composting bin and technique may speed or slow the decomposition process, but it will all turn into compost eventually. The most basic form of composting is an outdoor pile of green and brown wastes that grows over time as material is added to it. Though used by many home gardeners, this is not the best method for school gardens since it takes more time and space (piles spread out easily), and there is no way to control animals' or children's access to the compost.

Instead, many schools choose to contain their compost in bins. One popular format is a three-bin system. In this arrangement, the first bin is used to collect new green and brown material. The second bin stores it as it decomposes, and the third bin holds finished compost for use in the garden. The decomposing material is transferred from one bin to the next as it breaks down, and the process of transferring it helps to

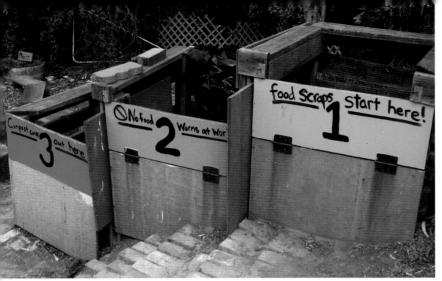

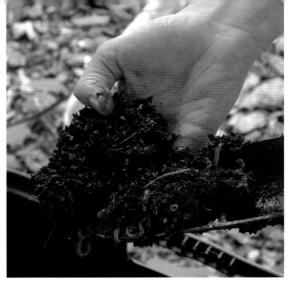

FIGURE 8.34 *Fairview School in Hayward, California, placed its three compost bins on a hillside and uses gravity to help move material from the top bin to the bottom. When the compost is ready to be turned, the wooden walls between bins slide out so the compost can be easily pushed to a lower level.*

FIGURE 8.35 *Red worms process food scraps in a vermiculture bin, turning it into rich compost.*

aerate the compost, speeding decomposition. (Figure 8.33 and Figure 8.34.)

Some schools use another style of composting called vermiculture, or composting with worms. The source materials for vermiculture are, commonly, food wastes and waste paper. Worms prefer a dark environment, so vermiculture takes place inside light-tight containers. The container's lid is only opened to add new materials or remove finished compost. Small "worm bins" can be used inside a classroom or larger boxes can be installed outside. The chief "engine" for this system are small "red worms" that work with microorganisms to pass the food and paper bedding through their systems, breaking down the organic material into "worm castings," which look quite similar to other types of compost. When it is ready, the worms are separated from the finished compost, so they can be added back to a fresh waste source. (Figure 8.35)

❀ Materials to Avoid

Schools can get very creative with what they re-use on their grounds; however, it makes sense to use caution when selecting materials. The following list is a sample of some things I avoid re-using in green schoolyards.

- **Avoid treated wood of all types:** Used railroad ties, telephone poles, and other types of treated wood should be avoided on school grounds and should *never* be used in edible gardens. Most railroad ties contain highly poisonous creosote, and many telephone poles contain arsenic and other known carcinogens.

- **Avoid using plastic lumber with wood fiber content:** Some plastic lumber contains pressure treated wood fibers,

so it should not be used in edible gardens or places where children may touch it.[36] This material is also not recyclable when its useful lifespan is over.

- **Avoid items with lead paint:** Use caution when reusing old painted wood or metal; test these items for lead before bringing them into the schoolyard.

- **Avoid using tires in edible gardens:** It is unclear whether used vehicle tires can leach toxins or heavy metals into adjacent soil, so I would recommend that they are never used for food gardens. (See chapter 10, tire sidebar for more information)

9 Lessons from the Landscape:
Weaving Teaching Resources into Schoolyard Design

Well-designed ecological schoolyards have many learning and play opportunities woven into their design, which may be continually reinterpreted as needs change over the years. When I work with teachers to develop curriculum connections to their own schoolyards, science is usually the first subject area they consider. While there are incredibly rich opportunities for schoolyard science studies, this is by no means the only area that is ripe for hands-on learning. With a little creativity, almost any academic subject may be taught outside.

The following examples are not meant to suggest that teachers should add additional topics to their teaching load— rather, the idea is to discover what teachers are *already* teaching that can be enriched by embedding educational resources in the schoolyard landscape. These carefully selected educational features become permanent additions to the grounds, available to the school's faculty members year after year.

Many outdoor lessons begin and end with a group discussion that focuses the class on the activity at hand. Outdoor classroom spaces make these gatherings much more comfortable and successful, so they are vital prerequisites for effective schoolyard teaching. (See chapter 13 for more outdoor classroom design options).

FIGURE 9.1 *Alphabet wall at Coombes School in England.*
Cam Collyer

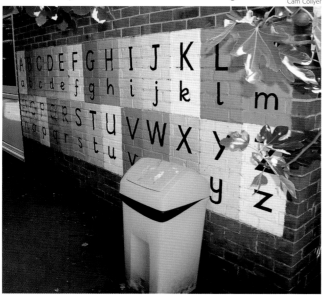

🍃 *Language and Literature Studies*

Some schools use their grounds to teach language studies, from simple lessons about the alphabet in kindergarten through complex language and literature curricula in upper grade levels. The schoolyard is the canvas for these explorations, with the addition of paint, seating, and signage.

Alphabet themes: Preschools and elementary schools paint playful alphabet murals outside to familiarize young children with letters. At Coombes School in England, upper and lowercase letters were used to create a colorful and instructive wall mural. (Figure 9.1) At other schools, the alphabet may be painted on the playground's asphalt in the form of a sinuous snake or within another playful graphic.

Story circles: Many British schools have designated "story circles" with a dramatic storyteller's chair, surrounded by places for children to gather within sight of the book. These comfortable

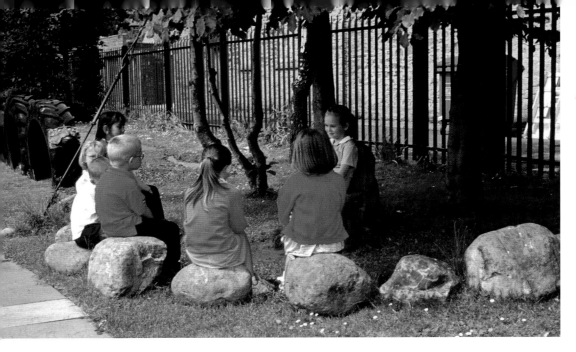

FIGURE 9.2 *A "story circle" at Leadgate School in England.*

seating areas make reading an even more enjoyable activity. (Figures 9.2 and 9.3)

Foreign language studies: Foreign languages may be practiced outdoors using role-playing activities or bilingual signage. For example, Royston High School in England sets up outdoor tables and chairs creating a temporary Parisian-style "café", when the weather is nice. Students pretend they are in Paris, and practice their French language skills while serving each other drinks and snacks.[1] (Figure 9.4)

Literature: Schoolyards may display poems or famous quotations from literature to expand students' literary horizons and reflect their teaching philosophy. At Tule Elk Park Child Development Center in San Francisco, California, the artist-in-residence worked with students to create a permanent ceramic mural explaining the history of books and writing around the world. The mural, called The Art and Evolution of the Written Word, is designed to look like a scroll and is organized chronologically. Its text is written mostly in English, but also includes examples of written Chinese and Greek, Aztec pictographs, Egyptian hieroglyphics, and other languages.[2] (Figure 9.5)

FIGURE 9.3 *A special story teller's chair at the Coombes School in England.*

Cam Collyer

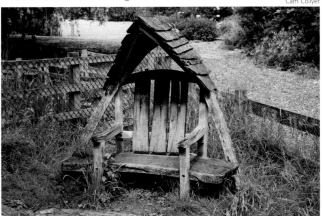

FIGURE 9.4 *Wall mounted artwork at Flynn School in San Francisco includes Spanish and English text.*

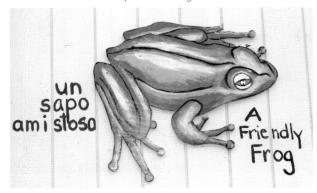

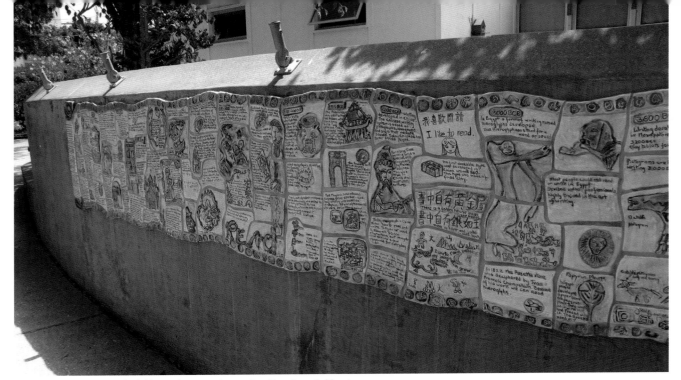

FIGURE 9.5 *Tule Elk Park Child Development Center, San Francisco, California*

FIGURE 9.6 *Children at Grattan School in San Francisco wrote poems that were incorporated into a brightly colored mural on a classroom building's wall.*

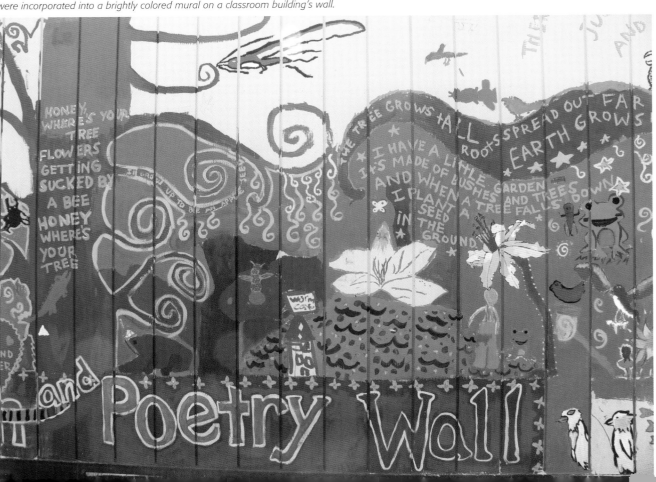

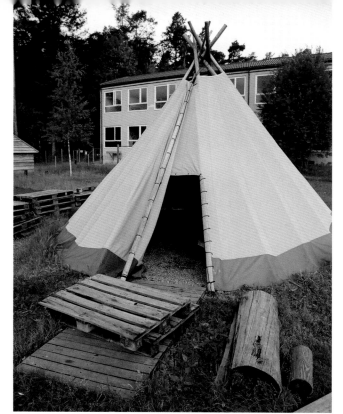

FIGURE 9.7 *The grounds at Manglerud School in Norway include a traditional Sámi-style, teepee-like dwelling (called a Lavvu) that students use as an outdoor classroom to study the architecture and culture of the Sámi people of northern Scandinavia.[3]*

Cam Collyer

History and Social Studies

History and social studies lessons are enlivened with hands-on outdoor resources that relate to what students are studying in their classrooms. (Figures 9.7 and 9.8) For example, schools with gardens may plant crops traditionally grown by cultures they are studying, and then cook meals inspired by these foods. Or, they may gather oral history about their grandparents' gardening experiences in their youth, and then grow these foods onsite.

Some schools extend their studies of world cultures or current events to include statements about the way countries—and neighborhood residents and students—relate to one another. "Peace gardens," murals, and other unity projects proclaim hope for a peaceful world. (Figures 9.9 and 9.10)

At Lampton School near London, England, a schoolyard "tree walk" celebrates the school's diverse student population. More than 70 trees native to the students' countries of origin are represented on the walk, which meanders around the perimeter of the school's large athletic fields. (Figure 9.11)

Lampton School also created a seating area near the school building that echoes the tree walk's multicultural theme. Each of five circular benches surrounds and protects a tree from a different continent. The arrangement of the circular benches

FIGURE 9.8

At Tenderloin Community School in San Francisco, students created a tile mosaic mural on the theme of "Women We Admire." Subjects range from women who are important to the students and school community to women who have changed the world.[4]

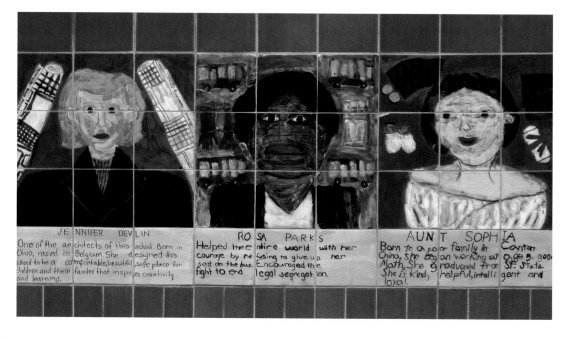

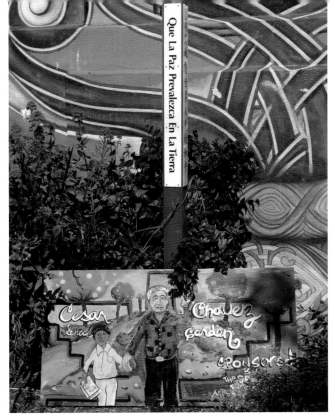

FIGURE 9.9 *This "peace pole" at Cesar Chavez School in San Francisco, California, is adorned with wishes for peace in multiple languages.*

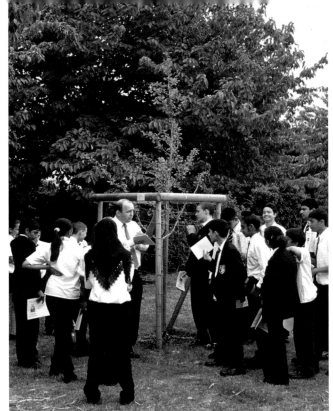

FIGURE 9.11 *The "tree walk" at Lampton School in England celebrates the school's diversity with trees from around the world.*

FIGURE 9.10 *This mural at Bret Harte School in San Francisco celebrates the school's annual tradition of holding a peace march in honor of Martin Luther King, Jr.*[5]

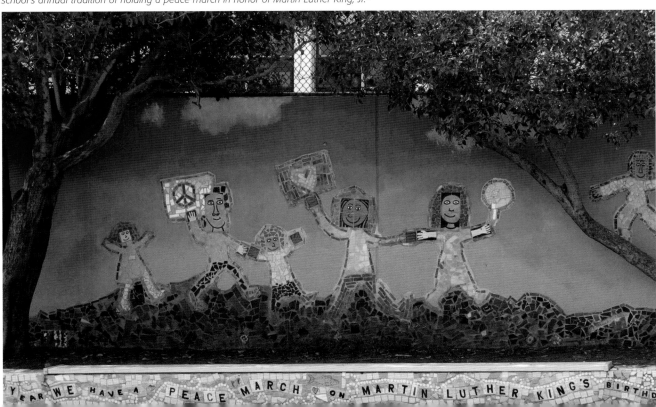

is reminiscent of the Olympic logo and is intended to symbolically unite the school community. The school also holds events during the year to honor major holidays in their students' home countries and to introduce the school community to their peers' traditions, foods, and cultures.[6]

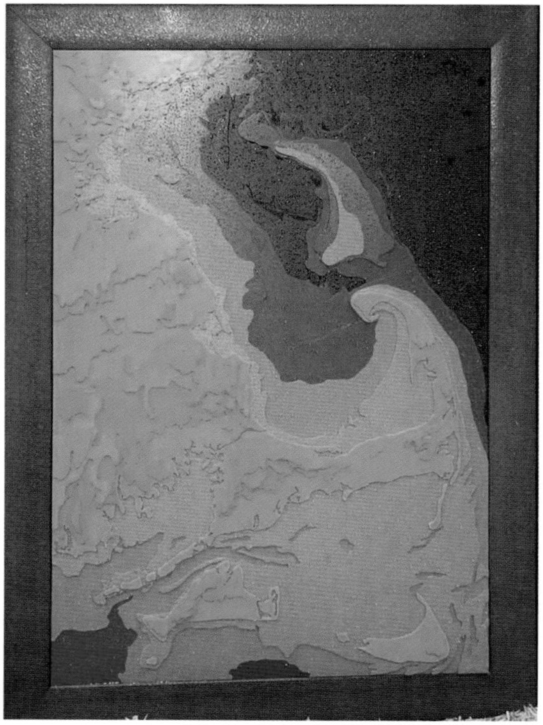

Geography

Geography studies are enriched using outdoor maps that depict local city streets, states, countries, continents, or the entire world. A compass rose that includes the cardinal directions is also a useful addition to the study of maps and geography.

The playground at Mullen-Hall Elementary School in Falmouth, Massachusetts, was designed with a nautical and science theme that reflects the school's local context. A relief map of the Cape Cod coastline, adorning a play structure, shows landforms above and below sea level. (Figure 9.12) Other related features include a lookout tower shaped like a lighthouse, a "Mini-Alvin submarine," referencing the nearby Woods Hole Oceanographic Institute, and a stage with a compass rose.[7]

Leathers and Associates

FIGURE 9.12 *Nautical relief map on the playground at Mullen-Hall Elementary School.*

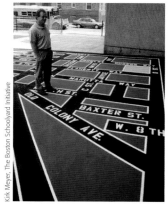

Kirk Meyer, The Boston Schoolyard Initiative

FIGURE 9.13 *Neighborhood map, painted on the schoolyard at Condon Elementary School in South Boston, Massachusetts.*[8]

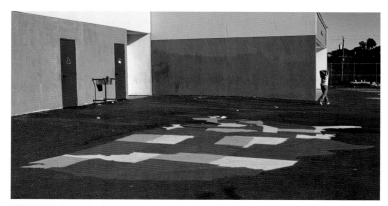

FIGURE 9.14 *United States map on the playground at Manzanita School in Oakland, California.*

FIGURE 9.15 *World map on the playground at Thousand Oaks School in Berkeley, California.*

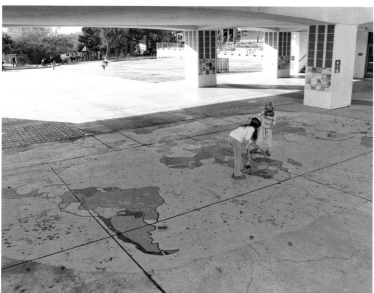

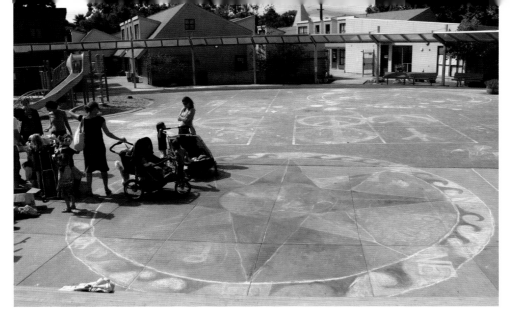

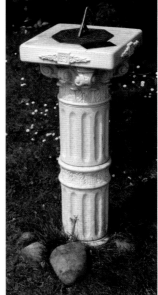

FIGURE 9.16 *A large, temporary compass rose, drawn with chalk, at Rosa Parks School in Berkeley, California.*

FIGURE 9.17 *This small, pedestal mounted sundial at Leadgate Infant School in England is placed so that children can examine it easily.*

🍃 *Curricula Related to the Passage of Time*

School grounds are ideal places to learn about the passage of time. Seasonal plantings, sundials, solar calendars and other outdoor installations make this topic relevant for students of all ages, in a manner they can observe first-hand.

Track the passage of time over a single day

Sundials: Schoolyard sundials help students track the passage of time over a single day. Many sundials are small table- or pedestal-mounted devices that use sunlight to cast a shadow on a fixed surface inscribed with the hours of the day. As the Earth turns each day, the shadow created by the gnomon—a vertical or angled pole—moves across the platform below and points to the time on the dial. Sundials range greatly in size and may act as small garden features, wall mounted "clocks," or schoolyard centerpieces.

Sundials offer many opportunities to reference school curricula: learning to tell time, discussions about seasonal change and sun angles, solar system lessons about the arrangement of the planets around the sun, and renewable energy systems. Sundials are also frequently adorned with the directional markings of a compass rose, which increases their educational value and extends their curriculum ties. (Figure 9.17)

Large sundials may be installed on school grounds as points of interest or integrated into the design of the school building itself. Mårten School in Sweden has a wooden obelisk on its playground that acts as a sundial. The wooden post, bolted in place, casts shadows onto an area of asphalt that has been inset with lines of rock, representing the hours of the day. At Georgina Blach Intermediate School in Los Altos, California, a sundial is integrated into the school building's design. The shade canopy at the main entrance acts as the sundial's gnomon by casting a shadow onto markings on the pavement below.[9] (Figure 9.18)

FIGURE 9.18 *The building's shadow points to the time at Georgina Blach School.*

Gelfand Partners Architects

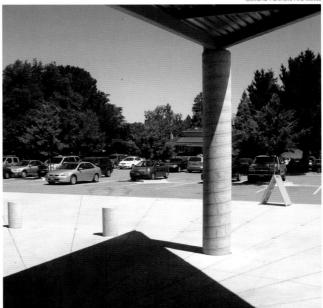

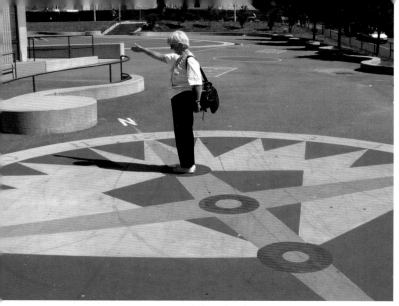

FIGURE 9.19 *Human sundial on the playground at Hennigan School in Jamaica Plain, Massachusetts.*

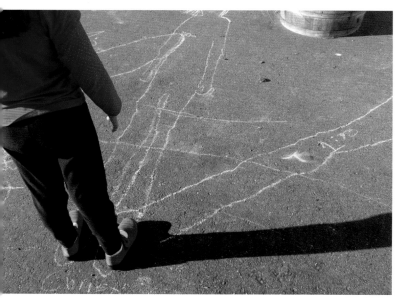

FIGURE 9.20 *Shadow study on the playground at Rosa Parks School in Berkeley, California.*

"Human sundials," without a fixed gnomon, work on the same principle as other sundials, but their shadows are cast by a person standing on the device. They are generally painted or otherwise inscribed on a large, flat, paved surface in a sunny location, such as schoolyard asphalt. To tell the time, a person stands in a designated place on the sundial with an arm raised over his or her head; the resulting shadow points to the time

on the "clock." Many human sundials, calibrated to account for seasonal changes in sun angles, indicate where a person should stand to cast the correct time based on the time of year. Any school that has a large (20-foot diameter) open stretch of asphalt that receives full sun all day can create a human sundial.

Hennigan School in Jamaica Plain, Massachusetts, has a beautiful, painted human sundial. The times of day are marked in large blue numbers on a yellow band around the rim of the sundial, and the compass directions are marked with white letters reading: N, S, E, W. To tell the time, a student stands on one of the three red circles at the center—determined by the time of year—and observes where his or her shadow falls.[10] (Figure 9.19)

Shadow studies: With the aid of a little chalk teachers can use simple, unadorned playground asphalt to engage their students in shadow studies about the passage of time. Students act as the temporary "gnomons" in these lessons and record their own shadow's movement throughout the day. This can be a useful exercise in connection with solar system studies, time-related lessons, and even tree planting projects.

Students from Rosa Parks Elementary School in Berkeley, California, went outside several times during the day and stood in the same place on the asphalt each time, so their partner could trace their shadow on the ground. At the end of the day, the children were able to see how their shadows had moved. (Figure 9.20)

Mark the days of the year and the seasons

Tracking days: Solar calendars use shadows to mark the passage of time over the course of a year, rather than the hours in a single day. This is possible because shadow length changes with the seasons, as the Earth's axis shifts in relation to the sun.

Many ancient civilizations used solar calendars to mark the equinoxes, solstices, and important holidays throughout the year, as displayed in architectural ruins across the globe. Some modern solar calendars imitate the ancient designs found in Stonehenge in England, Machu Picchu in Peru, and Chichen Itza in Mexico. In the United States, very old solar calendars can be found in many states, including New Mexico, Florida, Vermont, Wyoming, and Illinois.[11] Solar calendars work nicely with social studies and history lessons, or discussions about seasonal change and sun angles.

Schools can create basic solar calendars in their schoolyards using a design that is simpler than many of these ancient architectural pieces. One straightforward arrangement is to have an upright gnomon that casts a shadow on the ground below it. The playground surface is then marked with lines that indicate the placement of the gnomon's shadow at noon on different days of the year, including the solstices and equinoxes—and perhaps the first and last day of the school year.

Analy High School in Sebastopol, California, has a 9-foot-tall obelisk near the school's library that acts as a solar calendar. The obelisk's pointed top casts a shadow that falls on a pad of concrete, marked to indicate the shadow's position at noon on the summer and winter solstices and fall and spring equinoxes.[12] (Figure 9.21)

Two teachers at Vega School in Sweden created a more elaborate solar calendar, accentuated by the seasonal garden that surrounds it. The calendar includes a wooden "sun post" that serves as the gnomon. Small stones outline the planting bed and an additional line of stones through the middle of the garden indicate the placement of the post's shadow at noon throughout the year. (Figure 9.22. See yellow line on the drawing.) The short shadow at the summer solstice is very close to the post. At the spring and fall equinoxes, the tip of the shadow falls in the middle of the garden. At the winter solstice, when the schoolyard is generally covered with snow, the tip of the shadow is well beyond the garden, so its location is marked with a lone rock. The garden beds are planted with flowers that bloom in sequence through the year to help students track seasonal changes in a way that is intuitive, "a natural part of everyday life."[13]

Marking seasons: Schools in most climates can plant their yards to accentuate seasonal changes, creating an abundance of flowers in the spring, leafy greenery in the summer, bright red and yellow foliage in the fall, and deciduous trees with bare branches

FIGURE 9.21 *The solar calendar obelisk at Analy High School in Sebastopol, California.*
Analy High School

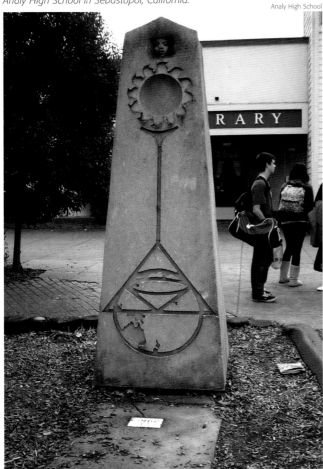

FIGURE 9.22 *Diagram illustrating the layout of a solar calendar garden at Vega School in Lund, Sweden.*
Karin Wingman and Britt Wall-Rydh

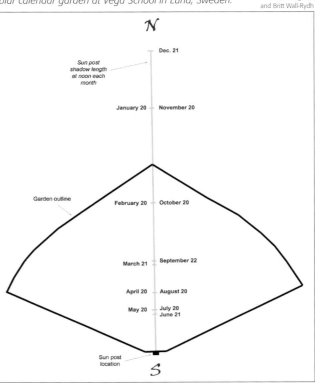

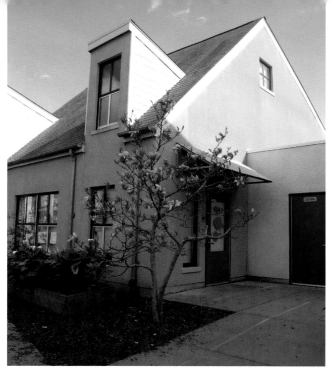

FIGURE 9.23 *At Rosa Parks School in Berkeley, California, teachers sometimes use a centrally placed magnolia tree as the subject of watercolor paintings in the fall, winter, spring, and early summer to help the children note the tree's changing appearance.*

FIGURE 9.24

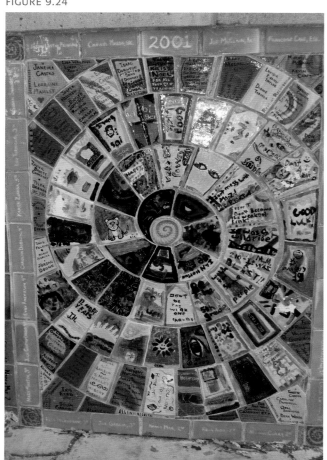

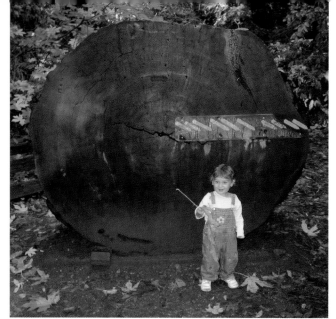

FIGURE 9.25 *This ancient tree in Julia Pfeiffer Burns State Park in Big Sur, California, was well over 500 years old when it was felled. The green arrows in the photograph point to dates of historical significance to make its age more meaningful for children and other park visitors. A similar display—with younger logs—would be instructive on school grounds as well.*

in the winter. Sometimes individual trees with dramatic seasonal foliage or flowers communicate this idea successfully on a smaller scale. (Figure 9.23)

Record the passage of years

Because the passage of years is often difficult for young children to grasp, it helps to visibly mark the passage of annual events or milestones that are important to the school community. At Cragmont School in Berkeley, California, for example, the art teacher and graduating fifth graders work together to create a unique mosaic that leaves their personal stamp on the school. The "mosaic quilt" that these panels collectively create grows as each artistic panel is added to the wall. (Figure 9.24)

Logs, which may be sanded or polished to show their growth rings, are also a good tool for illustrating the passage of years. Each ring represents one year of the tree's life and growth. Students can use tree rings as a timeline, calculating when that particular tree sprouted, and then mark important events that occurred during the tree's lifetime. The varied spacing of the rings also records wet and dry years, displaying changes in weather patterns over time. (Figure 9.25)

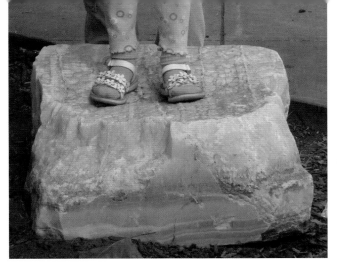

FIGURE 9.26 *A sedimentary rock on the playground at Rosa Parks School in Berkeley.*

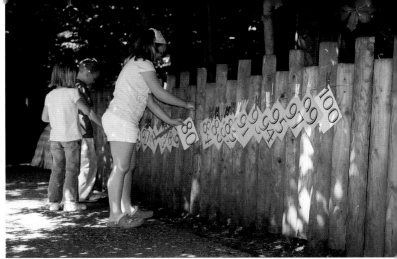

Cam Collyer

FIGURE 9.28 *At Coombes School in Arborfield, England, young students use a simple clothesline and moveable cards printed with numbers to practice arranging the numbers from 1 to 100.*

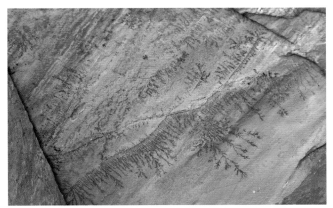

FIGURE 9.27 *Rocks that include fossils do double duty; they may be used to study ancient life forms as well as the passage of time.*

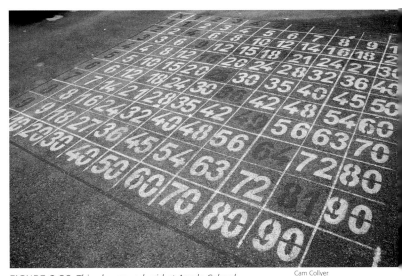

Cam Collyer

FIGURE 9.29 *This playground grid at Argyle School in England illustrates basic multiplication tables.*

Record the passage of millennia

Stone is a medium that records the passage of time on a much grander scale—thousands or even millions of years. School-yard boulders may assist teachers with discussions of geologic time—the amount of time it takes for layers of sedimentary rock to form, or for water to smooth the surface of a cobble-stone as it bounces along in a riverbed. (Figures 9.26 and 9.27)

🍃 Numbers and Mathematics

There are infinite things to measure, count, and calculate in an ecological schoolyard. Teachers might ask their students to calculate the following: the quantities of supplies needed to build new garden features; the length of hose needed to reach the farthest plant in the garden; the area of a new garden path, and the number of bricks needed to build it; or the volume of soil needed to fill a garden bed, and the amount of soil needed to fill it. As the schoolyard is growing, teachers may work with their students to build scale models of elements they wish to construct. (See chapter 2, Figure 2.6.) Some schools bring moveable numbers outside as portable lessons or paint them on the asphalt in charts as part of their numeracy curriculum. (Figures 9.28 and 9.29)

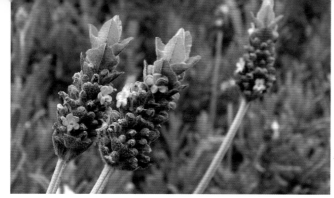

FIGURE 9.30 *Lavender plants add a distinctive floral scent to a school garden.*

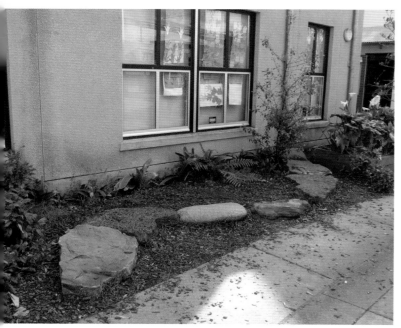

FIGURE 9.31 *One group of rocks at Rosa Parks, a student favorite, is arranged to look like the science teacher's popular pet corn snake, Cornelius.*

FIGURE 9.32 *Interpretive display for the geology trail at Coombes School in England.*

Cam Collyer

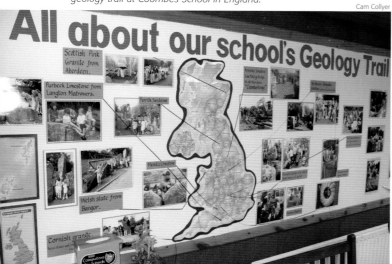

Science

There are countless ways to connect the k-12 science curriculum to the schoolyard landscape. (See chapters 4, 5, 6 and 7 for curriculum connections to ecology, wildlife habitat, water systems, energy systems, and edible gardens.) Other areas of science, such as sensory gardens, geology curricula, weather studies and astronomy, also lend themselves well to outdoor lessons

Sensory gardens

Preschool and kindergarten curricula often include studies of the five senses: tasting, smelling, seeing, touching, and hearing. To address this topic, some schools plant "sensory gardens" that include tasty food crops, fragrant flowers, a range of vibrant colors, plants with varying textures, and leaves or gravel that make sounds as they crunch underfoot. (Figure 9.30)

Geology

Geology is traditionally taught using small, hand-held examples of different rock types. This approach, however, makes it difficult to get a sense of what each material looks like on a large scale in nature. To make geology lessons come to life, some schools use much larger rocks, arranged outdoors, selected to correlate with their desired curricula. (See chapters 8 and 10 for additional examples of schoolyard stonework and geology curricula.)

I worked with the science teacher at Rosa Parks Elementary School in Berkeley, California, to add curriculum-tied boulders—from around California and western North America—to the playground. For most of the school year, the rocks are simply part of the landscape, acting as seats, points of interest, and play areas around the schoolyard's unpaved perimeter. When it is time to study geology, teachers bring their students outside for the "geology walk" to observe examples of igneous, metamorphic, and sedimentary rocks that are large enough for an entire class to examine together.[14] (Figure 9.31)

The Coombes School, in England, boasts the most impressive example of schoolyard geology curricula I have encountered.[15] Serving students between the ages of 3–7, Coombes School has been greening its large school grounds continuously since 1971. The geology trail they developed consists of more than ten distinct stone art installations, arranged throughout the site, to make a statement about the history and cultures

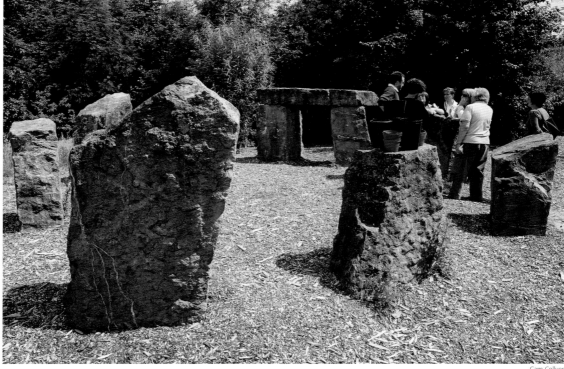

FIGURE 9.33
*"Coombeshenge"
is part of the
geology trail at
Coombes School
in England.*

Cam Collyer

FIGURE 9.34 *Red sandstone sculpture along
the geology trail at Coombes School in England.*

Cam Collyer

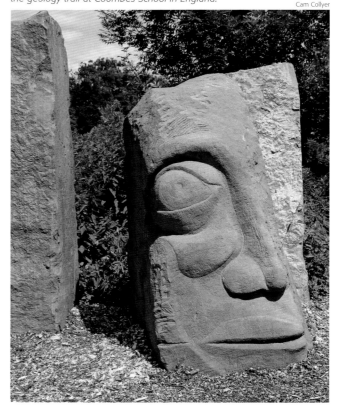

of England's residents through the ages. The school's detailed interpretive display shows each piece in its collection along with the type of stone and a map of the United Kingdom that notes where it was quarried. (Figure 9.32)

The stones used in the walk were shipped to Coombes School over time. Some of the rocks are in their natural forms; others have been shaped by artists or salvaged from previous uses. One art piece, "Coombeshenge," is a small scale Yorkshire limestone representation of the famous, historical landmark, Stonehenge. (Figure 9.33) Another cultural reference recreated in stone is "King Arthur's Chair" made from Purbeck limestone. The school grounds are home to several large pieces of red sandstone from the Lake District, one of which was carved into a giant face by an artist who allowed the students to observe the carving process.[16] (Figure 9.34) Large Mendip limestone boulders are provided as climbing structures in the preschool area. Three huge blocks of reclaimed Cornish granite have been stacked like bricks to create an exhibition space and interesting play feature, while three other large stones form a substantial playhouse. (See chapter 11, Figure 11.29.) The school also has an installation of crumbly Farringdon sponge rock filled with marine fossils, and an array of impressive Welsh slate boulders.[17]

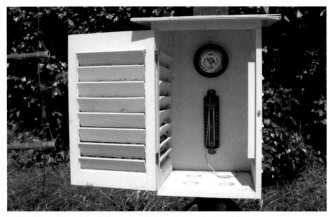

FIGURE 9.35 *Sidwell Friends Middle School in Washington, DC, has a rooftop weather station that collects weather data and transmits it in real time to the school's website, making it easily assessable to the students.*

FIGURE 9.36 *This school has their weather study equipment in a ventilated box to give it some shade and protection from vandalism.*

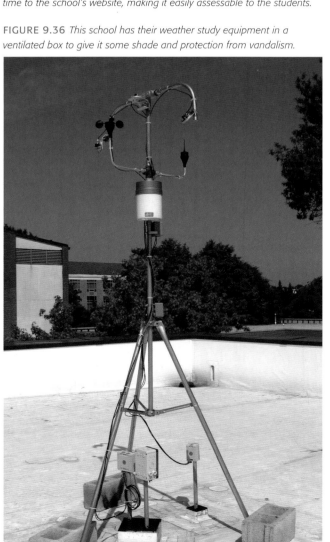

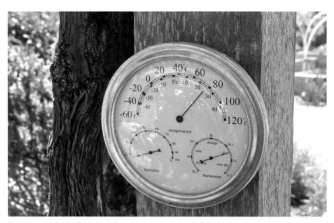

FIGURE 9.37 *This weather instrument at Edna Mcaguire School in Mill Valley, California, measures temperature, humidity and barometric pressure. It's mounted in a shady area of the garden.*

FIGURE 9.38 *Solar system model on the National Mall in Washington, DC.*

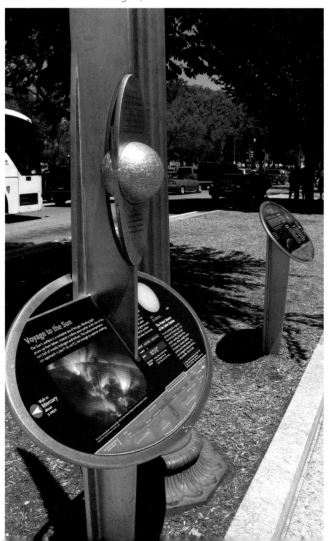

Weather studies

When students are outside on a regular basis, they naturally begin to tune in to the weather, observing sunny and rainy days and hot and cold temperatures firsthand. Some schools like to help their students quantify their weather observations by installing a range of tools to help them track the conditions in a more scientific manner. Schoolyard weather stations may be contained in a protective box that is opened to take readings, or the instruments may be installed in convenient locations throughout the yard. Some weather-related readings students might take include temperature, humidity, barometric pressure, wind speed and direction, and precipitation levels. (Figures 9.35–9.37)

FIGURE 9.39 *Scale model of the sun within the solar system model on the National Mall in Washington, DC.*

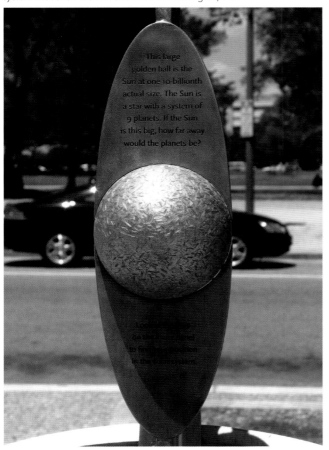

Astronomy: Solar system studies

Solar system studies are an important part of elementary school curricula, but it is difficult to study the night sky in a hands-on manner during daylight hours. Some schools incorporate solar system themes into artwork, paving patterns, or playground paintings to peak students' interest in this topic.

Many websites provide step-by-step directions on how to make a temporary or permanent scale model of our solar system; other examples are available from science institutions around the country. The elaborate solar system model on the National Mall in Washington, DC, created by the National Center for Earth and Space Science Education, is at a scale of one to 10 billion! It stretches along 2,000 feet of the Mall and contains representations of the sun and nine planets (including Pluto), as well as text on asteroids and comets. At this scale, the sun is less than six inches across, and the Earth is about the size of a pinhead![18] (Figures 9.38 and 9.39)

To make a less elaborate—and smaller—version of the solar system for a school playground, measure out the appropriate distances between planets and then paint the celestial bodies onto the asphalt. Some of the planets will be tiny, so be sure to mark them well! To make the planets more visible, some models increase the planets' scale; others represent the planets abstractly while keeping the distances between them to scale.

Marin School in Albany, California, for example, inlaid a simplified solar system model into the top of a concrete seat wall in their schoolyard. This solar system model represents the distances between the planets fairly accurately (1 inch equals 2,000,000 miles), but the planets themselves are not to scale. Instead, inlaid pieces of glass represent the approximate placement of each planet and capture the children's imaginations. (Figure 9.40)

FIGURE 9.40 *Marin School's solar system model includes this representation of the planet Saturn.*

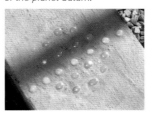

FIGURE 9.41 *The Fuller School in Jamaica Plain, Massachusetts, painted constellations on the playground.*[19]

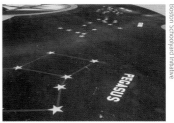

Boston Schoolyard Initiative

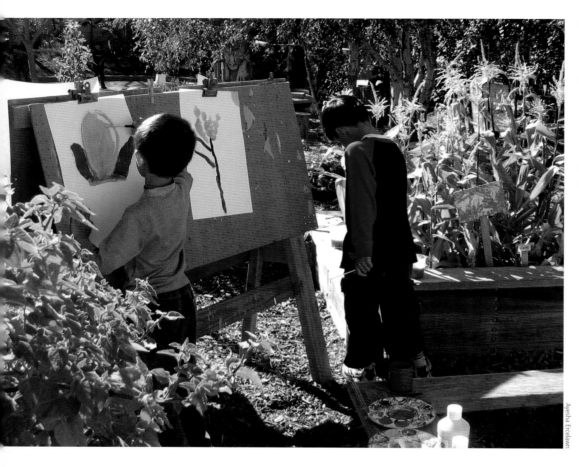

Portable art materials and informal studio space

FIGURE 9.42 *Tule Elk Park Child Development Center in San Francisco, California, offers portable painting easels during class time for supervised projects, and sometimes makes them available at recess, too. These first and second grade students celebrated their garden's corn harvest with a botany lesson that included painting pictures of the plants.*[20]

🍃 Outdoor Arts Instruction

Art, music, and the performing arts are easy to bring outside for academic studies and during recess. The following examples show how to incorporate these subjects into hands-on lessons that foster creativity and invite performances. (See chapter 12 for art "play" topics and chapter 16 for examples of student-created art installations.)

Visual art

Visual art is often, by nature, a messy undertaking. Yet, students of all ages benefit from art studio spaces that allow their creativity to blossom—and that are easy to clean, comfortable, attractive, and spacious. Creating an outdoor art studio accomplishes these goals while also increasing the available teaching space. Outdoor art studios may be temporary or permanent, formal or informal. They may allow collaboration between students or provide space for individuals to create their own works of art. They may be designed to serve one particular art form, or more broadly defined to allow students to explore many types of materials.

Sometimes a schoolyard landscape provides art materials as well as the inspiration for the finished work. Teachers may select garden plants intended to produce art supplies they need for their classes, such as fibers for basket-making or weaving projects, or plants useful for making natural dyes or pigments. (See chapter 12 for examples on this theme from Tule Elk Park Child Development Center in San Francisco.)

Dedicated art studio space

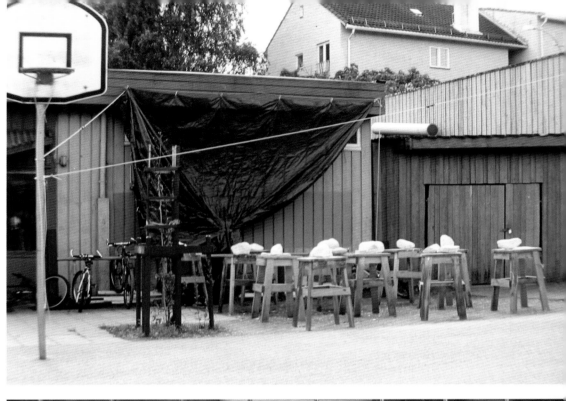

FIGURE 9.43 *Oslo Steiner School in Norway set up an outdoor stone-carving studio for its students.*

FIGURE 9.44 *Thomas Tallis School in England offers their high school students a courtyard art studio for a wide variety of painting and sculptural projects.*

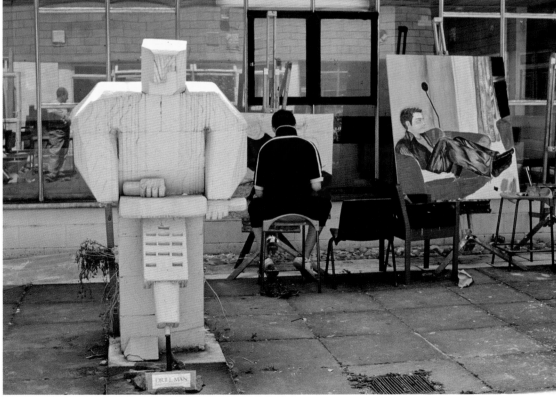

Music and performing arts

Music and performing arts lessons benefit greatly from an inspiring setting that motivates the performers to do their best work. Schoolyard amphitheaters, which provide comfortable settings for students to observe the performances, are valuable assets to these programs. The following examples illustrate how a few schools use their amphitheaters specifically for music and theater performances. (See chapter 13 for additional examples of amphitheaters and outdoor classroom spaces.) (Figures 9.45 and 9.46)

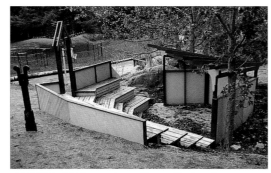

FIGURE 9.45 *The music pavilion at Skudeneshavn School in Karmøy, Norway, is nestled in a forested setting, providing an inviting venue for the students' music, dance, and theater performances.*[21]

FIGURE 9.46 *Students at Ravenstone Primary School in England perform plays in their schoolyard amphitheater. This 60-seat wooden venue has a gentle curving ramp that provides wheelchair access to the top tier. To "set the stage" for performances, the pupils at Ravenstone created a series of ceramic figurines depicting the characters from* Tales and Fables from Around the World, *and installed them in the perimeter railing.*[22]

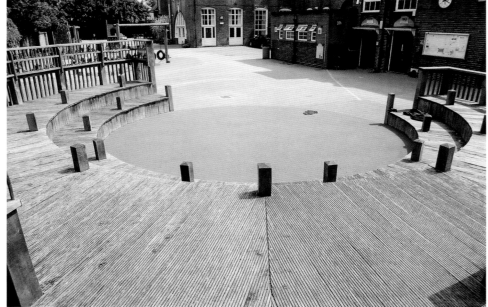

dents, and friends often find they have a wealth of knowledge and skills that can be harnessed to improve their grounds. Sometimes school communities design and execute schoolyard play projects on their own. In other cases, the school or school district hires outside professionals, who specialize in participatory design and construction, to help make the most of the community's talents and to ensure that the resulting playground complies with local and national safety standards.

Gathering input from the school community infuses the project with creative ideas and broadens the number of people who feel responsible for the site. Their ideas frequently translate into unique designs that reflect local cultures and the school's surrounding context. School districts often appreciate this community stewardship and, desiring to please their constituents, may be more likely to try new things if the project under consideration has widespread community support.

Professional designers, landscape architects, architects, artists, and other builders may help schools to harness the talents and enthusiasm of local volunteers to improve schoolyards through hands-on efforts. For example, Leathers & Associates, a design firm based in Ithaca, New York, specializes in creating community-built playgrounds. Each playground is one-of-a-kind and includes ideas from children and community members. Many of their projects incorporate special features related to local history and culture or science and educational themes. Their creative designs meet all federal guidelines for playground safety and accessibility. Over the last 38 years, Leathers & Associates has created over 2,000 community-built playgrounds in parks, schools, and other locations in the United States and abroad.[2]

Leathers & Associates worked with 'Aikahi Elementary School in Kailua, Hawai'i, to design and build a playground that also serves as a community space. First, they gathered ideas from children and adults during a festive "Design Day" and incorporated their ideas into the design. A few months later, members of the school community recruited hundreds of local volunteers and Marines to work side-by-side to construct it. The resulting playground includes themes that reflect the school's physical and cultural settings on this Hawaiian island. During school hours, children playing there expand their imaginations, stretch their growing muscles, and develop their social skills. After school and on weekends, it becomes a destination playground for local families to enjoy. (Figures 10.1–10.3)

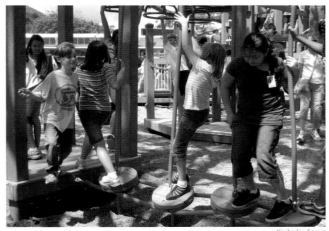

Kimberlee Eggers

FIGURE 10.3 *The playground at 'Aikahi Elementary School provides many opportunities for children to use their bodies and their imaginations as they play.*

FIGURE 10.4 *Volunteers build a new playground designed by Planet Earth Playscapes.*

Rusty Keeler

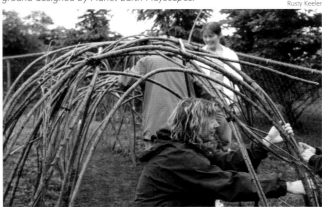

Planet Earth Playscapes, based in Ithaca, New York and Portland, Oregon, also specializes in community-built playgrounds. The firm has worked with many preschools, child care centers, and community groups around the country to create "natural playscapes" with rolling hills, sand and water play and a range of sensory experiences to delight children. Their projects are frequently built with help from local volunteers, who pitch in to sculpt the earth, lay pathways, build playhouses, and install other equipment. This process builds community around the new playground while keeping costs down. (Figures 10.4 and 10.5 on the next page)

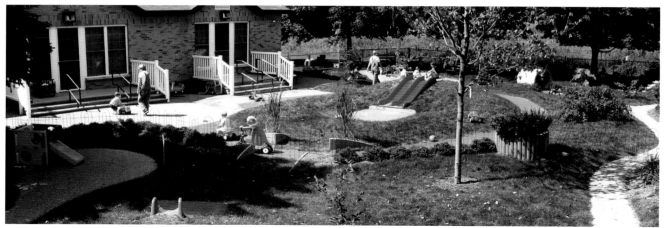

FIGURE 10.5 *Toddlers and infants have a range of active play choices at the art- and music-filled, community-built playground at Skaneateles Early Childhood Center in New York. Play choices include a tricycle path through a tunnel, grassy hills with a hillside slide, a sand box, and a wide array of plantings to explore.*[3]

Rusty Keeler

Research-Based Playground Design

Children's needs for "Real Play" are generally not being met on most standard playgrounds, argues Associate Professor Asbjørn Flemmen of Volda University College in Norway. Flemmen has been observing and researching children's spontaneous play behavior since the 1970s. His findings show that children need open-ended, stimulating environments that challenge their bodies with gross motor movements while simultaneously supporting their social development. He has observed that children's own spontaneous activities are different from adult-organized sports games and movement patterns. Flemmen defines Real Play as "a spontaneous and social activity, dependent upon its environment, where interaction takes place through extensive gross-motor movement."[4] He argues that children's Real Play is superior to physical education classes, because it allows children to incorporate physical exercise deeply into their lives in a way that is qualitatively and quantitatively more valuable to their overall level of physical fitness and development.

Flemmen says that Real Play can only occur when children are allowed to decide for themselves "what to play, where to play, how to play, and who to play with."[5] In his view, children develop key physical and social skills through play as they navigate complex, exciting play environments with their peers that include elements of perceived physical risk, uncertainty, and adventure. This helps them test their physical limits and work to achieve their goals. Stimulating play environments encourage children to explore their surroundings, solve problems collaboratively, and come up with rules for their own games in a manner that creates social order and fosters personal development.

Flemmen has helped to create more than forty playgrounds that reflect his research findings over the course of his career. All of his playgrounds are designed in accordance

---

The Challenging Playground at Skudeneshavn School Encourages Schoolyard Harmony

"The pupils themselves say that since the jungle was created there is no bullying in the school. Even if the bullying has not completely disappeared, teachers also see a clear tendency in a positive way in the pupil-to-pupil relation. Pupils who earlier just wandered around in the school ground during breaks have now found an environment that appeals to their urge to be active. One has also noticed a greater mixture of different age groups in play. This creates security among the children and ties the children together as a unit."[9]

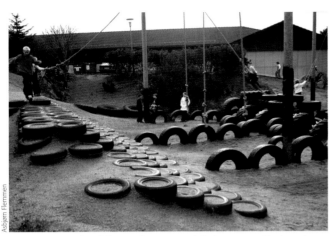

FIGURE 10.6 *The elaborate "Tarzan Jungle" play area at Skudeneshavn was built in the late 1990s. Securely placed telephone poles, topped by strong steel bars, create a framework for long ropes that children use to swing freely, pendulum-style, in dramatic arcs. The tires around the structure are arranged to make interesting places to land, perch, and traverse. The area under the ropes is padded with deep sand.*

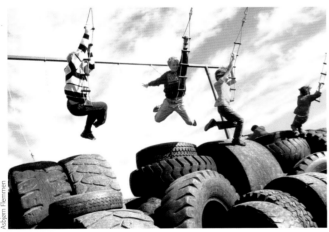

FIGURE 10.7 *This "jungle" playground at Øreåsen School in Rygge, Norway, is an ideal place for children to engage in Real Play, while experimenting with gravity. Research shows that children of different ages, genders, and skill levels play together in jungle playgrounds like this one.[10]*

with Norwegian and European safety standards. They are composed of materials that are securely fixed in place and use soft surfaces to cushion any falls.

In the late 1990s, Flemmen worked closely with Skudeneshavn Primary School in Karmøy, Norway, to help the school community create a highly diverse and challenging play en-

vironment for its 6–13 year-old students.[6] Skudeneshavn's grounds are now home to many open-ended play venues for children of all ages and abilities. They are designed to stimulate the children's "sensory-motor" skills and promote social interaction among the children as they play. They are also spacious, so the children have enough room to play without hindering each other's activities. The school has found that these design criteria help to reduce playground discord and bullying.[7]

Skudeneshavn's grounds include forests for nature play, tree climbing, and hide-and-seek games, areas for varied gymnastic activities, paved ball play zones with courts designed to encourage small groups to play together at their own varying skill levels, an area devoted to table tennis, sand and water play spaces, and an amphitheater for explorations in music, rhythm, and dance. In addition to these activities, their large campus has three areas for "Jungle Play" so children can hang from ropes in the trees and swing on ropes affixed to several dramatic play structures. This play environment is enjoyed by students of all ages, and is an asset for the surrounding neighborhood.[8] (Figure 10.6)

Tires are one of the primary building blocks for Flemmen's playgrounds. They are used to reinforce hillsides that take heavy use and serve as informal stairs that make the hillsides easy to climb. They are forgiving surfaces if the children fall on them; they are also good play props for balancing games and other ideas children invent. Asbjørn Flemmen's playgrounds are well loved in many other parks and schoolyards around Norway, as shown in the following photographs. (Figures 10.6–10.10)

FIGURE 10.8 *This playground is inviting for children of all ages. Volda University College's primary school, Norway.*

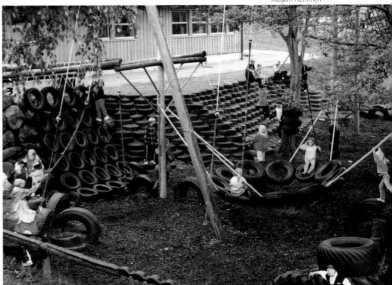

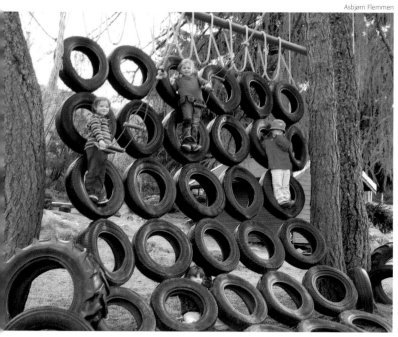

FIGURES 10.9 and 10.10 *Young children adore Asbjørn Flemmen's playground at Oppigarden Kindergarten in Volda, Norway.*

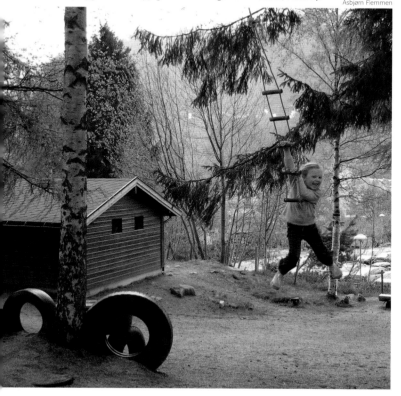

Young children at Oppigarden Kindergarten in Volda, Norway, enjoy climbing this dramatic wall of tires (Figure 10.9) and then swing away from it on ropes more than 30 feet long. (Figure 10.10) The ground surface under the tires and rope swings is softened with a deep layer of gravel.

Climbing Features

Climbing is an activity that many children enjoy, and that most of us experienced as we grew up at schools and parks and among the trees and rocks in our neighborhoods. It is a way for the smallest among us to feel "tall" temporarily, to see the world from a more elevated vantage point. Climbing is exhilarating and challenging, and the activity's perceived "riskiness" adds to its allure, even if the height a child has climbed remains a safe distance from the ground.

These days many schoolyards have commercial play structures with well defined "appropriate" places to climb—and fewer schools are allowing children to climb other things onsite. Each school, municipality, and country seems to define "safety" in a different way, resulting in vastly different regulations—and interpretations of those regulations—from place to place. This means that 5-year-old children abroad are often able to engage in more exciting schoolyard adventures than children twice their age in the liability-focused United States—without adverse injury rates. This section includes a range of schoolyard climbing walls and climbing adventures that allow children to test their skills to varying degrees in a manner that each school feels is appropriate and safe. I hope that more schools in the United States will follow their example.

Climbing walls

Commercial, parent-built, and custom-fabricated climbing walls encourage children to climb horizontally or vertically, creating physical challenges and an element of controlled risk. Because they are narrow and space-efficient, climbing walls are particularly useful for small school sites, whether they are free-standing or wall-mounted designs. (Figures 10.11 and 10.12)

Climbing-oriented schoolyard landscapes

Some schools integrate challenging play elements into their landscape design so children can choose to climb throughout the schoolyard and engage in more complex climbing activities. (Figures 10.13–10.15 on page 146)

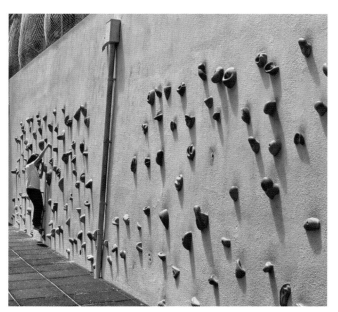

FIGURE 10.11 *This playground in San Francisco, California, used an existing cement retaining wall to create a space-efficient horizontal climbing challenge by bolting standard climbing holds onto the surface. A padded safety mat is located directly under the wall.*

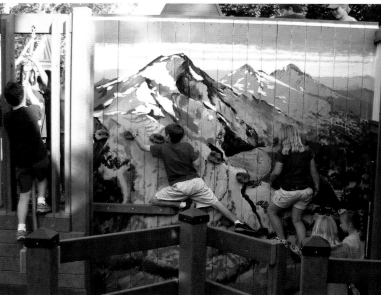

Leathers and Associates

FIGURE 10.12 *Children at Wildcat Park at Wilson Elementary School in Corvallis, Oregon, scale an artful climbing wall built by Leathers & Associates and the school community. The holds were applied in an ascending pattern on top of a mural depicting the nearby mountain range, allowing children to pretend they are "scaling mountains" without leaving the schoolyard.*

✿ Reusing Tires to Promote Active Play

Used automobile tires have been finding their way into schoolyards around the world for decades. I played on tire swings as a child and they are still present in some American schoolyards and parks thirty years later, although in reduced numbers. Tires can be used as building blocks for a range of play equipment that allows children to balance, swing, and climb. Whole tires add a myriad of creative play possibilities that challenge children physically, while still offering cushioned landings. Now, recycled tire rubber is also commonly used as a safety surface under manufactured play structures, as crumb rubber mulch in planted areas, and as underlying layers for artificial turf playing fields.

The widespread distribution of well-worn vehicle tires on playgrounds around the world suggests that this is a harmless and productive reuse of a material that challenges landfills worldwide. Tire-recycling advocates and playground safety surface manufacturers promote rubber safety surfaces as environmentally friendly options that put old tires to good use. However, there is some controversy surrounding the safety of this material that is important to consider. Some community members and environmentalists fear that small amounts of harmful chemicals may be released from tire rubber over time, during hot weather, or through repeated contact with children's hands. They are also concerned that the small particles of crumb rubber, used in some applications, could be inhaled or ingested by children as they play. Most studies on this subject conclude that these risks are not likely to result in adverse effects to children playing on tires or materials created with recycled rubber.[23] Because this issue has not been settled definitively, I suggest some caution in the use of tires and related materials on school playgrounds, particularly in applications that use crumb rubber. I do not recommend using tires in edible gardens.

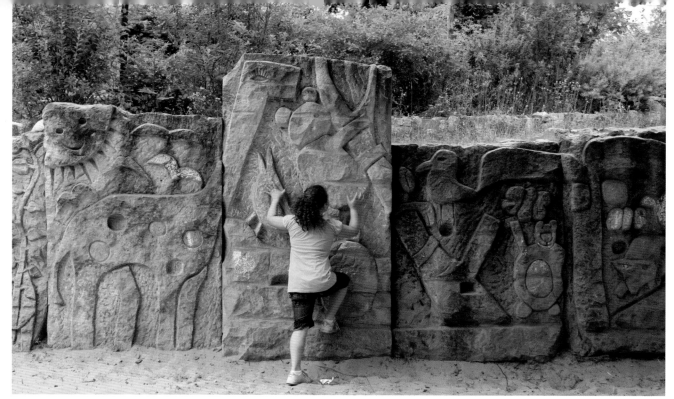

FIGURE 10.13 *Stone is an important part of the playground at Galeli Primary School in Berlin, Germany. The rocks give the schoolyard an attractive aesthetic and are intended to be scaled and enjoyed by the children as they play.*

FIGURE 10.14 *This unique boulder climbing sculpture delights children in a community park in Talkeetna, Alaska. The stones were collected from the local area, shaped, stacked, and anchored with steel rods running through the center of each pillar.[11]*

Leanne Gargett

FIGURE 10.15 *Children playing at recess enjoy the view from their high perch at Oslo Steiner School in Norway.*

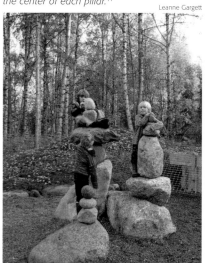

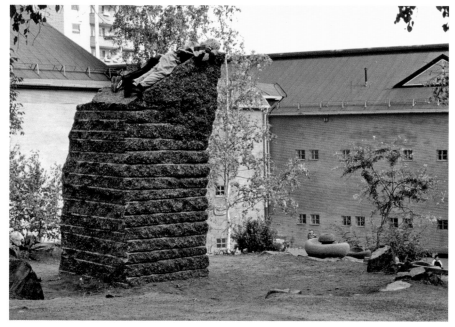

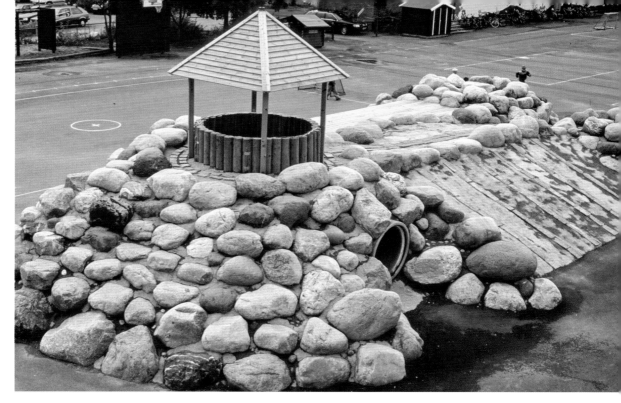

FIGURE 10.16 *The boulder mountain climbing structure at Manglerud School in Oslo, Norway.*

FIGURE 10.17 *Children descend into the boulder mountain at Manglerud School using ropes to rappel down the inside of a wooden tower entered from the mountain's peak.*

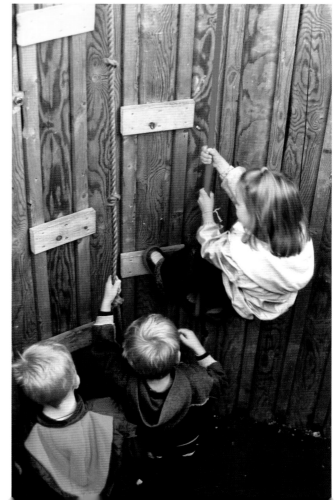

Manglerud School in Oslo, Norway, worked with local architect Frode Svane to create a monumental "mini-mountain" out of 350 boulders from the nearby Svelvick moraine, fulfilling the children's request for a "mountain" in their schoolyard. (Figure 10.16) The boulders from the moraine come in many colors, shapes, and sizes and represent rock types found throughout southern Norway. Over a period of three weeks and with the help of a crane operator, Svane carefully and securely arranged the stones into a "mountain" shape, mimicking the nearby rolling landscape. The resulting play structure has several different "peaks" and "valleys" as well as nooks in which children can sit, climb, and play imaginative games. The leftover boulders were used to create smaller rock piles around Manglerud's schoolyard, adding more places to sit and climb. Once the installation was complete, Oslo University's Geological Museum mapped the mountain's rock types, so they could be incorporated into the school's geology curriculum.[12] (Figure 10.17)

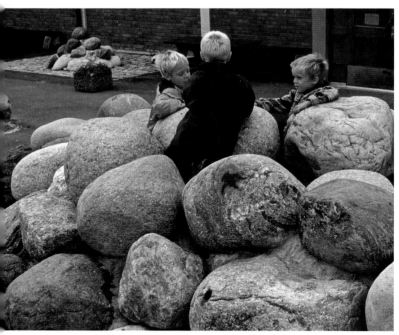

As I walked around Manglerud School in 2001, I noticed that none of the rocky mounds had safety surfaces around them, as would be required by American playground regulations—assuming a structure of this size would be permitted on a U.S. schoolyard at all. I toured the playground with the school's principal and asked him if he thought this unusual design was safe. He said the playground's injury rate had gone *down* after the boulders were added to their formerly empty asphalt yard. Because the children were now occupied doing *interesting* things, and actively climbing, jumping, and talking with their friends, they seldom got into arguments that resulted in physical fights or injuries. (Figure 10.18) They were also careful around the boulders, so they rarely tripped and fell while climbing.

This was a revelation to me, as a product of American liability-focused culture. Clearly, liability and safety are *not* the same thing—although they are often assumed to be in our country. I don't think that American schools should forgo their commitment to safety surfaces, but this safety *enhancing* play structure illustrates that we have gone too far in our own playground regulations. If a community provides interesting things for children to do, and is willing to trust them to play responsibly, many things are possible—and safe.

Man-Made Mounds for Active Schoolyard Play

Climbing is not the only way to get an elevated perspective. Some schools modify their flat schoolyards, building mounds to make them more interesting, and allowing children to safely ascend to new heights. Mounds may be made of earth and planted, paved with hard materials, or covered with soft safety surfacing.

This school in Copenhagen, Denmark, built a large earthen mound as an "island" in their otherwise flat, paved playground. (Figure 10.19) A path winds across the top through lush bushes and trees. When children walk along this magical path, they loose sight of their school and its urban surroundings just for a moment, and can imagine that they have been suddenly "transported" elsewhere. At some schools, dense plantings like these may make it difficult for teachers to supervise the playground. To improve adult oversight, while still preserving children's

FIGURE 10.18 *The boulder mountain at Manglerud School provides places for active play and for quiet conversation with friends.*

FIGURE 10.19 *A schoolyard play mound in Copenhagen, Denmark.*

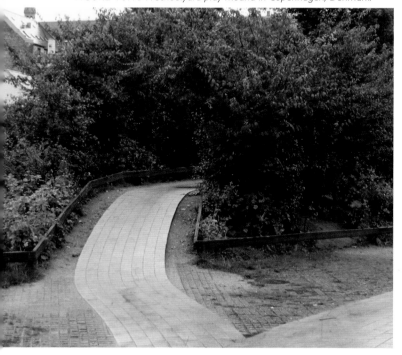

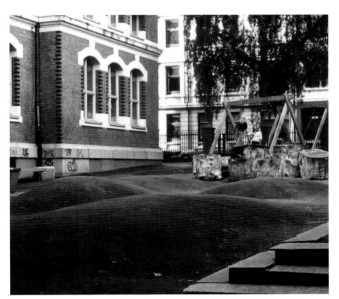

FIGURE 10.20 *Grünerløkka School in Oslo, Norway, enlivened its previously flat playground by creating asphalt-covered bumps. Students use the low mounds for skateboarding and other activities.*

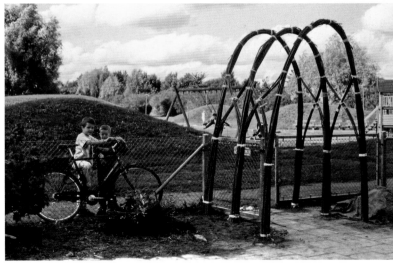

FIGURE 10.21 *At Mårten School in southern Sweden, undulating grassy hills, built to enhance the play space, are perfect for running up and rolling down.*

FIGURE 10.22 *A unique hillside slide at Bergen Steiner School in Norway.*

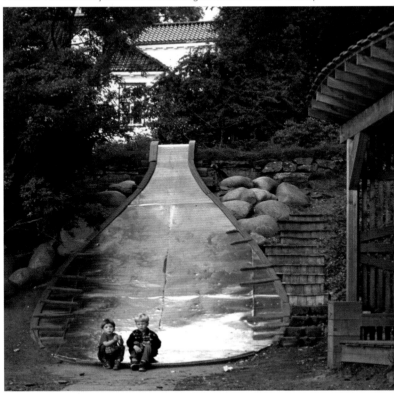

sense of "wilderness," such schools could prune the bottoms of the plants to make children's feet visible, if desired.

Hillside Slides

Hillside slides combine the excitement of climbing up high with the thrill of sliding down quickly, increasing the play value of hills. Even tall, exciting embankment slides are quite safe since the risk of falling off the side is minimized.

Tucked into a lush forested neighborhood, Bergen Steiner School on Norway's west coast is a gem. Over the years talented parents, using low-cost and natural materials, have helped school staff construct an incredible range of hand-made, custom play equipment, including two spectacular hillside slides. The unique tear-drop shaped slide in their kindergarten yard is approached from stairs that climb the hillside on each side of the slide. Its steep surface, made from sheet metal and trimmed with wood, widens as it reaches the bottom. (Figure 10.22) Across the school grounds, a second set of undulating, hand-made, sheet metal slides flow down a wide hillside. (Figure 10.23)

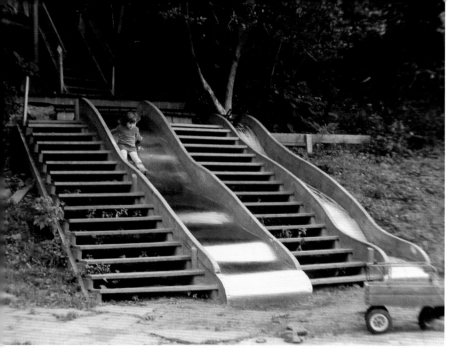

FIGURE 10.23 *A unique hillside slide at Bergen Steiner School in Norway.*

FIGURE 10.25 *This dramatic hillside slide at Svendstuen School in Oslo, Norway, rests directly on a hill at the playground's edge. It is exciting enough to be of interest to elementary or middle school students. Instead of stairs, children climb to the top using a rope ladder arranged on the hill.*

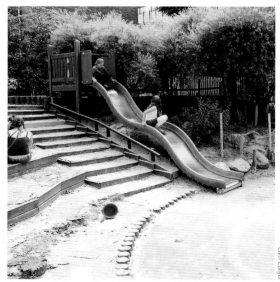

Cam Collyer

FIGURE 10.24 *The playground at Murergården Daycare Center in Copenhagen, Denmark, includes an undulating hillside slide. Children can choose to move from the playground's upper level to its lower level using stairs or the slide.*[13]

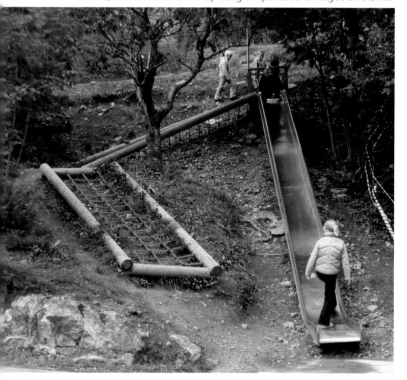

🍃 Tunnels to Crawl Through: Concrete Water Pipes Re-Imagined

Mounds let children climb *up and over*, slides allow them to come *down* quickly—and tunnels permit movement *through* the playground. Short tunnels also double as impromptu forts and comfortable hiding places for children that are still easily visible for supervising adults. Many schools around the world repurpose common concrete water pipes to build simple, enjoyable tunnels for students to play in. These pipes are widely available and are generally strong enough to support the weight of some earth—and children—on top of them. They can be used to form the core of small playground mounds that are built up around them, or serve as tunnels that connect separate play elements. (Figures 10.26 and 10.27)

🍃 Mazes and Labyrinths

Mazes and labyrinths are ancient designs found inscribed in thousand-year old rock art, included in classic stories like the Greek legend of the Minotaur and as part of meditation practices for some of the world's religions. Both mazes and

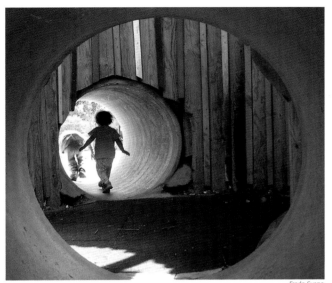

Frode Svane

FIGURE 10.26 *Large concrete pipes were used to form tunnels through the heart of the boulder "mini-mountain" at Manglerud School in Oslo, Norway.*[15]

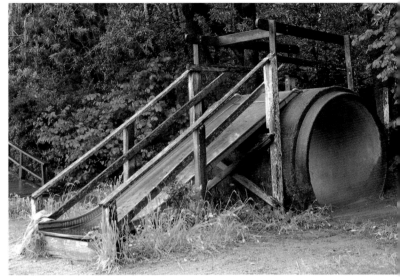

FIGURE 10.27 *Lagunitas School in San Geronimo, California, turned an unadorned, large concrete drain pipe into an enjoyable tunnel and slide combination for their playground.*

FIGURE 10.28 *Mass produced play elements like this "finger maze" may be incorporated into play structures to provide added play value in schoolyards or parks.*

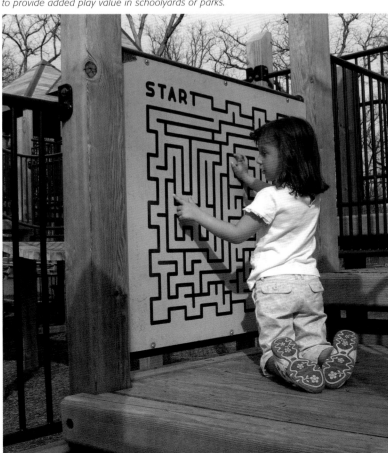

labyrinths are generally composed of winding pathways that follow circuitous routes from beginning to end. The designs used to create mazes include choices along the route, intended to make the pathway more challenging, while labyrinths generally have one meandering path that does not give the traveler any choices along the way.[14] With a maze, the goal is to find your way to the end; with a labyrinth, the purpose of following the path is the joy of the journey itself.

Many schools have wide-open, unadorned surfaces that could be enlivened with maze and labyrinth patterns to create low-cost active play opportunities. Painted mazes and labyrinths are particularly useful in places that need to remain unobstructed and are otherwise difficult to use. Planted mazes and labyrinths, carved from grassy fields or built using specially planted hedges, can be installed on open ground. Mazes and labyrinths may be almost any size—from tiny drawings intended to be followed using one's finger to larger creations, big enough for groups of children to explore together. They can be made from temporary sand mounds and chalk drawings or from materials permanently affixed in the desired pattern. (Figures 10.28–10.31)

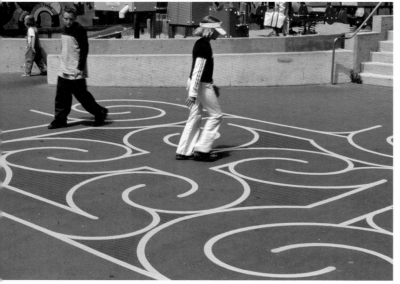

FIGURE 10.29 *This playground in San Francisco, California, includes a painted design that combines elements of both mazes and labyrinths. Children walking through this swirling pattern make choices along the way, but none of the choices result in a dead end. Since there are four entrance/exit points, many children can explore the design independently and simultaneously.*

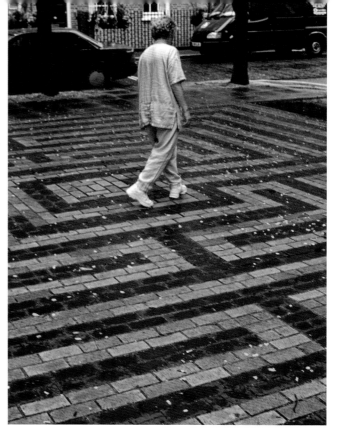

FIGURE 10.30 *The Warren Street Maze, located in a public square in London, England, was created using paving bricks with contrasting colors. This idea is easily transferable to a schoolyard context.*

FIGURE 10.31 *This temporary labyrinth at a California beach was built by hand-shaping sand into the desired pattern. Schools with large sandboxes or fields of bare earth could use this technique to make similar ephemeral constructions.[16]*

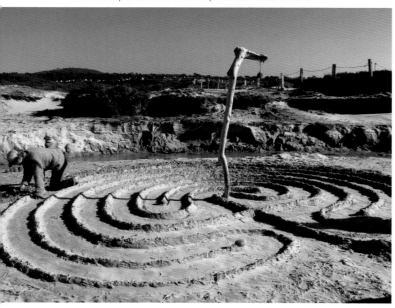

🍃 Unusual Swings

When I was in elementary school in the 1970s, swings were plentiful in American schoolyards. My school had tire swings that fostered group play and ordinary flat swings for individuals. Now, it seems that more and more American schools are removing swings from their playgrounds as safety regulations become increasingly strict—and the ever-increasing requirements for safety surfacing around the swings threatens to take over the entire available play space. While American regulations have children swinging alone, and farther and farther apart, European schools allow swinging children to play close together using clustered collaborative and "social" swings, designed to encourage interaction. I hope that these interactive swings will become more common in the United States in the future.

Nest-shaped swings, popular in Europe, are versatile designs that are enjoyed by people of all ages. They can comfort-

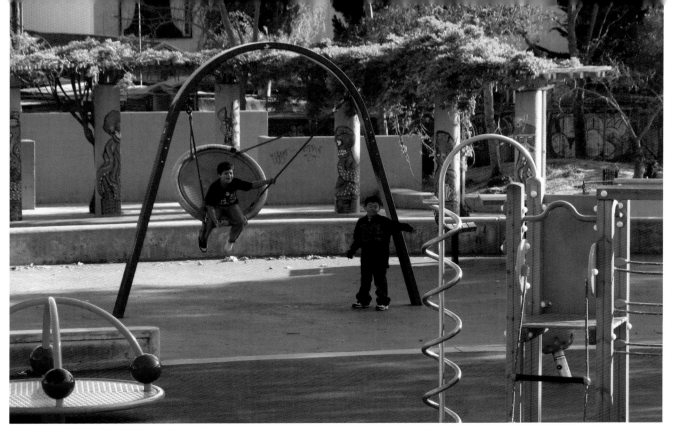

FIGURE 10.32 *A park in San Francisco, California, is home to a rare "nest" swing on American soil.*

ably seat a small group of children, an adult and child, or a reclining adult. Due to their large size, they require cooperation and collaboration between the swing riders and "pushers" to make the ride more enjoyable. (Figure 10.32)

Group-oriented social swings allow students to swing *toward* one another, at fairly close range, so they can talk, sing, and interact as they enjoy the swings together. This fosters social interaction and active play at the same time, and demonstrates that the schools using this design trust students to behave responsibly as they play. (Figure 10.33)

🍃 *Balancing Activities and Linear Play Structures*

Children love to test their balance as they play, whether they walk on a traditional balance beam or move across ropes or other challenges their school communities dream up. (Figures 10.34 and 10.35 on the next page)

FIGURE 10.33 *Social swings at Maridalen School in Oslo, Norway.*[17]

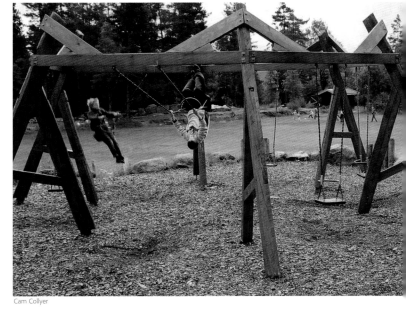

Cam Collyer

Chapter 10: Active Play in an Ecological Schoolyard **153**

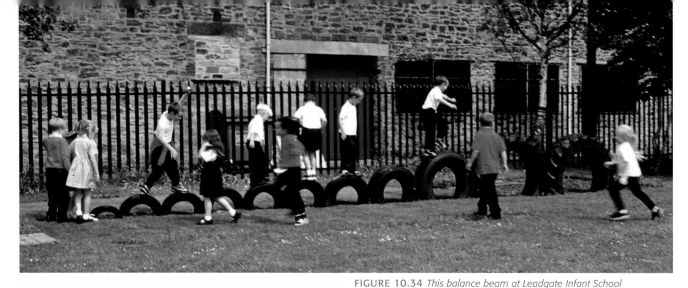

FIGURE 10.34 *This balance beam at Leadgate Infant School in northern England includes eleven recycled tires from different vehicles, large and small. The school calls this structure "the Lambton Worm," a reference to a British fairytale.*[18]

Some schools arrange their play areas in a linear format to accommodate narrow schoolyard spaces, or to give many children access to the play area at once. At Ravenstone Primary School in London, England, many students travel from one end of the yard to the other as they play along the linear climbing structure.[19] (Figure 10.36)

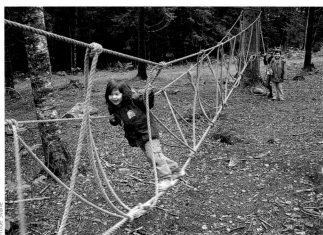

Frode Svane

FIGURE 10.35 *This Norwegian school used sturdy ropes to make a simple and entertaining balancing challenge for children to enjoy together.*

FIGURE 10.36 *Ravenstone Primary School in London, England.*

Cam Collyer

FIGURE 10.37 *Painted play elements may also be arranged in a linear format; in this case, a hopscotch-like game at a school in Japan.*

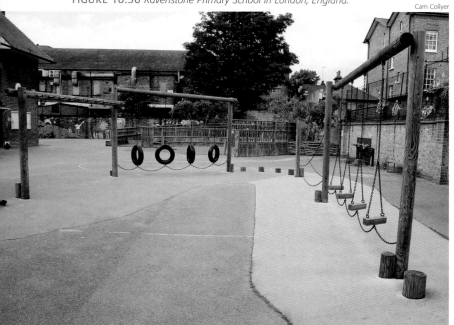

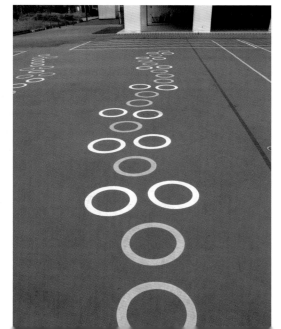

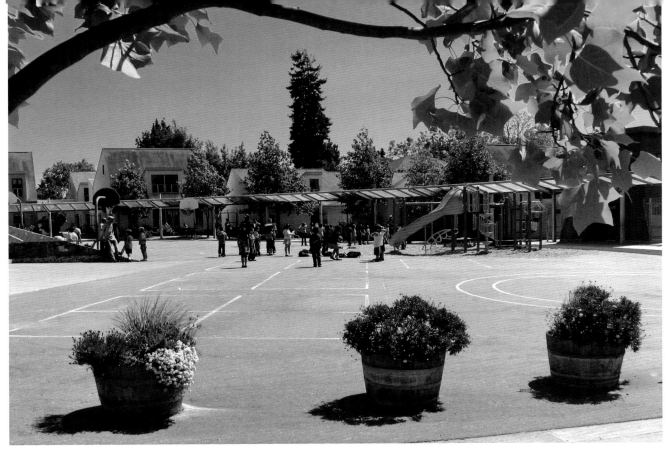

FIGURE 10.38 *At Rosa Parks School in Berkeley, California, a row of wine barrel planters separates ball games from an adjacent zone intended for imaginative play.*

FIGURE 10.39 *At Murergården Daycare Center in Copenhagen, Denmark, short fences are used to keep a small soccer pitch separate from the rest of the beautifully planted playground.*

Cam Collyer

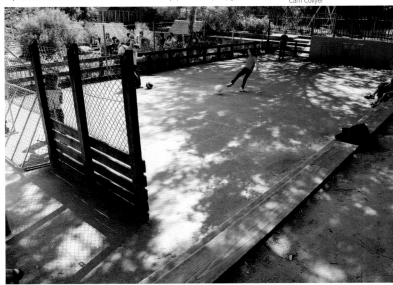

🍃 Ball Courts

Ball games are a vital part of most schools' playground culture. However, they are among the hardest play activities to integrate into a diverse and well-balanced green schoolyard, as balls sometimes travel great distances during children's games, impacting other activities. At some schools, it is almost impossible to walk across the playground during recess and not get hit by a ball. One solution is to create a "ball-free zone" on the schoolyard, defined by fences or other barriers, so children who aren't playing ball won't be disturbed. It is also helpful to have designated places in the yard that are strictly for ball games. (Figures 10.38–10.40)

Often, schools with small grounds find it difficult to accommodate large, regulation-sized courts for ball games and still have space "left over" for other activities. At the same time, many ball games only accommodate a small number of students

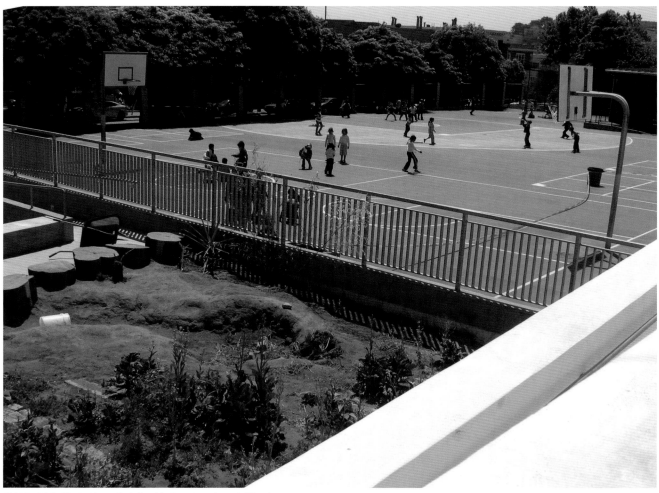

FIGURE 10.40 *At Alvarado School in San Francisco, California, the lower playground is used for most ball games, while the upper playground is home to the school's play structures. Several gardening areas are protected from these wilder activities by fences and beautiful, mural-covered concrete retaining walls.*

at a time on a given court—making them very space-inefficient. Some schools are addressing these two issues at the same time by creating a series of mini-courts in their schoolyards. These smaller courts can be designed to appeal to children of all ability levels, rather than just catering to the strongest and fastest children who often dominate a large single court. Temporary, movable courts can also be used to further diversify the playground. (Figures 10.41 and 10.42)

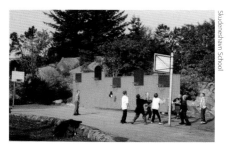

Skudeneshavn School

FIGURE 10.41 *Skudeneshavn School in Karmøy, Norway, installed a full size basketball court with five additional hoops, each at a slightly different height, along one side of the court. The full court may be used for physical education classes or basketball matches. The other hoops allow children of varying skill levels to practice shooting hoops, or to play many small games simultaneously during recess.*

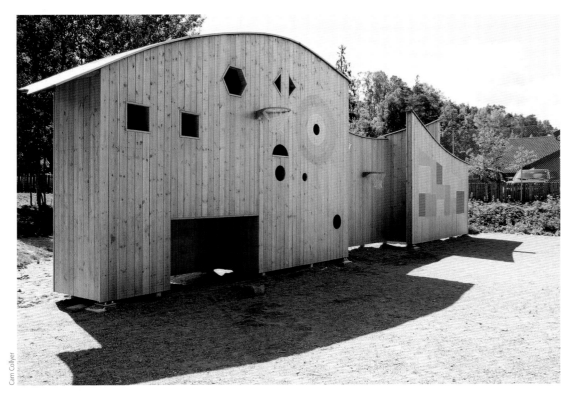

Cam Collyer

🍃 Winter Play Activities on School Grounds

Winter changes everything for schoolyards that receive snow. Growing up in suburban Chicago, I had a childhood filled with snow forts, snowmen, and sledding. This type of snow play didn't end when we went to school. Instead, the playground became more exciting in the winter since we could shape our play environment by building forts and fanciful snow crea- tures, and bravely make our way across semi-frozen "ponds" of melting snow. The grounds were even more enticing for climbing activities after the school had shoveled them, creating giant piles of snow around the perimeter of the yard.

Living in Northern California now, where our "deep" win- ters are warm enough to grow spring crops, my own children are missing this experience at school. My colleagues who live in colder climates, though, report that their local schoolyards are still filled with snow-filled exuberant winter play, as Figures 10.43–10.45 illustrate.

FIGURE 10.43 *The boulder "mini-mountain" at Manglerud School in Oslo, Norway, remains a great place to play and climb when covered with snow.*[20]

Frode Svane

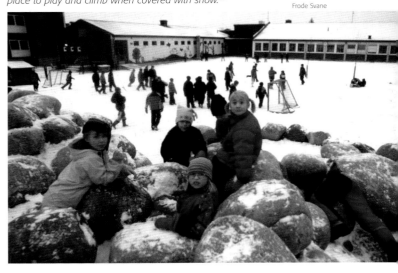

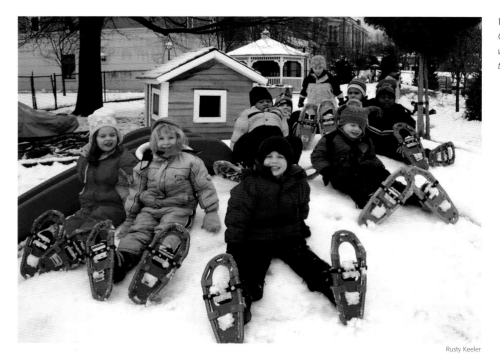

FIGURE 10.44 *Children at Mercy Cares for Kids in Albany, New York, enjoy winter snow shoeing and sledding in their nature play-oriented schoolyard.*[21]

Rusty Keeler

🍃 *Diverse Schoolyards are Active Schoolyards*

As the examples in this chapter illustrate, many forms of active play are possible on school grounds. Effective ecological schoolyards include a wide variety of active play activities, including ball games and creative play structures, that let everyone play at their own skill levels while they engage with their peers. This balance between creativity and social interaction along with physical challenges and adventure promotes play environments that are engaging and safe. Playgrounds that include unusual play features that reflect the local environment and culture reinforce the school's sense of place and make each playground unique. All of these factors contribute to making exciting playgrounds that children will enjoy and remember for many years.

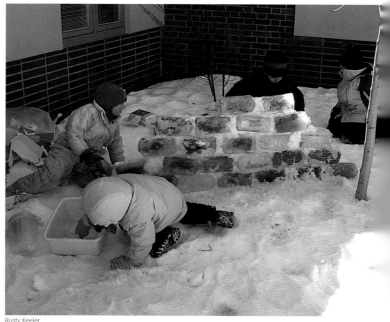

FIGURE 10.45 *These young children at Mercy Cares for Kids built a colorful fort using ice blocks they created by filling milk cartons with water, food coloring, toys, and other items—and letting them freeze outside.*[22]

Rusty Keeler

11 *Creative Play on School Grounds*

Every school is different—shaped by its local culture, geographic location, and ecological context. Rich, creative play environments spring from these differences and celebrate them, while also allowing children to influence their own play experiences. Playgrounds designed for these activities typically place less emphasis on games with rules and fixed climbing structures than traditional schoolyards, and foster more open-ended explorations that drive children's curiosity and spark their imaginations.

Successful creative play environments are flexible; children use them differently each day as launching points for the games they dream up. They offer a wide range of potential activities suitable for all age ranges and temperaments and frequently include semi-private, restful spaces where children may nestle comfortably, while still being easily supervised by their teachers. Creative play elements on school grounds might include natural materials, settings for fantasy and dramatic play, movable play props to build with or incorporate into games, and board games built into the physical structure of the schoolyard.

🍃 *Natural Materials Encourage Active and Imaginative Play*

The diversity of the natural world is an enormous asset for creating successful creative play environments on school grounds. Playing among trees, shrubs, soil, sand, and water is simple, inexpensive fun for children—and presently an underutilized opportunity in American schoolyards. Children's open-ended play scenarios in these environments blend both active and imaginative play, and change each time they go out for recess, bringing much needed variety to settings that are otherwise static and connecting children to the world around them.

Nature play activities can be integrated into existing schoolyard designs—or provide the larger framework in which other play activities occur.

Living play environments and natural materials have a great array of textures, colors, and movable pieces that lend themselves well to games children make up on their own. Trees and other plantings—used to create unique "forts" or selected for their pinecones, acorns, or other "play props"—diversify climbing and play activities. Sandboxes and "digging beds" encourage imaginative play that engages children's muscles and creative minds at the same time, as they "dig to the other side of the world," build dramatic castles, or construct miniature landscapes they envision. Water play in the form of hand pumps and movable channels allows children to explore the physical properties of this liquid. Water can also be combined with sand boxes, mud play, or other elements to further increase play options.

Existing trees and bushes as play options

Trees are one of the most time-tested children's "climbing structures." Their branches have welcomed children's hands and feet for thousands of years and created challenging, imaginative play environments for people of all ages. Children are often happy to explore the existing vegetation around a school site, if they are allowed to do so. Sometimes all that is needed to create an inviting play environment is a good tree and permission to climb it. Both living and dried tree branches may also be shaped into fanciful playhouses, tunnels, and forts. Tree leaves, pods, and twigs lend themselves easily to children's imaginative games. (Figures 11.1 and 11.2 on the next page)

Existing shrubs and other vegetation on a school site may function, too, as play environments for young children, who

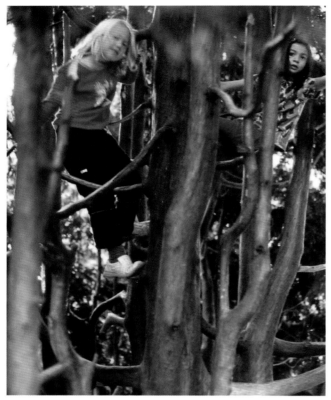

are endlessly fascinated by creating "dens" and forts to sit in while they talk with their friends. A few well-placed clips from pruning shears make the plants more transparent, enhancing supervision yet still allowing children to feel the sense of enclosure they desire.

Two informal "dens" nestle under tall bushes at the perimeter of the paved playground at Rosa Parks School in Berkeley, California. I worked with the school community to trim flowering shrubs to create "forts" with leafy walls and arched "roofs" that invite children to relax in their embrace. We also placed large eucalyptus tree rounds and boulders under the branches to make these spaces more comfortable. These niches are very popular and almost always occupied during recess. (Figure 11.3)

Playful living willow structures[1]

Whimsical play elements, crafted from live willow tree branches, are common in many schools and parks throughout England, Scandinavia, and other parts of Europe, where they are a relatively recent adaptation of traditional agricultural crafts. Many of these projects—including play houses, archways, domes and other structures—use *salix viminalis* (Osier willow) but other willow species will work, too. Similar techniques are now being used by some schools in the United States.

FIGURE 11.1 *At the schools I visited in Norway, children often played in schoolyard forests and climbed trees onsite at recess.*

FIGURE 11.2 *Branches and other loose forest materials become inviting forts for imaginative play.*

FIGURE 11.3 *Children enjoy their shady, easily-supervised "fort" in the bushes at Rosa Parks School in Berkeley, California.*

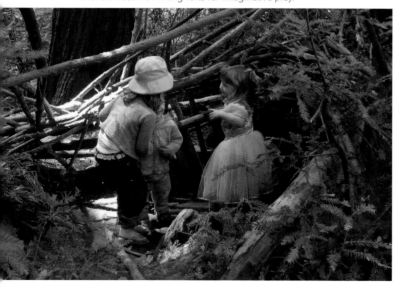

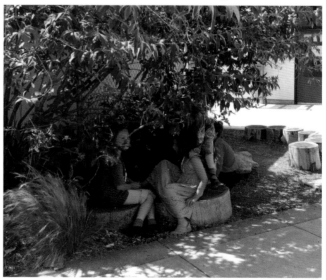

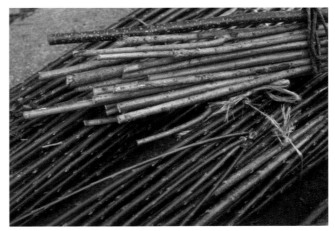

FIGURE 11.4 *Willow whips are found at some plant nurseries in the United States and, often, through organizations that supply materials for creek restoration. They can also be gathered by hand from riparian parks—with permission—in areas where they grow abundantly.*

Dynamic living willow constructions offer dramatic focal points for school grounds. Their flexible branches bend into eye-catching shapes that spark children's interest and invite them to climb inside. The deciduous willow branches showcase seasonal changes with varying leaf and twig colors, and foster varied year-round play experiences.

These living play features, made from natural, sustainably harvested materials, are inexpensive and straightforward to create. Simple forms can be designed and built by teachers, children, and community members. Some schools hire local artists, who specialize in basket weaving or fiber arts, to help them create more complex forms.

To create teepees, archways, domes, tunnels, mazes, and sculptures, freshly cut whips (long, straight willow branches) are planted in the ground in tight holes that outline the desired form. They are woven or tied together into the desired shape, then watered thoroughly. The ground under the structure is usually mulched to prevent weeds from growing between the newly planted whips as they form roots and become trees. As these structures age and leaf out, their translucent walls become increasingly opaque and sturdy. Annual or semiannual pruning is required to maintain the desired form and level of transparency. If additional visibility is desired for proper supervision, the leaves and branches may be pruned to let teachers see children inside, while maintaining a comfortable sense of enclosure for the students. Larger structures have proportionally bigger

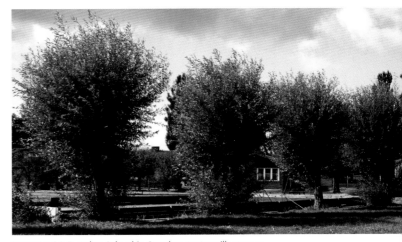

FIGURE 11.5 *Palett School in Sweden grows willow trees onsite—to provide shade and to produce long, flexible willow whips, which are harvested every two years.[2]*

annual pruning, watering, and maintenance requirements. (See chapter 15 for examples of sculptural willow forms.)

During playtime, students use leafy, semi-enclosed domes and teepees as "playhouses" for dramatic play or to talk quietly and relax. When it's time for class, these spaces become meeting places for outdoor lessons. Leafy tunnels and mazes invite active running games, hide-and-seek, and other activities. (Figures 11.4–11.9)

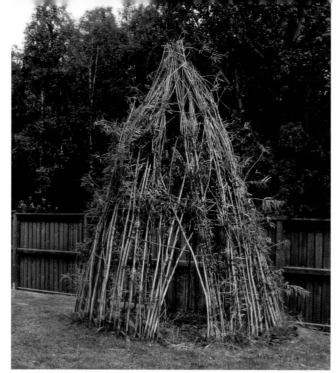

FIGURE 11.6 *Östra Mölla Gård Preschool in Sweden built a small living willow hut at a comfortable scale for their preschool students. The tiny entry purposely prohibits adults from entering the children's private domain.*

FIGURE 11.7 *The living willow dome at Cowick First School in southwest England, photographed after five years of growth, was constructed by students and teachers as a playhouse and meeting area for outdoor lessons.[3]*

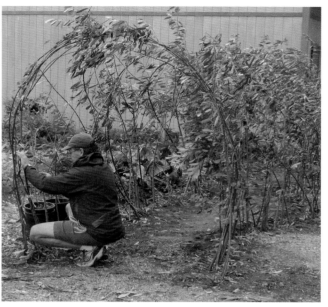

FIGURE 11.8 *This photograph shows a living willow tunnel at San Francisco Community School in California on planting day.*

FIGURE 11.9 *Curving, living willow tunnels like this one at St. Peter Chanel Primary School in England can be vibrant playground centerpieces. During my visit to the school, only five months after the tunnel was planted, children darted in and out of the branches and delighted in running its length.*

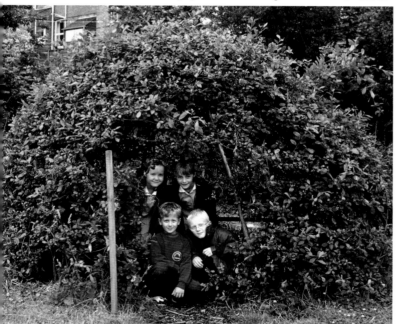

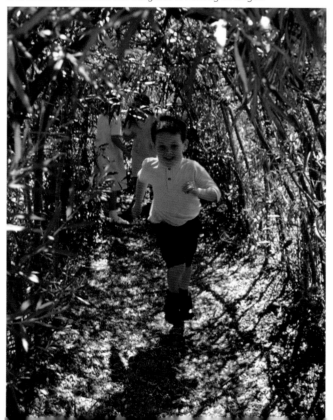

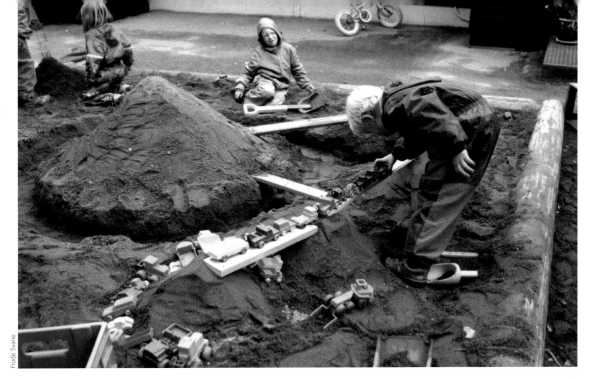

FIGURE 11.19
Small toys enrich imaginative sandbox play at this school in Norway.

Frode Svane

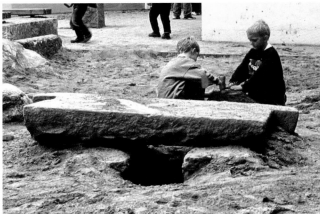

FIGURE 11.20 *This school in Norway, has a large sandbox that incorporates boulders around the edges and in the midst of the sand. The children use these rocks as they play, sometimes digging around or under well-supported stones.*

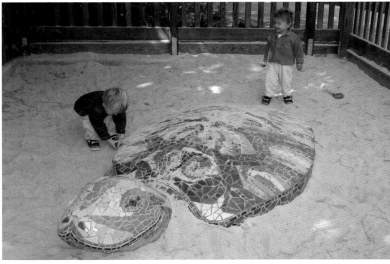

FIGURE 11.21 *Sandbox at F.R.O.G. Park in Oakland, California.*

cars and trucks animate and populate this imaginary landscape, and help the children bring it to life.

Sandboxes may also be enriched with educational and artistic elements that provide additional dimensions to fantasy play. For example, San Francisco Community School's sandbox, in California, includes interesting "archeological dig" features, including "bones" and other "finds" affixed to the bottom and side walls of the sandbox. Children dig into the sand to find these "treasures" and then cover them back up so others can find them. At F.R.O.G. Park in Oakland, California, a giant, mosaic-covered turtle sculpture inhabits the sandbox. As children move the sand around the enclosure, the turtle appears and disappears. His feet are almost always buried, just waiting to be discovered by curious toddlers. (Figure 11.21)

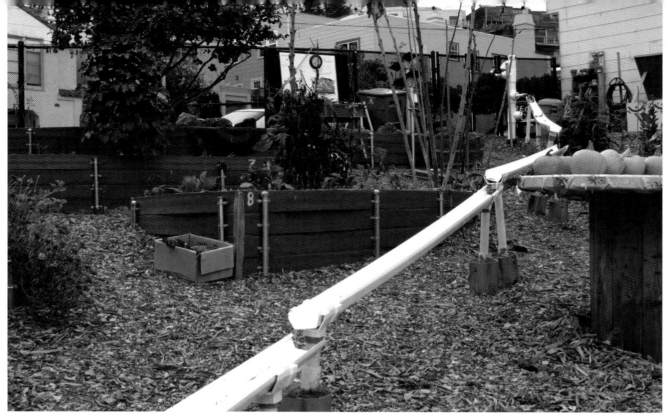

FIGURES 11.22 and 11.23 *Creative watering system at Alice Fong Yu School in San Francisco, California.*

Schoolyard water play

Children are fascinated by moving water, whether it comes from the faucet or a natural source. In addition to sandbox water play, some schools use their irrigation water to amuse their students as it flows to garden plants.

A large edible garden on a hillside overlooks the classroom buildings at Alice Fong Yu Alternative School in San Francisco, California. Raised garden beds step down the slope, but the water source is only at the top. Instead of installing expensive drip irrigation for the entire site, the school's creative garden coordinator and founder, Arden Bucklin-Sporer, developed a system for conveying the water from the source to the beds. Her idea puts all 30 children from a single class to work watering the garden simultaneously.

This cooperative garden irrigation system has a wonderful "building toy" quality that the children adore. (Figure 11.22) The system is composed of movable gutter segments and vertical supports that students set up, rearrange, and remove each time they water the garden. The movable "footings", made by filling empty paint cans with concrete, each hold a piece of

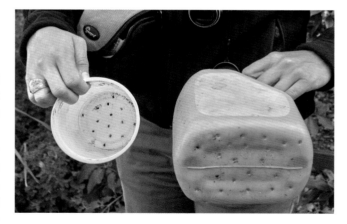

plastic pipe upright, which in turn supports a rain gutter segment on a bracket. When a class comes to the garden, students arrange this set to create a path for the water to follow from the water source to the chosen bed. As the water flows down the gutter channel, children gather at the end to catch it as it spills out. To do this they use empty plastic containers with holes drilled in the bottoms. (Figure 11.23) As soon as one child's container fills, it begins to drip, and the child has

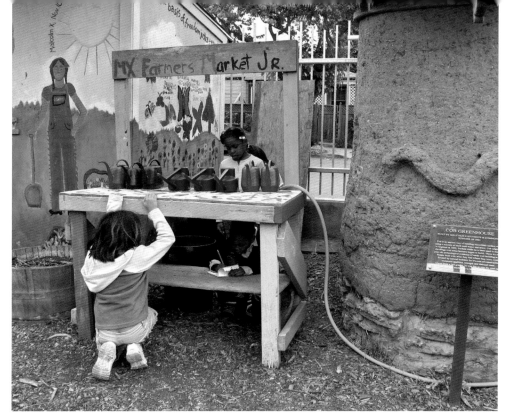

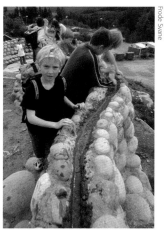

FIGURE 11.26 *Lørenskog Steiner School in Norway has a beautiful, sinuous stone wall that forms the edge of the schoolyard at the peak of a steep grade change. (See chapter 8, Figure 8.20) The wall is topped by a narrow runnel that channels water along its length and into a pond at one end. Designed by architect Frode Svane and built by students with his help, this water play feature is enjoyed by children of all ages.*

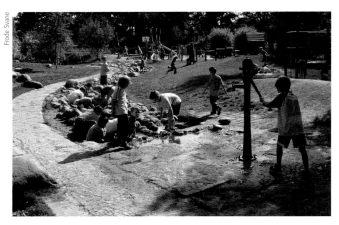

FIGURE 11.24 *"Water store" game at Malcolm X School in Berkeley, California.*

FIGURE 11.25 *In this German schoolyard's water play area, children use a hand pump to fill a shallow, rocky channel and then play with the water as it moves slowly past them.*

to move away from the water source to spread it on the garden—giving the next child a turn. Meanwhile, other children amuse themselves exploring the properties of moving water by floating small sticks and leaves in the channel.

Garden educator Rivka Mason developed an innovative "water store" game at Malcolm X School in Berkeley, California, that engages the elementary school children in enjoyable gardening tasks during recess and cleans up the garden at the same time. The garden includes a small "farmer's market" stand that becomes the "watering station" during the game. To play, a few children work behind the stand, filling small watering cans from a hose. Other children—"the customers"—walk through the garden picking up sticks, stones and litter to trade for full watering cans. When the water is gone, they return to the stand for a refill, along with an additional food wrapper or other piece of garbage to "pay" for it. (Figure 11.24)

Sometimes schools create artificial creeks or other water channels for students to play in at recess. These water features may recirculate or simply flow downhill to a sandbox or moisture-loving planting bed. (Figures 11.25 and 11.26)

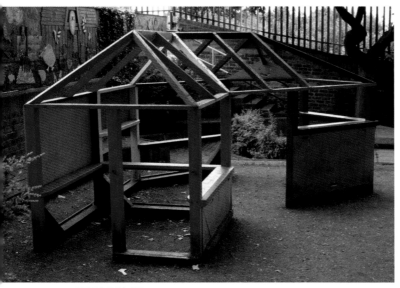

FIGURE 11.27

🍃 *Fantasy and Dramatic Play*

Preschool and elementary school children often enjoy using playhouses, tree houses, and puppet theaters as backdrops and props for role-playing games. Older children also enjoy similar but larger forts, "dens," and tree houses used as special meeting places. These structures come in a variety of sizes, shapes, colors, and designs suitable for inclusion in school-yard play.

To offer these imaginative social environments, some schools install commercial playhouses, while others build them with their school communities—or allow their students to have a hand in the construction process. "Off the shelf" playhouses are often quite nice, but are frequently less open-ended in their design; they are usually painted in particular styles to suggest one type of use or another, or with colors that appeal more to one gender than the other. If given a choice, it

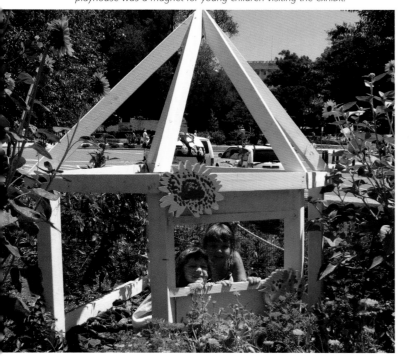

FIGURE 11.28 *This playhouse with a puppet theater window was part of the Sustainable Schoolyard display my firm designed for the **One Planet, Ours!** exhibit at the U.S. Botanic Garden in Washington, DC (May-October 2008). Nestled in a flowerbed, the playhouse was a magnet for young children visiting the exhibit.[7]*

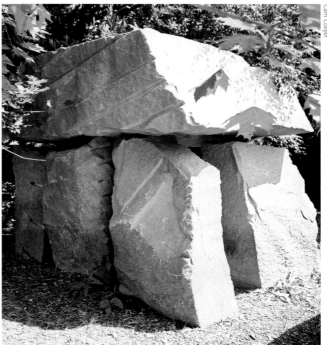

FIGURE 11.29 *There are numerous playhouses at Coombes Infant and Nursery School in England and each is a unique, vibrant school-yard focal point.[8] This sturdy stone playhouse, made of massive pieces of Scottish pink granite, also serves as part of the school's geology trail.*

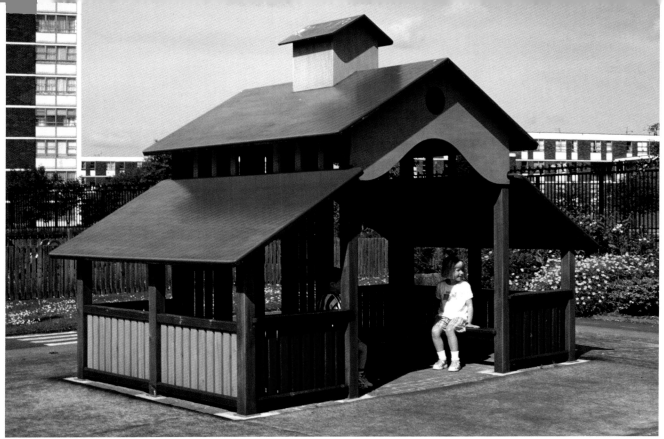

FIGURE 11.30 *The playground at West Walker Primary and Nursery School in Newcastle, England, includes a series of commercially made playhouses, artfully arranged to look like a small village with buildings, streets, and street signs.*

is a good idea to build or select playhouses with fewer design details, so children can fill these in with their imaginations.

Playhouses are versatile structures that fit almost any schoolyard context. They may be placed directly on the ground or raised slightly to create "tree houses"—with or without a tree present—and entered through doorways, openings, or tunnels. Some have an enclosed roof and/or walls to provide protection from the elements; others are open-sided to facilitate supervision. They can be draped in fabric or plants or finished with other materials. Some also double as outdoor puppet theaters.

The simple, open-sided playhouse at Ashfield Nursery School in England is one of the most versatile designs I have seen. (Figure 11.27) Made of wooden beams, its open-ended design may be imagined as a castle, doctor's office, market, or whatever else the children decide on a given day. Built by the school community, it provides hours of fantasy play for their preschool students. It is large enough to accommodate a group of children playing together, but is also a comfortable size for one child to play in alone. The open sides make supervision straightforward. The half walls give the structure a sense of comfortable enclosure and may be used for puppet shows. The playhouse is painted bright, cheerful colors that welcome children of both genders.

Vine-covered playhouses

There is something very appealing about sunlight filtered through leaves that blow in the wind, vines that hang down to enclose a space, and the sense of being tucked into a small, living nook. The living willow play structures described earlier in the chapter fulfill this desire to be sheltered among leaves and branches, as do bean teepees and other vine-covered shelters.

Small teepees are very easy and inexpensive to build. Directions are as follows: (1) purchase long, bamboo poles or harvest some, with permission, from a willing neighbor's yard; (2) push one end of each pole into the ground at an angle to form

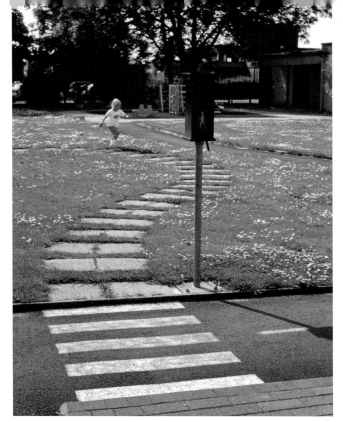

FIGURE 11.31 *A bicycle track surrounding the play area at West Walker is striped like a street to teach children about road safety; it even has "traffic lights" and signs to complete the educational model.*

FIGURE 11.33 *This Oslo Steiner School has a number of creative playhouses, including this retired boat.*

Cam Collyer

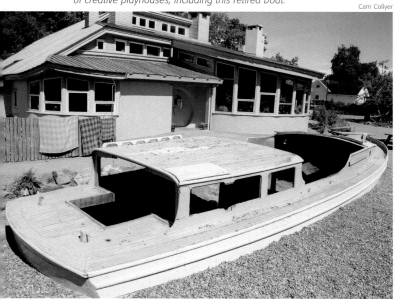

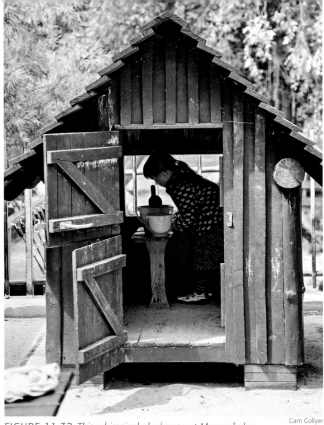

Cam Collyer

FIGURE 11.32 *This whimsical playhouse at Murergården School in Copenhagen, Denmark, is perfect for a single child.*

FIGURE 11.34 *The "chatter box" at Cowick First School in England is a small, rustic playhouse that invites children to sit and talk with their friends. Two sides of the chatter box are open so adults can supervise the children from afar.*

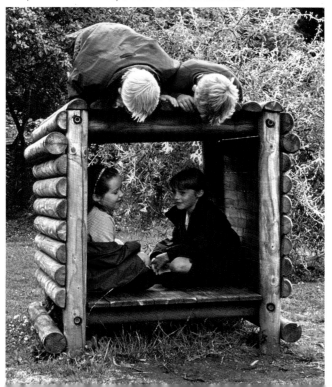

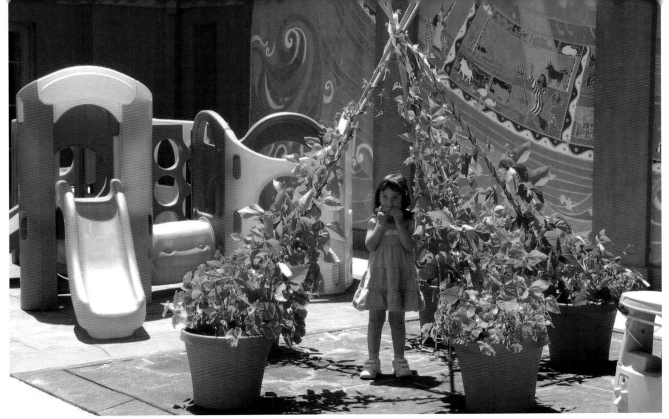

FIGURE 11.35 *This bean teepee at the Jewish Community Center became a leafy, inviting play space just 6 weeks after planting.*

FIGURE 11.36 *This attractive tunnel at Fairview Elementary School in Hayward, California, which runs the length of the edible garden, invites children to stop and play among the plants. Shown here in early spring soon after construction, the tunnel will soon be covered by exuberant plant growth.*

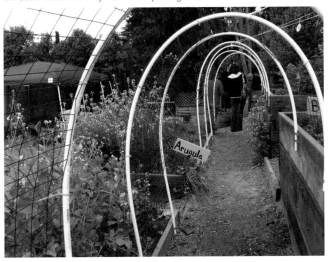

a circle with the tops gathered together at the center; (3) tie the top of the poles with strong, natural twine or thin rope; and (4) plant vines at the base of each pole. As the vines grow, train them up the poles to create a leafy space. Some schools also add bamboo crossbars or rope netting to the sides of the teepee to encourage the vines to fill in the spaces between the poles.

In 2004 I worked with the Jewish Community Center of the East Bay, in Berkeley, California, to create a leafy bean tee-pee in their paved courtyard play space. We used large sturdy pots to create the base of the teepee and arranged them in a circle. Each eight-foot long bamboo pole was pushed to the bottom of one of the pots to make this temporary, seasonal structure more stable. We planted the five pots with edible nas-turtiums and scarlet runner beans. These two types of plants exhibited lush growth quite quickly, were fairly tolerant of rough handling by the young children, and produced colorful blooms for the children and staff to enjoy. On hot days, the teachers occasionally tied a sprinkler to the top of the teepee, adding a cooling water play feature. (Figures 11.35 and 11.36)

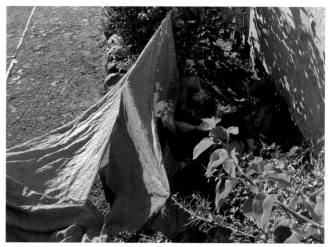

Impromptu "dens" and forts

Sometimes, the best "playhouses" are temporary ones, built by children to suit their needs of the moment, rather than formal playhouses built or purchased by adults. These ephemeral dens and forts are built from materials such as old bed sheets, fabric, sticks, branches, leaves, and mud, and, typically, fulfill the play needs that arise on a single afternoon. Materials are put away after they are used or rearranged on an ongoing basis. (Figures 11.37 and 11.38)

FIGURE 11.37 *Elementary school children constructed this simple, temporary fort on their own, while attending the after-school program at the Jewish Community Center of the East Bay in Berkeley, California. After building their fort, the children crawled inside to enjoy it for the afternoon.*

FIGURE 11.38 *When my daughter attended preschool in Berkeley, California, I added some brightly colored nylon fabric to the ordinary, commercial play structure in the schoolyard to encourage the young children to use the area underneath for imaginative play. The inexpensive fabric lasted about a month, through rainy weather and tugging hands, before moving on to another use in the art room, but the children loved their "fort" while it lasted.*

🍃 Movable Play Elements and Construction-Oriented Play

Children seem to find something very magical about shaping their own environment and then dreaming up stories to describe what they have created and the fanciful creatures that "live" there. I think many of us played "hot lava" games as kids, joyfully hopping from one stone to another, taking care not to step in the pretend "hot zone" on the ground. We also often shaped soil and other found objects into "castles" that we knew were "really" in far away lands.

Most of our modern playgrounds are built around the idea of fixed play structures and other elements that stay exactly the same every day, thwarting children's desire to explore and create. Schools that find themselves in this situation can improve the play value of their landscapes by giving their students moveable elements to play with during recess. For more information about natural play props, I recommend *Plants for Play* by Robin Moore. This well-written book includes a detailed list of trees and other plants that produce useful, non-poisonous pods, cones, nuts, and flowers that enhance children's outdoor play options, and other topics related to children's planted play environments. (Figures 11.39 and 11.40)

Some schools give their students larger movable parts in the form of building materials—and, sometimes, tools—that they may use to construct their own playhouses on a temporary or permanent basis. This type of construction-oriented play seems to be particularly well suited to upper elementary and middle school students who are old enough to handle tools confidently. Many schools also give their students art materials to use at recess, so they can create works of art in the schoolyard. (Figures 11.41 and 11.42) (See chapter 12 for more art play ideas.)

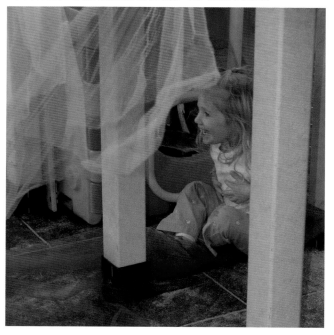

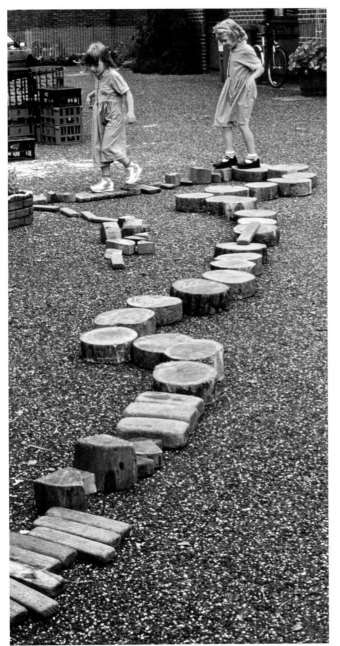

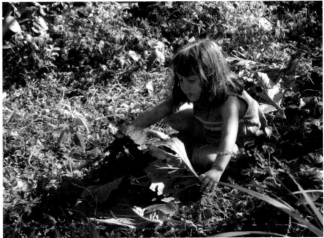

FIGURE 11.40 *This child made a temporary "home" for a garden snail, with great care.*

Skudeneshavn School

FIGURE 11.41 *At Skudeneshavn Primary School in Karmøy, Norway, one area of the school grounds is dedicated to construction activities. Students are given lumber, saws, hammers and nails to build creations that*

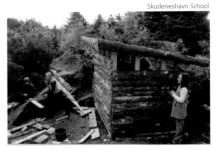

spring from their own imagination. Students of all ages are allowed to build huts for themselves (and younger children) to play in.[9]

FIGURE 11.42 *This Oslo Steiner School in Norway gives students a wooden construction kit to play with at recess. Each piece of wood is notched, so the pieces fit together easily and the logs are large enough for use in building temporary forts or other structures. After they are finished playing, their buildings can be disassembled so that others may take a turn.*

Cam Collyer

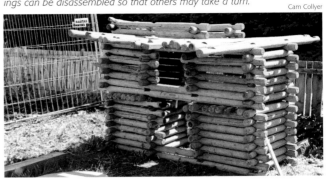

FIGURE 11.39 *At recess time, children at Cowick First School in southwest England are given the usual balls, jump ropes, and other standard play equipment, along with crates filled with wooden tree rounds and blocks. These movable pieces can be used for building, as blocks, or assembled into pathways across "large swamps" or other imagined environments. Contact your local tree-trimming company for left-over tree rounds, which can frequently be obtained free of charge or at low-cost.*

✿ Outdoor Board Games

One of the easiest ways to diversify schoolyard environments is to add board games. Board games encourage social interaction, logical reasoning, and cooperation among small groups of children—and many kids really enjoy them. Some schools have incorporated game boards into their school grounds as markings for the tops of tables and chairs or as portable elements that travel outside each day with the children during recess. Schools can also create oversized game boards by painting them on the ground or incorporating them into paving patterns.

Mary Jackson

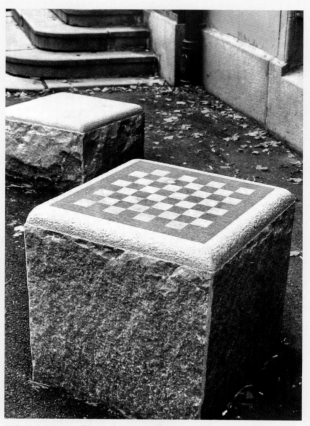

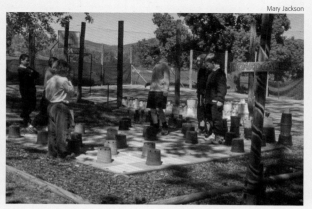

FIGURE 11.43 *This chessboard at Brungle Public School in New South Wales, Australia, was assembled using concrete pavers in alternating colors. The children shown here are playing their game using overturned garden pots.*[10]

FIGURE 11.44 *The yard at Grünerløkka School in Oslo, Norway, includes striking granite cubes, scattered on the schoolyard to provide informal seating and work surfaces. Some of the cubes are inscribed with game boards to encourage play.*

12 *Outdoor Art and Music Play in an Ecological Schoolyard*

Outdoor art and music play are underutilized resources on most school grounds; yet, they are rewarding, enjoyable, enriching activities for students of all ages. Some schools across the United States and around the world are weaving art and music into their students' free time by making creative materials and resources available outside at recess. Students at these schools enjoy the freedom of personal expression and artistic experimentation in contexts that are not tied to classroom instruction, grading, or their teachers' approval.

In my experience, preschools seem to offer these activities more often than elementary schools, and elementary schools more often than middle and high schools. Perhaps this is due to the increasing pressure on schools to adhere to traditional academics during the school day, and the dwindling free time students are allowed outside as they ascend through the grade levels. However, many of the ideas presented in this chapter, illustrated with examples of young children engaging in art and music play, could be easily implemented with older age groups. Some of these activities can be accomplished with older students just as they are presented, while others might need some simple modifications to the materials or techniques to make them more interesting to older students. I hope that the following examples will inspire more schools to put art materials and musical instruments at their students' fingertips during their free time, and, in so doing, encourage children to move beyond classroom lessons to explore their own creative passions.

🍃 *Outdoor "Art Play"*

Some schools give their students an array of informal, outdoor art options among the range of recreational choices available to them during their outdoor breaks. Unstructured "art play," using a wide variety of inexpensive materials, allows students to get their hands dirty and express themselves creatively in ways that are not always possible during class time. Activity choices may even include finding and using natural materials onsite, such as flower petals, leaves, or soil, as painting and drawing pigments. (See chapter 15 for more art-related play options.)

"Art at Recess" programs

Parent volunteers at Rooftop School in San Francisco, California, run an innovative "art at recess" program several days a week during lunch recess. They bring a rotating selection of materials for children to use and supervise the distribution and clean-up of the projects the students create. On one of my visits to the school, for example, students were creating a "chalk quilt" in a shady corner of their asphalt playground. Each child made his or her own drawing within a larger framework established by the parent supervisor. This orderly arrangement lets the children collaborate in making a large project, while freeing them to draw what they like in their own individual spaces. (Figures 12.1 and 12.2 on the next page)

FIGURE 12.1

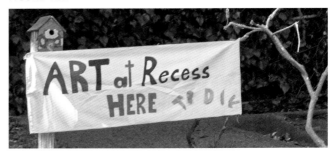

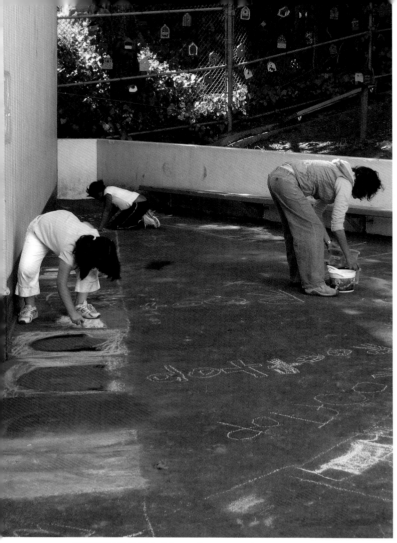

FIGURE 12.2 *"Art at Recess" program at Rooftop School in San Francisco, California.*

This successful program at Rooftop School inspired Rosa Parks School in nearby Berkeley, California, to start a similar program in spring 2008. The Rosa Parks program started with parent volunteers and is now staffed by a paid recess supervisor. Projects include chalk days as well as water painting (see Figure 12.6) and other projects. (Figures 12.3 and 12.4)

Outdoor painting with water or colorful paints

Water painting is a simple, inexpensive, and easy way to bring artistic expression to the schoolyard. Painting with water only requires a few supplies: a dark, uniform, accessible surface to act as the painting "canvas" (an outdoor chalkboard or a wall painted a solid color), some paint brushes, and small buckets of water. Students dip their brushes in the water and "paint" the water on the dark surface to create temporary designs. When the water dries, other students take a turn. Unlike working with paint, there is no mess to clean up when the children are finished (unless water *play* becomes the focus!), and there are no supplies that get "used up" during the activity, so the cost is minimal. (Figures 12.5 and 12.6)

Regular painting supplies and traditional easels can also be brought outside for students to enjoy at recess. Younger students typically use watercolor sets, washable poster paints, or natural materials. Older children may also use more durable materials, including acrylics and oil paints, as the school's budget and level of supervision allows. Painting outside often changes the subject of children's artwork to include what they see around them. (see chapter 9, Figure 9.42)

FIGURE 12.3 *Some schools supply their students with outdoor chalkboards to encourage artistic expression at recess.*

FIGURE 12.4 *Rosa Parks School in Berkeley, California, uses the asphalt playground as a "giant chalkboard" for art play at recess.*

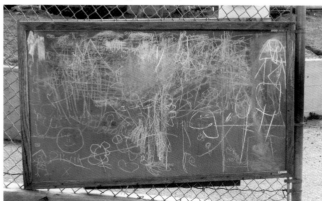

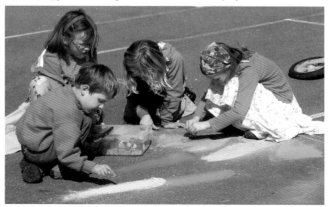

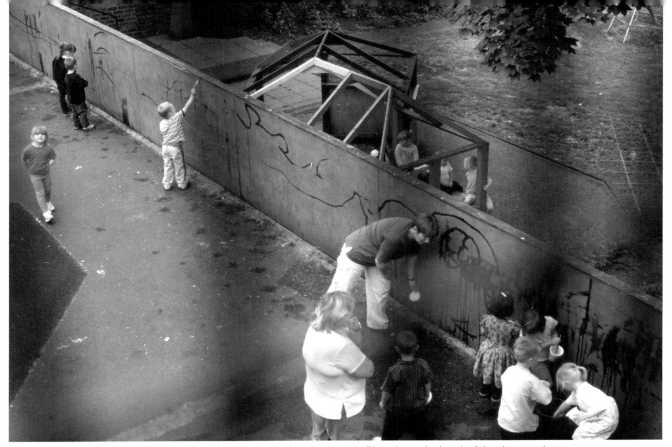

FIGURE 12.5 *At Ashfield Nursery School in northern England, a large outdoor chalkboard runs the length of the playground fence and is often used for water painting. This substantial "canvas" has plenty of space for each child's expressive drawings.*

FIGURE 12.6 *Rosa Parks School added two water painting boards to the playground fence for students to enjoy at recess. The boards were cut from a sheet of plywood and painted with weatherproof exterior primer and chalkboard paint.*
Michelle Contreras

FIGURE 12.7 *This portable painting table set up outside at a preschool in England allows the young students to paint when they want to, without instruction from their teachers.*

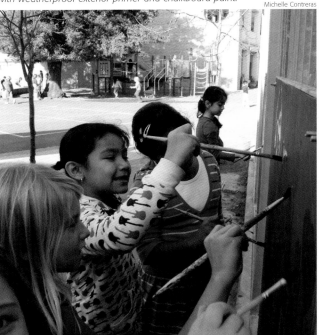

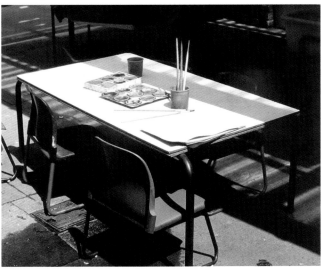

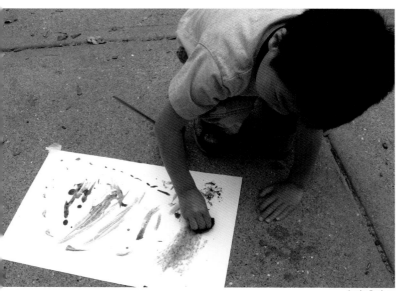

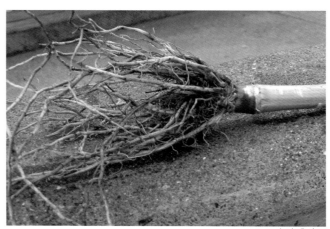

FIGURE 12.10 *Plant roots can become brushes for applying paint.*

FIGURES 12.8 and 12.9 *Children enjoy drawing and painting with natural materials at Tule Elk Park Child Development Center in San Francisco, California.*

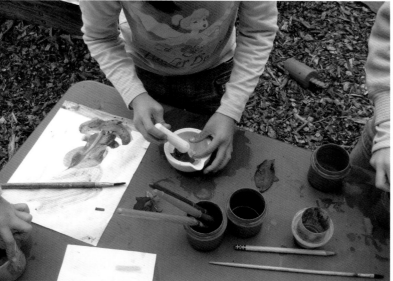

Outdoor art play with natural materials

Natural materials found in school garden settings have a range of interesting colors, textures, and forms. With a little creativity, these resources may be harnessed as freely available supplies for children's artistic explorations.

Garden educator Ayesha Ercelawn, at Tule Elk Park Child Development Center in San Francisco, California, offers her young students a wide variety of enriching outdoor play opportunities at recess and after school. The children sometimes use flower petals, leaves, soil, and other natural materials found onsite as art pigments for painting and drawing. To use the colors directly, children rub a vivid petal or leaf on a piece of white paper to make lines. (Figure 12.8) They also use small mortars and pestles to grind these materials into "paints" that, with the addition of a few drops of water, are applied with a brush. (Figure 12.9) Sometimes the "brushes" they use for their paintings are themselves natural materials, such as twigs, grasses, and roots. (Figure 12.10)

Weaving, using natural materials, is another one of Ercelawn's many creative and impressive ideas. To prepare the children to participate in collaborative weaving projects, she prepares the warp strings for a large, shared outdoor loom and weaves a few rows using long leaves, vines, and other natural materials from the garden. Ercelawn teaches the children how to use the loom and where to find the supplies in the garden, and then lets them work on their own during recess. Popular weaving materials from the site include long, green *Dietes* leaves (African iris) that dry to an attractive brown as time passes, vines of all shapes and sizes, flowers, branches, and fallen leaves.[1] (Figures 12.11–12.13)

FIGURE 12.11
This young girl is just starting a new weaving project on a freshly prepared loom.

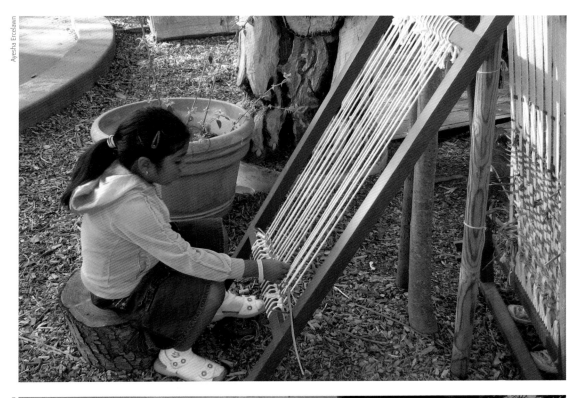

FIGURE 12.12
This child is adding flowers and other finishing touches to a completed weaving project, which will soon be displayed in the school building for all to enjoy.

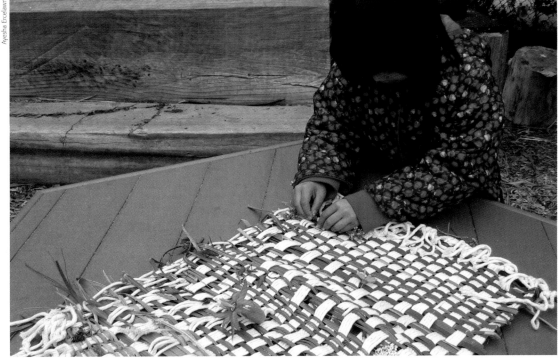

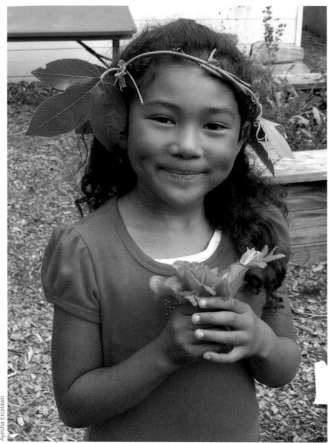

Ayesha Ercelawn

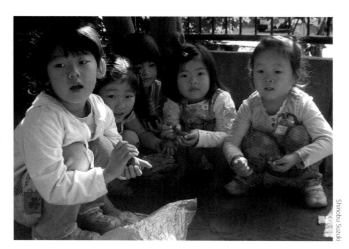

Shinobu Suzuki

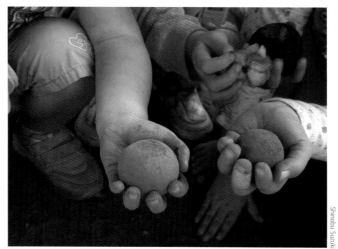

Shinobu Suzuki

FIGURE 12.13 *Ayesha Ercelawn's students enjoy gathering natural materials to make free-form sculptural creations. After studying birds in class, one child used a pile of garden trimmings to make a "nest" for imaginary creatures. Another (shown), used a leafy green passion vine to create a crown and flowers she picked onsite to make a bouquet.*

FIGURES 12.14 and 12.15 *Children make Japanese mud balls* (hikaru dorodango) *at Little Lamb Kindergarten in Japan.*

Hikaru Dorodango: Special Japanese mud balls. Preschoolers at Little Lamb Kindergarten near Tokyo, Japan, spend part of their outdoor play time making carefully crafted mud balls with very smooth surfaces. This mud ball-sculpting activity, called *hikaru dorodango,* is a traditional children's pastime in Japan that has grown in popularity over the last decade.[2]

These are not just ordinary balls of mud! The children work hard, for days or weeks at a time, to carefully sculpt perfectly shaped, smooth, and shiny spheres using their playground's soil. To make a beautiful mud ball, each child picks up some of the clay-rich soil from their school site and lovingly squeezes a handful of it into a round ball shape. Next, they alternate additional layers of dry and moist clay soil and press it firmly in place. (Figure 12.14) When the ball has reached the desired size, they gently shape the surface so that it will be as round as possible, and then burnish the outside of the ball to make it smooth; some of the finished creations may be as shiny as billiard balls. (Figure 12.15) The children put their mud balls aside as revered treasures and show them off to their parents with pride.[3]

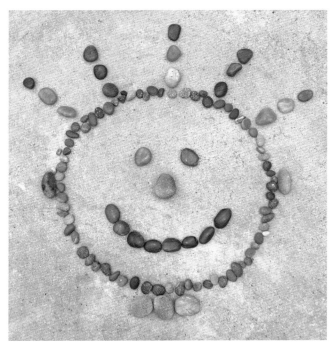

FIGURE 12.16 *Small stones of varying colors are used to create temporary mosaic pictures on paved surfaces.*

FIGURE 12.17 *Leaves from fast growing nasturtium plants were used to create a picture of a flower garden. Leaves move in the slightest breeze, so this type of project is most suitable for a windless day.*

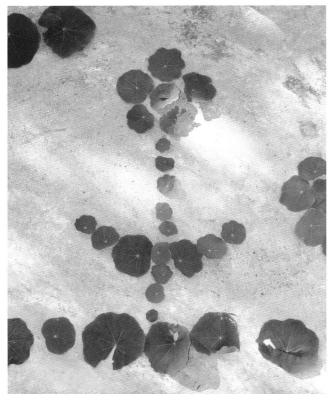

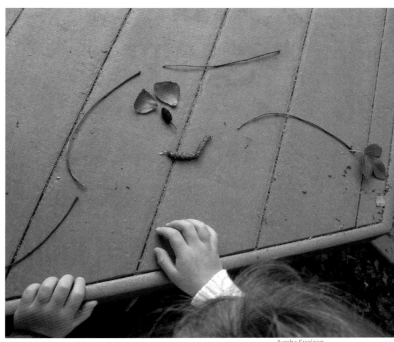

Ayesha Ercelawn

FIGURE 12.18 *Students at Tule Elk Park Child Development Center make expressive faces, and other temporary pictures, using materials from the garden.*

Temporary schoolyard mosaics. "Temporary mosaics" are another low-cost art project to offer students at recess. Schools either provide students with a set of small pebbles or cobbles, or allow them to gather leaves, flowers, wood chips, or other schoolyard materials. Students use these materials to create ephemeral pictures on smooth paved surfaces in the yard. When recess is over, students clean up their mosaic materials and put them away. (Figure 12.16–12.18)

🍃 Outdoor Play with Music and Sound

American schoolyards are filled with ambient sounds that surround children as they play: the distinctive "smack" of rubber balls bouncing on paved surfaces, children's voices yelling to one another across the yard or cheering on their friends as they play a game, the murmur of nearby traffic and honking horns in the neighborhood, teachers' piercing whistles used to get children's attention, and the predictable, periodic ring or buzz

Messy Play

Outdoor spaces are ideal for messy art activities since they can be hosed off when the projects are complete, if dramatic clean-up is needed. At the Jewish Community Center of the East Bay in Berkeley, California, preschool teachers often set up temporary art studio space in their courtyard to accommodate messy art projects like papier-mâché.

FIGURE 12.19

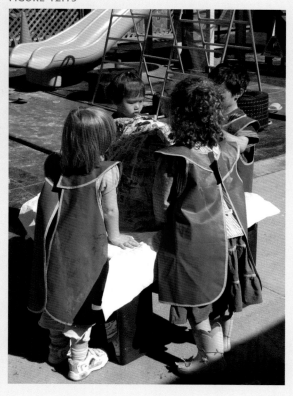

of the school bell at the beginning and end of class times. In an urban or suburban schoolyard environment, these sounds make quite a cacophony—sometimes drowning out bird calls and other softer sounds of the natural world, and making it harder to engage in quieter, creative activities that require concentration or collaboration.

One way to change the aural dynamics of the playground is to design each area of the yard so that it is sonically unique, adding a subtle diversity and sense of place to each portion of the play environment. In addition to zones of the schoolyard devoted to boisterous games, green schoolyards might include quieter nooks with the soothing sound of falling water in a fountain or the soft music of wind chimes hanging in a tree branch. Wildlife habitat areas, set apart from noisier zones, become places to listen to chirping birds, rustling leaves, and mulch crunching underfoot. Physically changing the schoolyard landscape with earthen mounds or thick walls will dampen unwanted street noise or separate different playground zones from one another.

Adding outdoor musical instruments to the play environment is another easy option, and it encourages musical experimentation while also diversifying children's creative play opportunities. Some types of durable, weatherproof musical instruments and sound-related toys may be permanently installed outdoors. Smaller, portable instruments may be carried inside and outside as needed. Schoolyard-appropriate instruments range from simple chimes and xylophones to more elaborate drums, marimbas, "talk tubes," and listening devices. Many instruments produce sounds that are quiet enough to blend in with the schoolyard environment without special placement considerations. Others, designed to produce louder notes, should be carefully sited so that they do not disturb classrooms or neighbors.

Schoolyard "Soundscapes"

Playground designers Rusty Keeler and Leon Smith of Planet Earth Playscapes developed a three-pronged approach to working with sound in young children's environments. They use sound as (1) "an ambient 'backdrop' to the play yard" to shape the mood and react to natural forces, such as the wind or rain, (2) "a 'by product' of play" that occurs when chimes or other instruments hidden in the environment move as children bump into them, and (3) "the 'goal' of play," using permanently installed musical instruments to encourage experimentation with sound while outdoors.[4]

Planet Earth Playscapes put these ideas into practice in an elaborate "Soundscape Project" for preschoolers at Cornell University's Early Learning Center in Ithaca, New York.

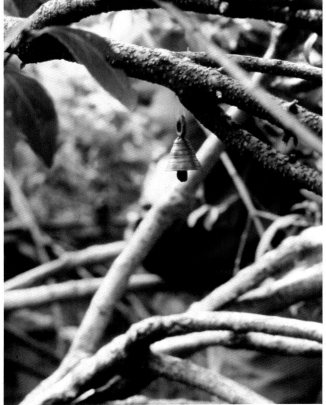

FIGURE 12.20 *Bells hung in the bushes make soft sounds as children walk by.*

Rusty Keeler

marimba and set of tongue drums were made by Sound Play of Georgia. Inspired by Sonic Architecture, the enormous Thunder Drum is the booming attraction in the far corner of the yard. Six softball mallets allow a group of children to play the 48 inch diameter galvanized steel drum at once.[5]

Artists Bill and Mary Buchen (Sonic Architecture), based in New York City, create exciting, playful soundscapes that captivate children, allowing them to experiment with rhythm, music, and sound. Their sculptural outdoor instruments and intriguing, interactive speaking and listening devices often change children's perspectives on familiar sounds, which are bounced through underground chambers or focused with parabolic reflectors. Many of their sound sculptures are installed in group settings to encourage collaborative play, but they are also enjoyed by individual children playing alone.

At their "Global Rhythms" playground at Green Valley Ranch Park in Denver, Colorado, visitors make music together using sleek metal instruments based on traditional musical forms from around the world. Green Valley Elementary School, adjacent to the park, also benefits from this installation; they use a curriculum guide developed by the Buchens, tailored to this site.[6] (Figures 12.21–12.23)

After observing the site and listening to the sounds on the playground, they decided which types of new sounds to include and where they should be placed within the yard. In Keeler's words:

The sounds range from delicate twinklings in quiet areas to loud resonating booms in active areas. Because too often children get stuck with clanky, non-harmonious instruments and toys, all the materials we used were chosen for their rich, deep sounds. We added a variety of wind chimes of wood and of metal, including a set of four chimes by Woodstock Windchimes tuned to Vivaldi's Four Seasons. (The children and staff have a ceremonial "changing of the chimes" at the start of every season.) We hung tiny Tibetan bronze bells in a huge forsythia bush (Figure 12.20) and cow bells from India in existing trees that the children climb. "Listening Cones" were fastened to the outer fence. Children put their ears to the cones to hear the sounds of the forest that borders the play yard. Beautifully tuned "Entrance Chimes" were mounted in an existing railing just outside the door to help mark the transition point from indoors to outdoors. A huge set of 3 inch diameter tuned standing chimes with rubber hammer mallets let children "pound out a song." A giant wooden

FIGURE 12.21 *A set of three metal drum seats, designed to resemble* **djembe** *drums from West Africa, surround an earth drum buried underground in the center. The earth drum can be played with hands or feet and is based on West African pit drums and Native American powwow drums that are played collaboratively.*

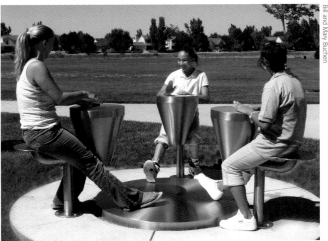

Bill and Mary Buchen

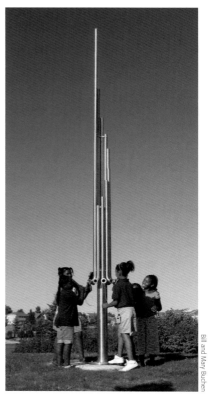

FIGURE 12.22 *A tall spiral of "slapped pipes" rises from the park with steel cylinders tuned to a 2-octave pentatonic scale. Based on bamboo percussion instruments from Micronesia, this metal version of the instrument is played using beach sandals to hit the openings of each tuned pipe, producing a tone. Longer pipes produce lower notes and shorter pipes produce higher ones.*

Bill and Mary Buchen

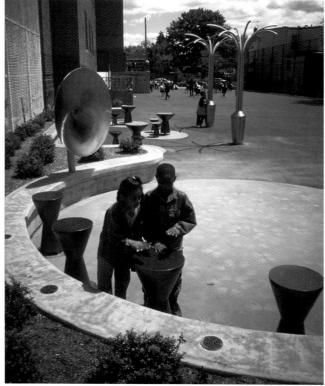

Bill and Mary Buchen

FIGURE 12.24 *"Sound Carnival" playground at Public School 224 in Brooklyn, New York.*

FIGURE 12.23 *The Global Rhythms playground includes parabolic dishes that "reflect and concentrate sound and create an acoustic feedback loop that is started with a clap and ended with a wave of the hand."*[7]

Bill and Mary Buchen

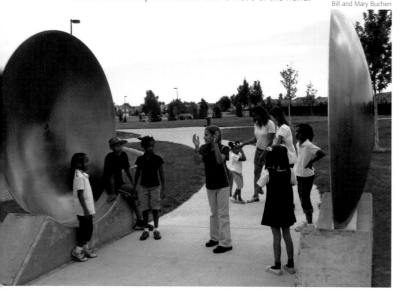

The Buchens' "Sound Carnival" playground at Public School 224 in Brooklyn, New York, includes a drum circle (foreground, Figure 12.24) with two adjacent, stainless steel parabolic dishes. "When children speak into the dishes or play the bronze drums in the circle, the sounds travel into a large underground tank below and emerge from grates in the concrete benches."[8] The same site also has bronze drum tables and seats, as well as two palm-tree shaped "slapped pipes." (background, Figure 12.24) (Figure 12.25)

Sound Play, Inc. based in Parrott, Georgia, makes a wide variety of hand-crafted, durable instruments often used to create children's outdoor musical landscapes. Their marimbas, metallophones, amadinadas, drums, chimes, and other instruments adorn schoolyards, parks, and children's centers across the United States, Canada, and the United Kingdom. Sometimes their instruments are used alone, as focal points, or they may be arranged in a cluster so children may play

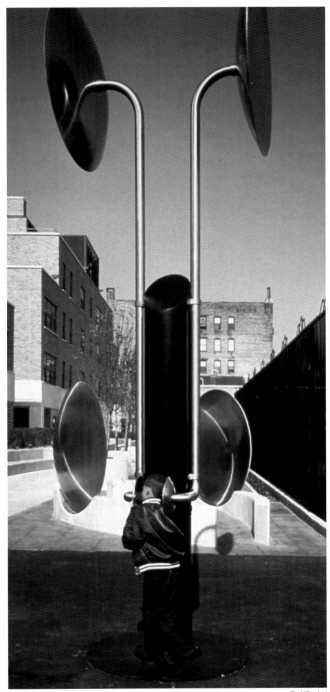

FIGURE 12.25 *At Public School 23 in New York City, the Buchens created a piece called "Big Eyes-Big Ears" that uses parabolic dishes and a periscope to allow the user to experience sounds and sights present at a higher elevation.*[9]

Paul Warchol

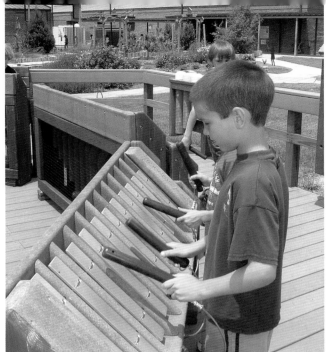

FIGURE 12.26 *Children at Worth County Primary play a soprano metallophone together outside their school.*

Bond Anderson, Sound Play

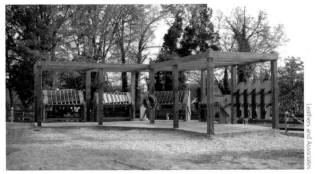

Leathers and Associates

FIGURE 12.27 *The grounds at Summit School in Winston-Salem, North Carolina, include an array of instruments to encourage students' musical collaboration: (from left) a tenor marimba, a bass metallophone, a blue rain wheel, a diatonic amadinda, a soprano metallophone, and four tongue drums. Sound Play made the instruments from wood, recycled plastic lumber, and aluminum with PVC resonator tubes.*[11]

them together, in their free time or during classes and concerts. The outdoor music studio at Worth County Primary School in Sylvester, Georgia, for example, is filled with Sound Play's instruments, including tongue drums, a soprano marimba, and soprano metallophone. All of the instruments are built low to the ground to accommodate preschoolers as well as older children.[10] (Figure 12.26)

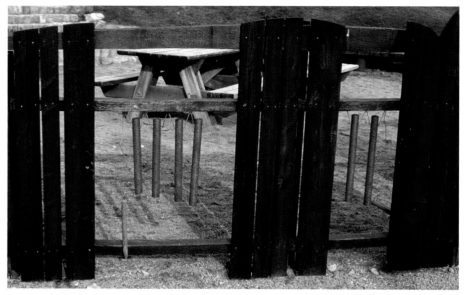

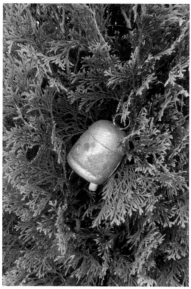

Rusty Keeler

FIGURE 12.28 *The lovely, unique, parent-built wooden fence at Maridalen School in Oslo, Norway, defines the edge of an outdoor classroom space. Metal chimes and wooden mallets, hung from openings in the fence, invite children to play a tune as they pass by.*

FIGURE 12.29 *When children brush up against this arborvitae tree, the cowbell nestled in its branches makes a pleasing sound.*

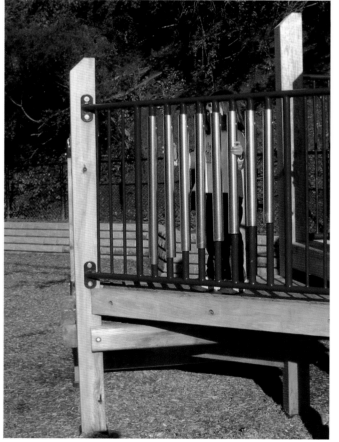

FIGURE 12.30 *This set of built-in chimes on a commercial play structure is a nice gesture toward musical play, but seems somewhat less successful than other designs. Here, metal tubes are each strung on a railing bar and cannot be removed. Children push the swinging outer tubes against the railing's bars to make musical tones. This arrangement, while theft-proof, makes them much less resonant than other types of chimes.*

Outdoor percussion instruments for schoolyard landscapes

Chimes. Simple chimes or bells add pleasing, musical tones to school grounds. They can be hung in places where they will be blown by the wind or positioned so children can play with them. (Figures 12.28–12.30)

Xylophones, marimbas and more. Large percussion instruments with a wide range of musical pitches, covering at least a full octave, have greater musical possibilities for students'

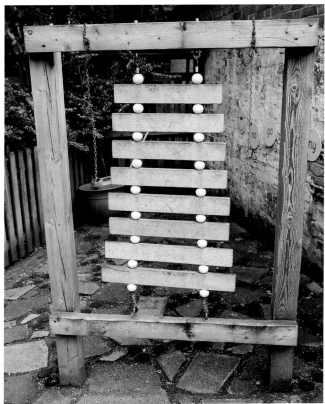

Cam Collyer

FIGURE 12.31 *This simple xylophone at Argyle School in England is hung low to the ground to encourage children to try it.*

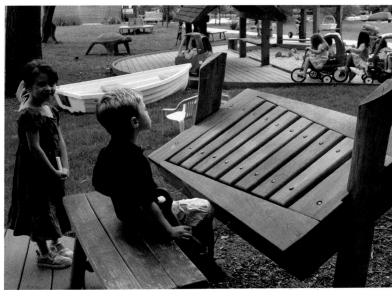

Rusty Keeler

FIGURE 12.32 *This beautiful xylophone, made from durable black locust wood, enlivens the leafy playground at Garden City Community Church Preschool in Garden City, New York.[12]*

FIGURE 12.33 *This metallophone has tuned metal bars that are amplified by the red plastic pipes within the instrument's screened stand.[13]*

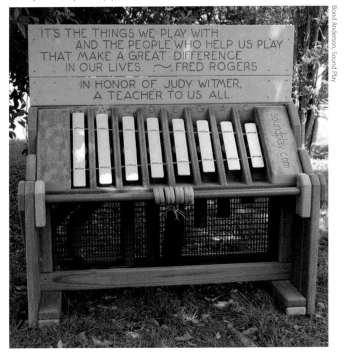

Bond Anderson, Sound Play

creative expression than smaller instruments. Large sets of chimes, marimbas, xylophones, or other instruments (made from metal, wood, or plastic) can be fairly durable in the schoolyard landscape and stand up to a variety of weather conditions and active use.

Xylophones are percussion instruments consisting of an array of tuned bars of various lengths that produce a range of tones when struck by a mallet. (Figure 12.31 and 12.32)

Marimbas, like xylophones, include an array of tuned wooden bars. However, each bar gets a richer and louder sound from a resonator tube placed below it. The instrument is usually played with mallets, tipped with a soft material such as rubber. Metallophones are similar to marimbas and xylophones but their bars are made from metal. They can be built with or without resonators. (Figure 12.33)

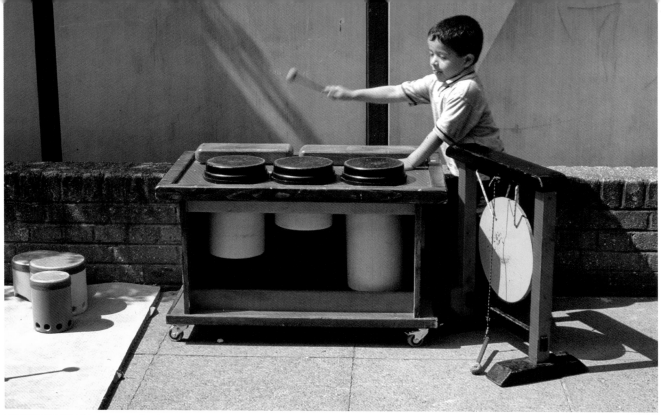

FIGURE 12.34 *This nursery school near London, England, sets up a small group of portable musical instruments for students to enjoy outside when the weather is nice. The instruments, including a variety of hand drums, are not weatherproof so they are stored indoors at the end of each day.*

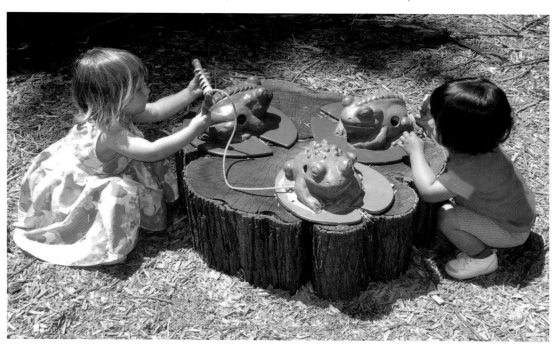

FIGURE 12.35
These plastic frogs are permanently installed in the beautiful outdoor playground at the Bay Area Discovery Museum in Sausalito, California. Children make the frogs "croak" by stroking the bumps on the frogs' backs with tethered wooden dowel rods.

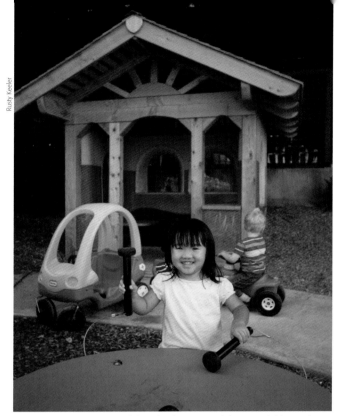

FIGURE 12.36 *This metal thunder drum at Joyful Noise Child Development Center in Portland, Oregon, draws children in with its deep, pleasing tone. The drum is played with rubber-tipped mallets, attached to its side.*[14]

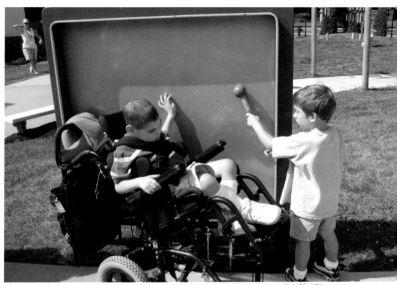

FIGURE 12.38 *The thunder wall at Alternatives for Children in East Setauket, New York, is a flat panel drum made from a thin sheet of stainless steel freely hung in a sturdy metal frame. It responds with a satisfyingly loud "boom" even when gently struck. This drum is large enough to be played by several children at once. It is located in the school's Sound Garden, a music therapy playground for young children with disabilities.*[15]

FIGURE 12.37 *This handsome, alligator-shaped box drum produces four tones when the wooden tongues on top are struck with rubber-tipped mallets. Created by Sound Play, it was a popular focal point for my firm's 2008 Sustainable Schoolyard exhibit at the United States Botanic Garden in Washington, DC. Children couldn't resist playing with it as they walked by.*

Drums. Drums are also very popular additions to schoolyards, parks, and other children's play areas. Like other percussion instruments, they may be either permanently installed or temporarily placed in the schoolyard using portable equipment. Simple drums can also be made from recycled materials, or improvised using whatever materials are on hand. (Figures 12.34–12.39)

Children and playground staff members at the City of Berkeley Adventure Playground in California built this substantial drum tower using materials that were otherwise destined for a local landfill. The drum set rests on a wooden structure made from industrial cable spools, stacked on top of

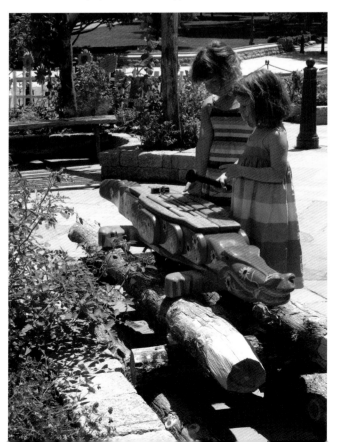

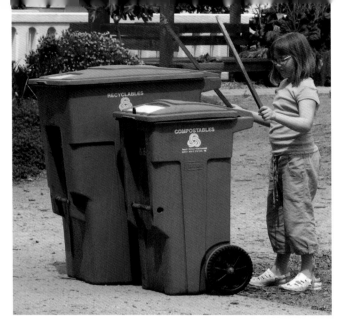

FIGURE 12.39 *This girl, playing after school in the lovely garden at Sherman Elementary in San Francisco, California, used wooden sticks to play an impromptu rhythm on the resonant recycling and compost bins she found in the yard.*

Outdoor wind-driven instruments

Outdoor wind-driven instruments use air movement to make sound. Chimes, for example, produce sound as they blow in the wind and their component parts knock together. Other wind instruments produce tones as the wind blows over resonating tubes of different lengths. Sound Play, Inc. creates outdoor wind instruments using these methods to generate musical tones.

One installation at Nevils Elementary School in Georgia includes wind played fipple flutes (block flutes) and percussion instruments. The wind-driven flutes are oriented towards the prevailing breezes from the southeast and southwest, created by the "U"-shaped adjacent school buildings.[18] (Figure 12.44)

FIGURE 12.40

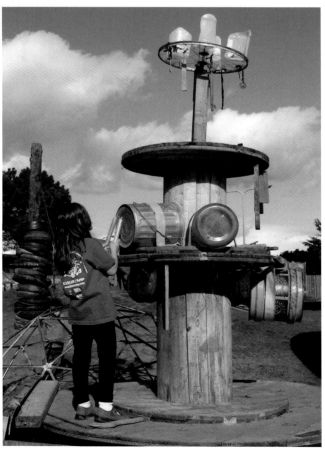

one another and bolted securely together. (Figure 12.40) The top is crowned with plastic jugs that have been split in half so that they catch the wind and cause an elevated wheel to spin, making some hanging wooden chimes knock together. The lower levels include empty plastic water jugs, a metal trash can, and other elements that are played using simple wooden dowels as mallets.[16]

Sound tubes and other tools for making and listening to sounds

Musical instruments are not the only sonic elements that students can play with in a schoolyard environment. "Talk tubes," often attached to climbing structures at schools and parks, are a more common device.

The idea is simple: a plastic or metal tube is routed through or around a play structure so that its ends are not within sight of one another. The opening on each end of the tube is positioned within children's reach. Kids then talk or sing into one end of the pipe, and their playmate at the other end of the pipe hears what they are saying. Children find these simple devices "magical" as their voices are transmitted to places they can't see, and their friends' voices come to them by invisible means, too. (Figure 12.41–12.43)

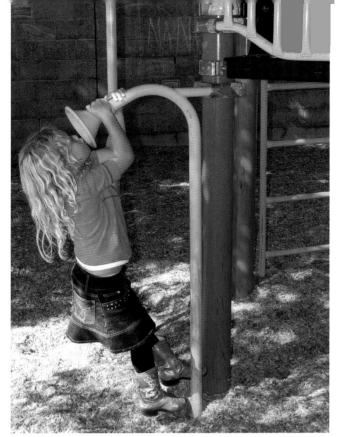

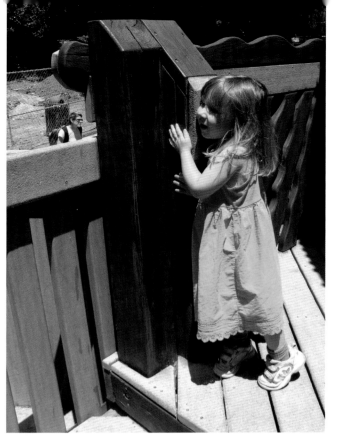

FIGURE 12.41 *The metal talk tubes at Rosa Parks School in Berkeley, California, were installed as part of a commercially produced play structure. Similar devices are widely available from many manufacturers.*

FIGURE 12.42 *The talk tubes at the community-built playground called F.R.O.G. Park in Oakland, California, are disguised within wooden boxes.[17]*

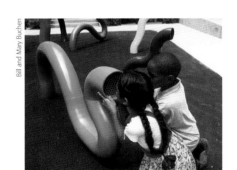

FIGURE 12.43 *An artful set of steel "telephone tubes" at Public School 244, by Bill and Mary Buchen, let children listen and speak to each other through interconnected, color-coded pipes that pass through the ground.*

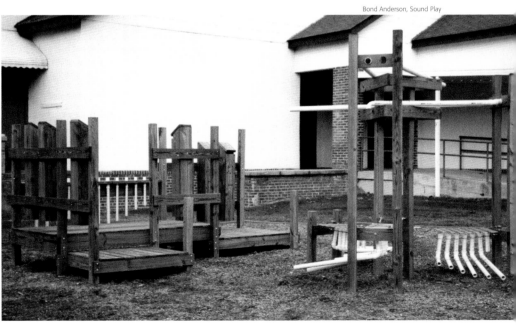

FIGURE 12.44

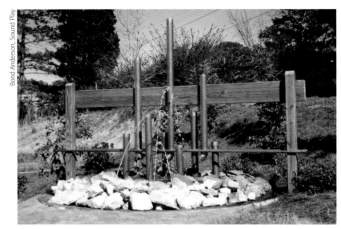
FIGURE 12.45 *This fountain turns wind and water into musical tones.*

An art piece that Sound Play designed for Oconee Regional Medical Center in Georgia translates the motion of the wind and the water in the fountain into musical tones. Some of the copper pipes act as flutes, making sounds when the wind blows over their open ends. Other pipes are capped and act as resonators, amplifying the sound of aluminum tone bars that are played by the fountain's water jets. (Figure 12.45)

Sound buffering to reduce nearby urban noises

Some school grounds receive more noise than they would like, either from nearby busy streets or simply from their own playgrounds filled with hundreds of children. When designing a green schoolyard, consider selecting areas of the grounds that are already the calmest spaces for activities that benefit from silence. Sound buffering and masking techniques also are useful for separating noisy areas from zones intended for quieter purposes.

Thick walls, made of sound absorbing materials such as earth or straw bales, dampen loud sounds. Dense structures made from stone or concrete can block sounds from traveling beyond their boundaries. Sturdy school building walls may dampen street noise, making interior courtyards ideal refuges for quiet outdoor classrooms and gardens. Walls or berms on the perimeter of a schoolyard will also dull noises from nearby traffic and make the yard quieter. (Figure 12.46)

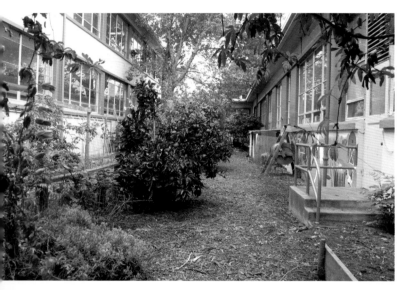

FIGURE 12.46 *LeConte Elementary School in Berkeley, California, has a serene courtyard garden, sheltered from the street by thick classroom walls on all sides.*

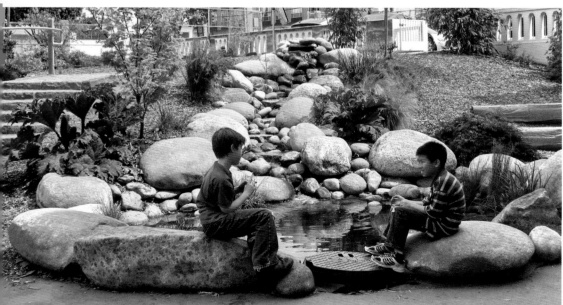

FIGURE 12.47 *The sloping terrain at Sherman School in San Francisco somewhat shelters the school's beautiful garden from the sounds of busy streets nearby. The splashing water in their two ponds also helps to mask urban noises and create a calm, quiet mood in the garden.*

PART 4 *Shaping Schoolyard Infrastructure to Create Comfortable, Effective and Memorable Places*

INTRODUCTION

Ecological schoolyards spring from the creativity of their school communities and reflect each school's unique needs for outdoor learning and play. The most effective examples are not only useful for academic lessons and recreation, but are also comfortable, well-organized, and memorable spaces that are a joy to spend time in. Their success depends on the effectiveness of the infrastructure—thoughtfully considered physical elements and systems that keep the yard running smoothly.

Most successful ecological schoolyards are arranged around a central core of permanent infrastructure that acts as a flexible framework for the schoolyard's site design. Once established, the site's infrastructure framework remains the same over the years, while the programming for the individual "outdoor rooms" within it shift as the school community's needs change over time. For example, an outdoor area that is originally designed as a vegetable garden can be easily converted to hold wildlife plantings, down the road, while the associated infrastructure of seating, irrigation, and pathways remains unchanged.

The ecological schoolyard infrastructure discussed in the book includes key features: a variety of options for outdoor seating areas; shelter from the sun and rain; pathways that direct movement throughout the site; low walls and ornamental fences to define the edges of each special place; tool sheds and other storage areas; and comprehensive signage that welcomes visitors and communicates the purpose of important features. Although topics such as irrigation systems, drainage networks to manage precipitation, electrical systems for night lighting, and maintenance roads or pathways are also important schoolyard infrastructure elements, they are beyond the scope of this book.

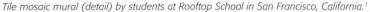

Tile mosaic mural (detail) by students at Rooftop School in San Francisco, California.[1]

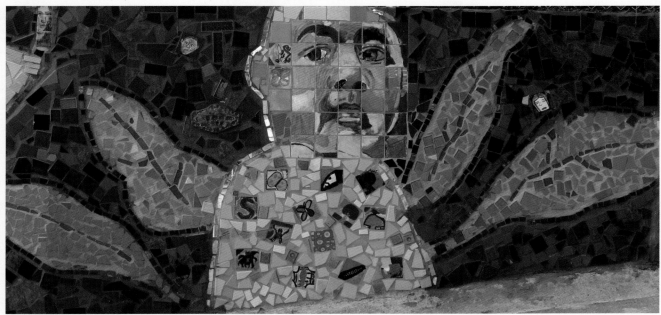

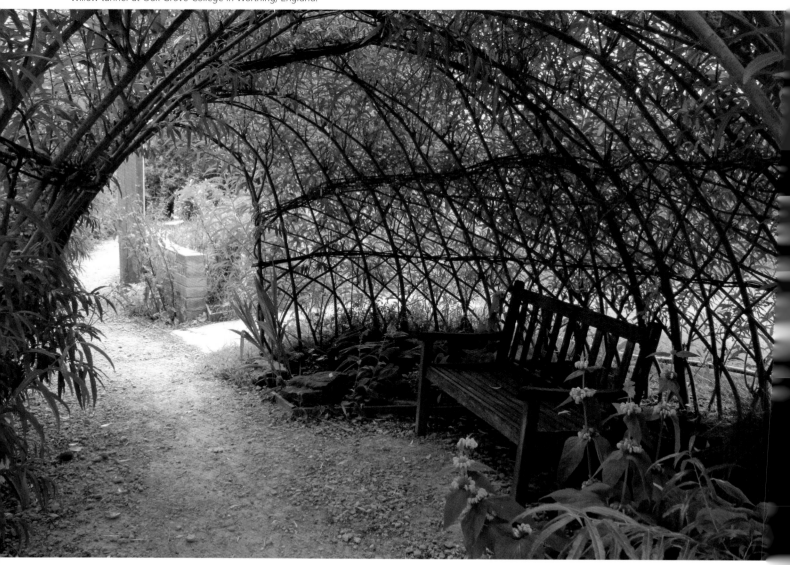

Willow tunnel at Oak Grove College in Worthing, England.

13 *Comfortable Schoolyards: Seating, Microclimates, and Protection from the Elements*

The asphalt playgrounds and grassy fields of most schoolyards are not particularly comfortable places; they offer little protection from sun, wind, and rain, and very little microclimate variation. Most have minimal seating, so students perch where they can, whether or not the space is comfortable or inviting.

Ecological schoolyards address these issues of physical comfort, while also making school grounds more useful for academic lessons and for fostering social interaction. Outdoor classrooms and seating areas of all different sizes enhance teaching and learning and provide inviting venues for class and recess activities. Green schoolyard design increases the diversity of microclimates onsite by providing shady areas as well as sunny ones—allowing students to find the places where they feel most comfortable each day as the weather patterns and seasons change. (Figure 13.1) Some schools also create outdoor rain shelters that allow classes to meet outside or children to play in fresh air, when the weather is not ideal. Some schools may also install a bubbling fountain to cool a warm space or a windbreak to shelter cool, breezy locations.

FIGURE 13.1 *This schoolyard at Jefferson School in San Francisco, California, includes varied microclimates, so students can choose to be in sunny or shady areas.*

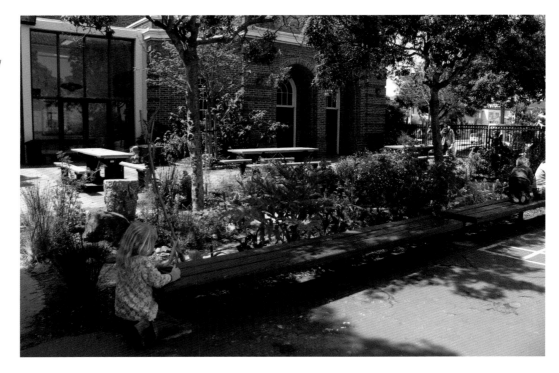

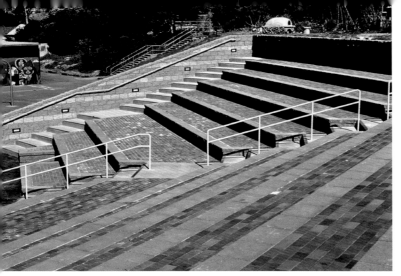

FIGURE 13.2 *Large outdoor amphitheater at Martin Luther King Jr. Middle School in Berkeley, California.*

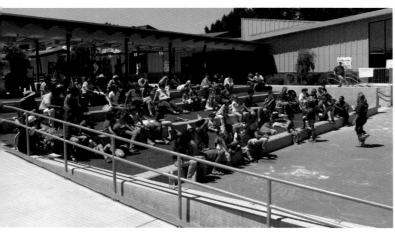

FIGURE 13.3 *The amphitheater at Prospect Sierra Elementary School in El Cerrito, California, creates a graceful transition between the upper portion of the grounds and a playground on its lower level. The wide, flat, artificial turf-covered terraces can seat the entire school—250 children and adults.*

🍃 *Outdoor Classroom Seating*

Outdoor classrooms are designated schoolyard gathering places. Teachers use them to bring their students together to work on academic lessons. Students use them informally at recess, and the school community also uses these areas after school and for special events.

The largest outdoor classrooms and amphitheaters are venues for performances and large assemblies—seating several classes at a time or even the entire school. Most schools find that they need at least one gathering place that can ac-

commodate thirty students, so an entire class can sit comfortably outside together. Equally important are small seating areas with tables, which encourage students to collaborate on projects and provide places for children to eat outdoors during nice weather. Some schools also scatter small seats and benches around the yard to promote relaxation and quiet reflection and to provide a place for individuals to work alone on their lessons.

The principal outdoor classroom space in a given schoolyard should be conveniently located close to the school building to make it easy for faculty members to bring their teaching materials outside. It should be protected from the wind and direct sunlight, so everyone will be comfortable when seated. Some schools nestle their outdoor classrooms under leafy trees, and others use shade or rain canopies to provide shelter. Gazebos and other open-walled structures lend a sense of enclosure to outdoor seating areas, making them feel inviting and special. Outdoor classrooms, like their indoor counterparts, should be wheelchair accessible and connected to pathways that comply with standards set by the Americans with Disabilities Act.

Commercially made benches are available, but there are also countless inexpensive and simple ways to build seating. Thick tree trunks can be cut into rounds to create individual, movable "chairs" or sliced in half lengthwise and laid on the ground as massive benches. Boulders from a local quarry, while not inexpensive, are very sturdy and easy to arrange into almost any seating configuration. Straw bales are useful, too, as inexpensive, temporary seats.

Experiment with temporary seating arrangements by using inexpensive materials, such as logs and straw bales, to determine the ideal seating configuration for a given site before committing to more expensive, permanent solutions. Sometimes schools find that they like the rustic feel of straw and wood and decide to use "temporary" materials on a permanent basis—replacing individual bales or logs as they decay over time.

Designed to reflect and enhance the overall atmosphere or theme of schoolyard spaces, seating areas reinforce their school's unique sense of place. For example, rustic building materials such as rough-hewn logs or boulders lend an informal, nature-oriented atmosphere to an outdoor learning space. Brick pavers, metal, and concrete, on the other hand, make the environment feel more formal and urban. Sculptural

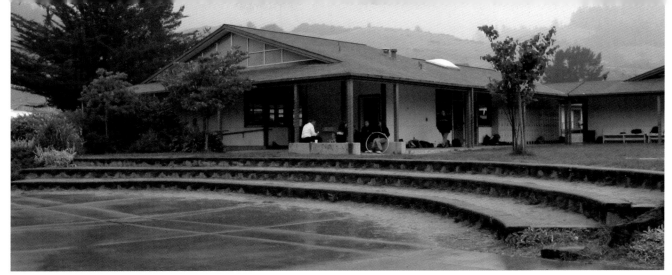

FIGURE 13.4 *The curving amphitheater at Lagunitas School in northern California is nestled in a gentle grade change near the classroom buildings. Parents used concrete blocks to construct it and filled the tiered seats with firmly-tamped decomposed granite (similar to course sand).*[1]

materials, such as cob (a mixture of clay, straw, and sand) and "earthbag benches" (filled with sand or soil), can be shaped by students into almost any form they imagine. (See chapter 8) A simple bench sculpted into a fairytale dragon, a school mascot, or a familiar animal transforms an ordinary schoolyard space into a memorable place.

Amphitheaters and other seating areas for large groups

Schoolyard seating areas vary greatly in cost, depending on the materials used and the design's complexity. Because they require a relatively large amount of space, amphitheaters should be worked into a schoolyard master plan early in the design process. It is important to position them for easy access to the school's entrances and exits along wheelchair accessible pathways, and to take advantage of local conditions onsite, such as topography and shade provided by mature trees.

Large seating areas: The large concrete amphitheater at Martin Luther King Jr. Middle School in Berkeley, California, was constructed along a steep hillside between the school's playground and garden. (Figure 13.2) The top seating tier is at the same level as the school's entrance and the bottom is flush with its lower playground. This wheelchair accessible amphitheater, built just before the school underwent a substantial renovation in 2001, served as the primary outdoor assembly space when the indoor facilities were under construction. It is now used for a variety of outdoor gatherings.

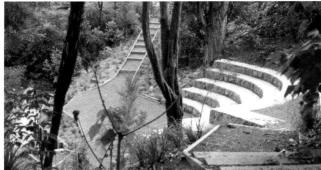

Mary Jackson

FIGURE 13.5 *This beautiful forest amphitheater at Meadowbank School in New Zealand takes advantage of a natural hillside and its inviting shady setting.*[2]

FIGURE 13.6 *This amphitheater at Ebchester Church of England School in Great Britain was carved directly into the hillside. The seats are planted with grass and the space between the tiers is the natural soil onsite.*

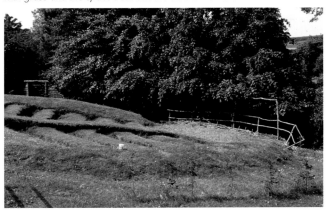

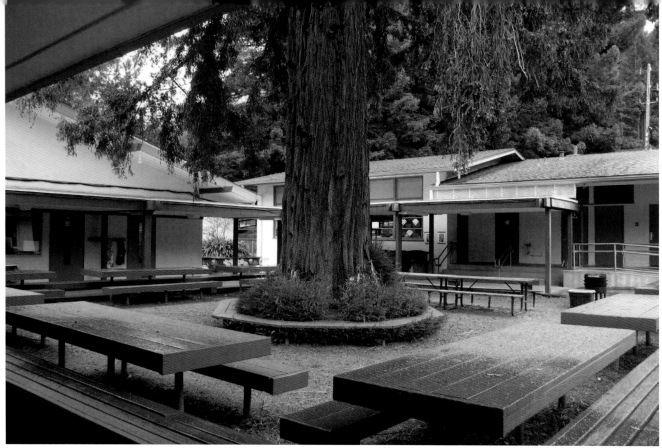

FIGURE 13.7 *At Bonny Doon School in Santa Cruz, California, a serene central seating area composed of large picnic tables is sheltered under a giant redwood tree. It serves as a gathering place for the school community, and can seat up to 100 people.*

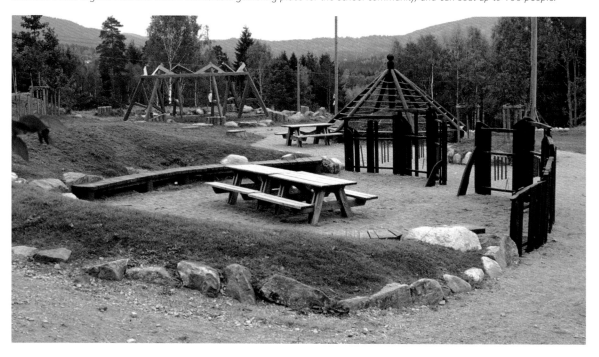

FIGURE 13.8
This hillside at Maridalen School was shaped to form a grassy amphitheater.

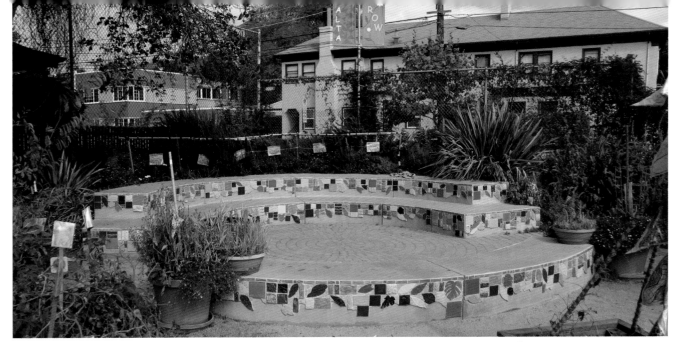

FIGURE 13.9 *This inviting amphitheater at Peralta Elementary School in Oakland, California, is composed of two wide, curving concrete tiers, topped by a built-in flower bed. Children created the hand painted tiles that brighten the surface.*[3]

Seating for several classes: Some schools find it useful to build smaller amphitheaters and gathering places that only seat a few classes at a time. These spaces are useful for small school assemblies, performances, and presentations, and are also comfortable places for individual classes to meet.

Maridalen School in Norway shaped a grassy hillside to act as an amphitheater and ringed the base of the hill with a wooden bench. The thoughtful design is a comfortable size for a few students, seated at the central picnic table, a single class, seated on the inner circle of benches, or for several classes, seated on the surrounding hill. A curving, hand-crafted fence completes the seating circle and defines the small amphitheater's "stage." (Figure 13.8 and 13.9)

Single-class seating

Space is at a premium in many schoolyards and there often isn't enough room to build an amphitheater. Most schools, however, have space for at least one outdoor instructional area that can seat 30 students, or a smaller space that can seat half a class. These seating areas may reflect the teachers' preferred instructional style—set up in a circle to encourage collaborative group discussions and eye contact among class members, or forward-facing to mimic a traditional indoor classroom, complete with a chalkboard. (Figures 13.10–13.12)

FIGURE 13.10 *Nyvång School used cut log rounds to create an inviting, rustic, outdoor classroom in a natural setting.*

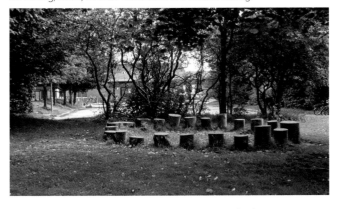

FIGURE 13.11 *Garden classes at Edna Maguire School in Mill Valley, California, sometimes meet in a simple seating circle made from painted pieces of concrete, sheltered by fruit trees.*

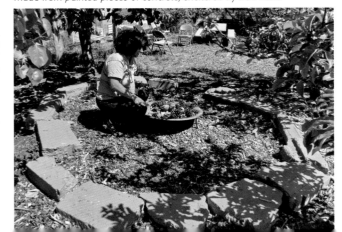

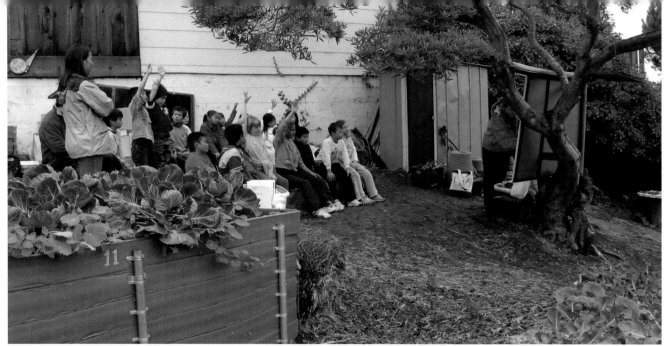

FIGURE 13.12 *The garden classroom at Alice Fong Yu Alternative School in San Francisco, California, has forward-facing seats and a white board at the front under a tree. The seats are made from unadorned straw bales, arranged in two rows, placed directly on the woodchip-covered ground. At the beginning of each school year, new bales are purchased to refresh the seats and the old bales become garden mulch.*

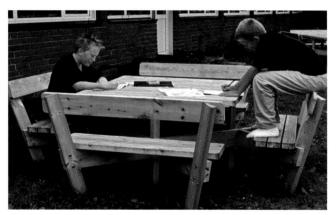

FIGURE 13.13 *Picnic tables, large and small, are good places for students to work on outdoor projects or to collaborate in small groups.*

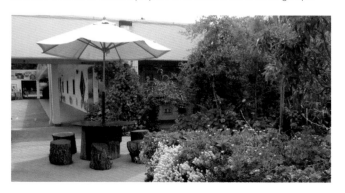

Seating areas for small groups

At many schools, outdoor lessons are carried out in small groups of 5–10 students. Cozy meeting spaces for these groups can be tucked in among school garden beds or comfortably placed under trees or shady trellises. They can take the form of story circles (See chapter 9), large benches, picnic tables, and other clustered seating arrangements.

Small seating areas. Students who work on academic lessons outdoors appreciate small seating areas, particularly if they include a table or similar surface that can be used for writing. It is helpful to include a range of seating choices so several groups of students can work independently. (Figures 13.13–13.15)

Pocket-sized seating areas. Informal seating areas, intended for 2–4 people, invite conversation among students or school staff members. A single bench located in a comfortable and in-

FIGURE 13.14 *This attractive table and chair set at Peralta School in Oakland, California, was made with an industrial cable spool for the table top and tree stumps for the table support and "chairs." An umbrella provides shade and makes the setting more inviting.*[4]

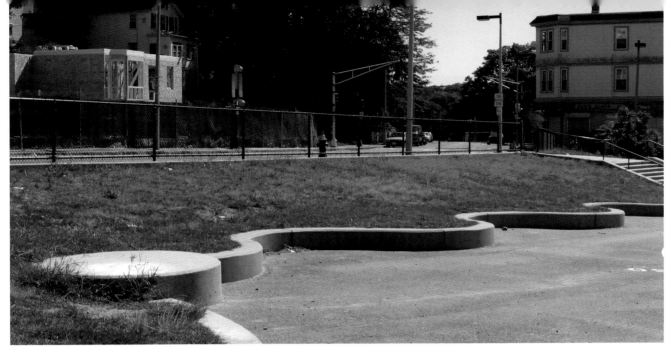

FIGURE 13.15 *An undulating concrete seat wall at Hennigan School in Jamaica Plain, Massachusetts, is punctuated by well-placed circular forms that serve as worktables or impromptu stages.*

viting place will serve this purpose—as will a loosely grouped collection of tree stumps, boulders, or benches. The smallest seat groupings fit nicely into peaceful, leafy corners or under arbors. (Figures 13.16–13.20)

FIGURES 13.16 and 13.17 *These seating nooks, made from clustered benches, invite small groups of children to gather for conversations with their friends. They are each positioned so the seated children can see the schoolyard and each other while they talk.* Cam Collyer

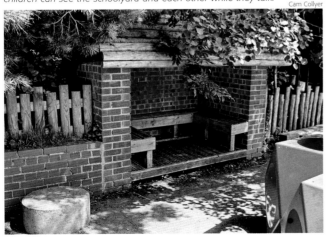

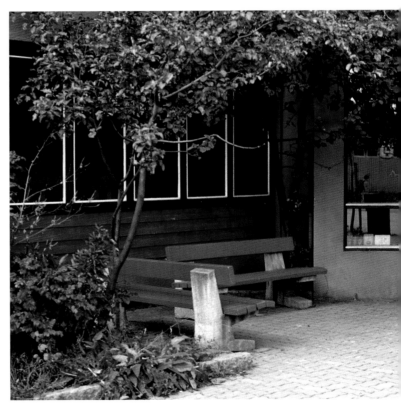

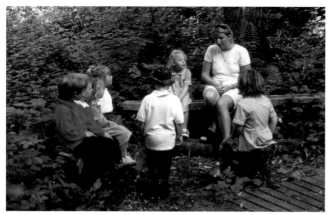

FIGURE 13.18 *This charming, rustic meeting space at Ebchester Church of England School is composed of two well-placed benches along the school's forested nature trail.*

FIGURE 13.20 *A playful flower-shaped, concrete seat wall doubles as a raised planter at Grattan Elementary School in San Francisco, California. The curving edge of the planting bed, built by the school community, creates inviting niches that beckon small groups of children to gather informally during recess. As the tree grows and its branches extend out farther, this space will become even more comfortable and welcoming.*

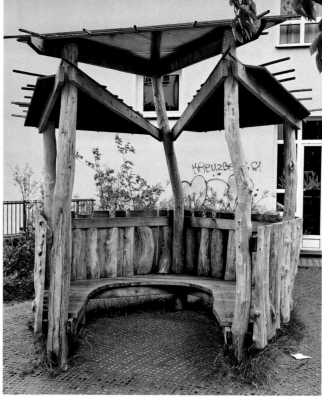

Cam Collyer

FIGURE 13.19 *The grounds at Galelei Primary School in Germany include this hand-crafted, cozy, wooden seating alcove that can accommodate a small group of children.*

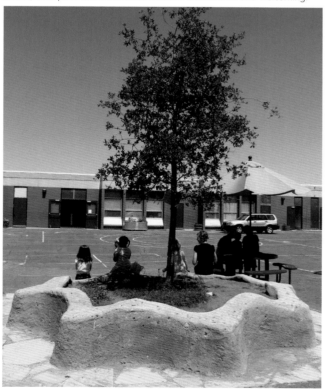

Whimsical seating

Sculpted creatures are "magnets" for children—and are almost guaranteed to inspire creativity within a school community. Mid-sized seating areas lend themselves well to sculptural forms, as do smaller benches. Some schools find local artists to help them create exciting benches— storybook characters, imaginary beasts, wild animals—and may involve the students in the building process. (Figures 13.21–13.24)

🍃 Outdoor Seating Areas that Promote Rest, Relaxation, and Remembrance During the School Day

Most American schoolyards are designed with wide open spaces, perfect for ball games and other types of lively activities that involve running, yelling, and exuberant play. While physical activity is something to encourage among today's sedentary student population, not every child feels equally comfortable in this type of play environment—and there are times when even

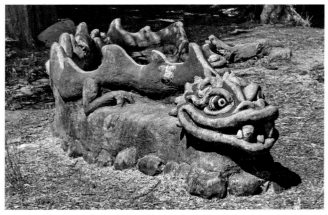

FIGURE 13.21 *With the help of teachers and a local artist, students at Salmon Creek School in Occidental, California, built a stunning cob bench in the shape of a dragon.*[5]

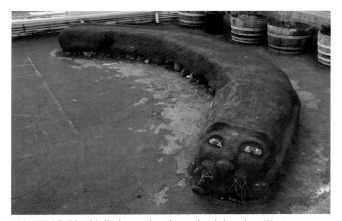

FIGURE 13.22 *This lively, panther-themed, cob bench at West Portal School in San Francisco, California, was created by school volunteers, with the help of a local non-profit organization.*[6]

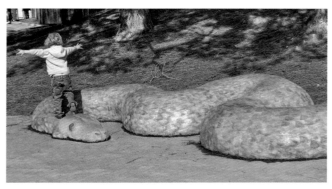

FIGURE 13.23 *The Oakland Zoo in California is home to a curving concrete snake bench, whose sinuous form invites passing children to use it as a balance beam. The graduated thickness of the snake's body results in a bench with varying heights, so both adults and children feel comfortable when seated.*

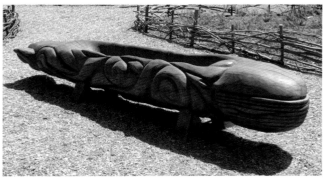

FIGURE 13.24 *This carved wooden bench at the Bay Area Discovery Museum in Sausalito, California, beckons children to climb into the open cavity and play imaginative games.*[7]

FIGURE 13.25 *A leafy arbor shelters a small bench at Cowick First School in England. Fragrant flowering vines cascade around it, providing a sense of privacy and calm within the busy schoolyard.*

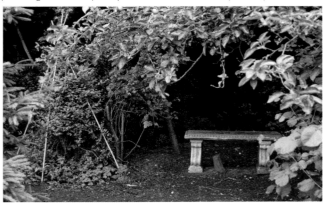

the most energetic child needs some quiet "down time" to recharge. Teachers, too, benefit from the addition of quiet refuges in schoolyard settings—places to relax while eating their lunch, supervising children, or preparing for a lesson.

Quiet zones

Creating a relaxing environment that allows a few moments of respite from a chaotic playground need not be complicated. The simplest quiet zones may be a comfortable chair or bench in a leafy garden space, somewhat off the beaten path or away from active play areas. (Figure 13.25)

Some schools have developed special school gardens specifically intended to promote reflection and allow peaceful activities. These spaces usually have comfortable seating, and they are often set apart from the rest of the yard in some way. Many of them also create a sense of enclosure through the judicious use of overhanging plants, arbors, and choice of location. (Figures 13.26 and 13.27)

Memorial gardens and other spaces for quiet reflection

Some schools commemorate the passing of a student, teacher, or class pet by planting a memorial garden. The somber tone of memorial gardens promotes quiet reflection and offers a place for rest and relaxation as well. (Figures 13.28–13.30)

🍃 Shelters for Outdoor Classrooms and Playground Spaces

Outdoor shelters enhance learning and play environments, enabling students to seek the most comfortable outdoor places as the weather changes. Year-round protection from the sun's rays is a priority for schools in many countries, who seek to

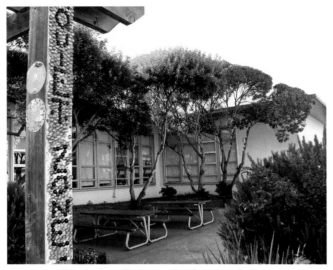

FIGURE 13.26 *The large "quiet zone" at the edge of Ulloa School's busy playground in San Francisco is filled with thriving plants and picnic table seating. Students and teachers who need a break from the fast paced action on the rest of the schoolyard step inside this peaceful garden to relax.*

FIGURE 13.27 *Peralta School in Oakland, California, removed a large portion of playground asphalt to create an area for nature play activities and gardening. This green space includes informal places for students to comfortably sit and talk, as well as garden beds for bug hunting and grass to run their fingers through.*[8]

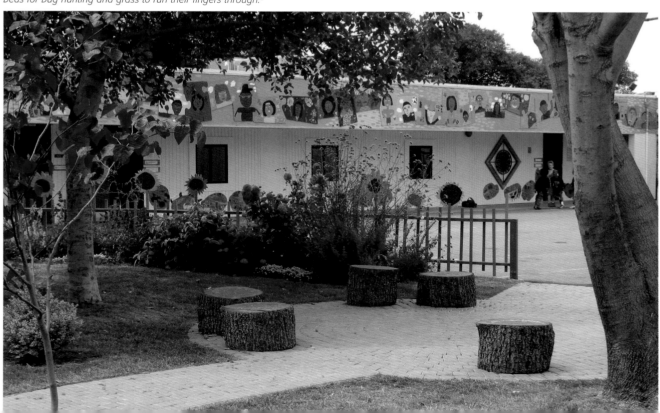

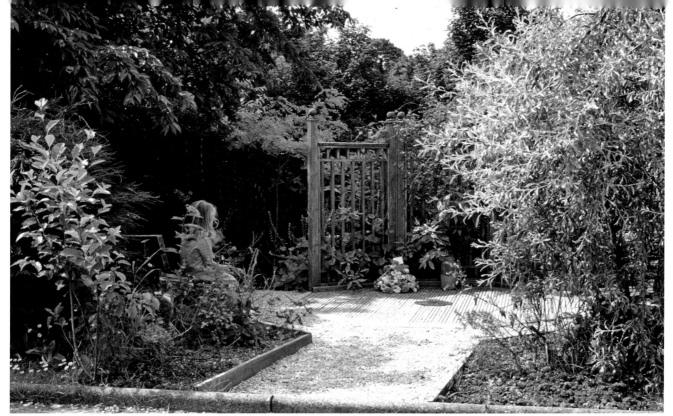

FIGURE 13.28 *This peaceful memorial garden at Ebchester Church of England School in England is a lovely place for quiet reflection and small group gatherings.*

FIGURE 13.29 *Leadgate Infant School planted a tree as a memorial to a student who died. The circular bench around the tree provides a restful seating area for the schoolyard, and also protects the young tree.*

FIGURE 13.30 *Tuna School in Sweden has a small, peaceful garden space dedicated to remembering class pets. This sign reads, "Hero Marcus," in honor of the class's pet rabbit.*

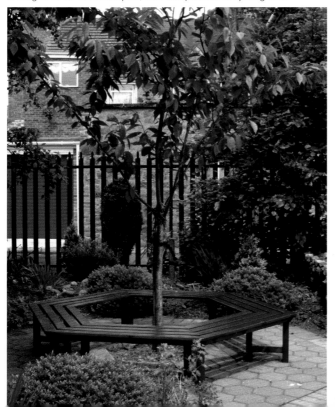

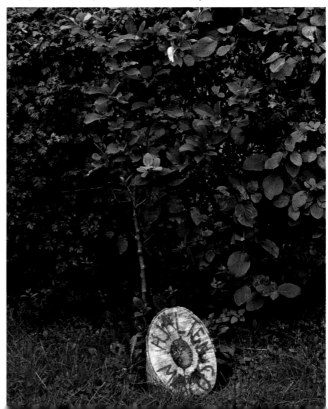

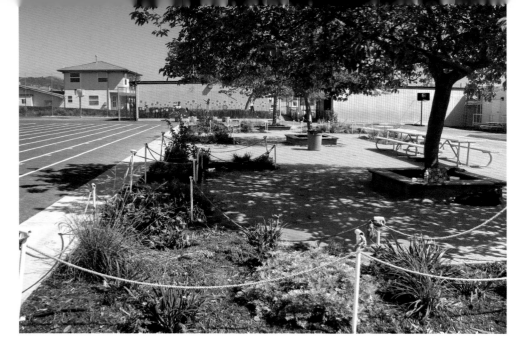

FIGURE 13.31 *This shady patio at Sequoia Elementary School in Oakland, California, includes mature, deciduous trees. Seat walls under the trees offer a cool retreat on warm days; sunny picnic tables offer a warmer environment on cooler days.*

shield their students from skin cancer risk. The simplest solution is to create more shade by planting trees with wide, leafy canopies. Trees take a long time to grow, however, and schools often need more immediate sun protection. To address this concern and improve comfort on hot days, some schools use shade structures over their seating and play areas. They range from simple, portable umbrellas to more elaborate, permanently installed canopies and roofs. The permanent shelters are also useful during rainy and even snowy weather.

Shade trees

Deciduous trees are particularly helpful in creating comfortable microclimates as they provide shade when it is warm and let the sun in during cooler months. (Figures 13.31 and 13.32)

FIGURE 13.32 *Brookside School in San Anselmo, California, shelters its outdoor classroom in deep shade provided by a small grove of redwood trees. This cooler location is particularly pleasant during hot spring and fall days.*

FIGURE 13.33 *Leadgate School in England uses portable shade umbrellas to cast shade around their picnic tables.*

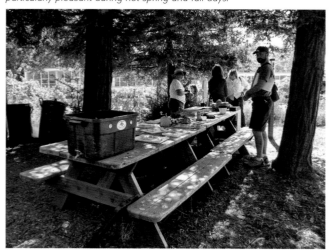

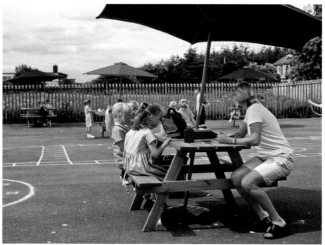

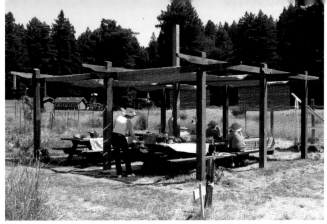

FIGURE 13.34 *Salmon Creek School has a large seating area with four picnic tables, sheltered by a permanent structure of heavy wooden beams. During warm spring and fall weather, the school hangs temporary bamboo screens on top of the canopy to cool the classroom space below.*

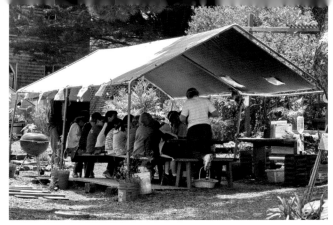

FIGURE 13.35 *Rooftop School in San Francisco, California, uses a lightweight canopy to shelter an outdoor teaching space from the sun and light rain. Shelters like this one are intended to be portable, but some are sturdy enough to leave in place for years if the weather is mild.*

Portable shade

In some climates, warm days alternate with cooler ones, making it useful to have movable shade canopies to shelter outdoor classroom spaces when needed. (Figures 13.33–13.35)

Open-sided gazebos

Airy gazebos are useful schoolyard amenities. Many have open walls and trellises overhead for growing vines or hanging shade cloths when needed. Vine-covered structures bathe the seating areas below in dappled light and light shade, adding variety to onsite microclimates. Gazebo structures are particularly comfortable and appealing because they offer both an inviting sense of enclosure and the ability to see and enjoy the surrounding landscape through the open walls. (Figures 13.36–13.38)

Some outdoor classroom shelters are made from permanent, solid roof materials that provide protection from both

FIGURE 13.36 *This small gazebo at Rosa Parks School in Berkeley, California, was built by parent volunteers. The redwood structure can accommodate ten elementary school students and gives the garden teacher a cozy place to assemble her class.*[9]

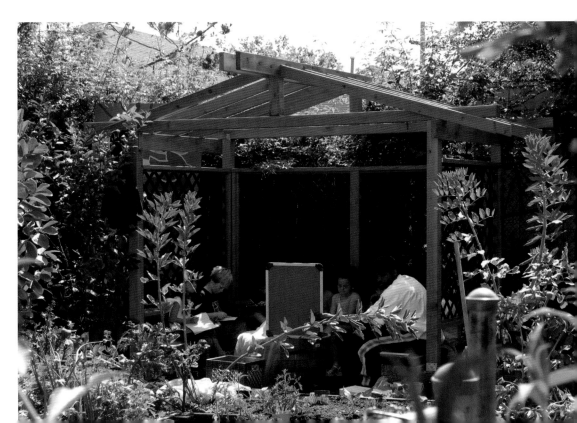

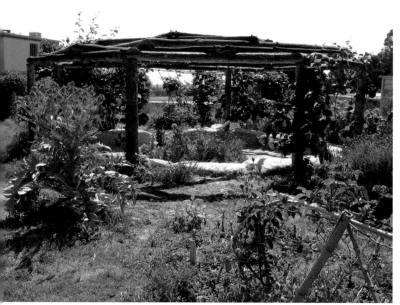

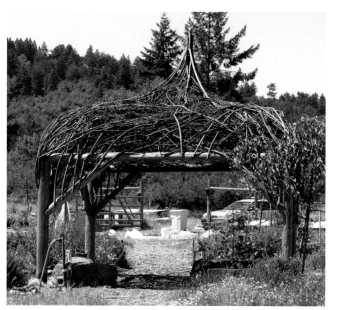

FIGURE 13.37 *In 2003 the Edible Schoolyard at Martin Luther King Jr. Middle School in Berkeley, California, built a "ramada" (gazebo) from heavy, round wooden beams. Its open walls and ceiling are lushly covered with vine crops including kiwis and squash, which create a comfortable sense of enclosure and dappled light.*

FIGURE 13.38 *This graceful domed gazebo inside the garden at Salmon Creek School shelters a ring of cob benches. Handcrafted by a local artist, the shade structure is supported by sturdy logs harvested from the school site. Its peaked top is woven from a collection of artfully arranged branches shaped to form a distinctive rounded roof with a pointed top.*[10]

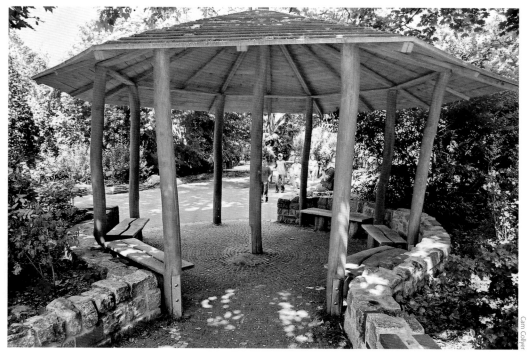

FIGURE 13.39 *This attractive, covered seating area is an asset to the school grounds at Neumark Primary School in Germany.*

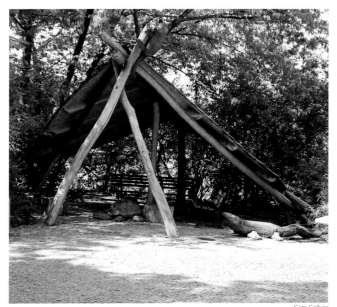

Cam Collyer

FIGURE 13.40 *This handcrafted, artful shelter on the grounds of Peter Joseph Lenné School in Germany has a peaked roof that protects several seats and benches.*[11]

sun and rain. In some climates, the sturdier structures may also shelter the seating areas from snow. (Figures 13.39 and 13.40)

Shade sails for sun protection

One of the fastest ways to produce a shady playground is to erect "shade sails" in places where students spend most of their time. Shade sails are typically made from durable cloth, metal, or plastic, and are attached to tall poles or building rooflines to cast shade onto the schoolyard's play or seating areas. Shade sails can significantly cool the schoolyard and they protect students from the harmful effects of intense sun exposure. (Figure 13.41)

The Jewish Community Center of the East Bay, in Berkeley, California, has a paved preschool playground in a large, interior courtyard. The concrete building, walls, and ground surface intensify heat in the yard when the sun is shining during the warmest months. To protect the young children from sunburns and high temperatures, the school hangs a large cloth shade sail across half of the courtyard when the weather begins to heat up around May, and keeps it there until the weather cools down in September. (Figure 13.42)

Mary Jackson

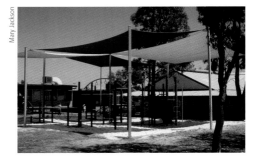

FIGURE 13.41 *Middle Swan Primary School in Australia erected a substantial permanent shade structure over their playground, supported by tall poles, to protect students from the sun and cool the surrounding area.*[12]

FIGURE 13.42 *A seasonal shade sail cools the preschool playground at the Jewish Community Center of the East Bay in Berkeley, California.*

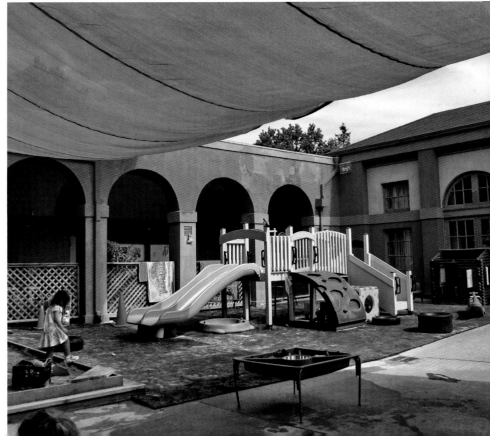

Rain shelters for outdoor classroom and play spaces

In some climates, it rains so frequently that it is often difficult to use outdoor spaces to their full potential without some protection from the rain. Schools in these areas sometimes build substantial, open-sided rain shelters that allow children to get fresh air and meet outside for classes, even during wet weather. (Figures 13.43–13.45)

🍃 Comfort is Key for Long-Term Enjoyment

Schoolyard comfort is a key factor that determines how frequently a green schoolyard will be used by teachers and how much it will be enjoyed by students during their lessons, recess,

and after school. Creating school ground environments with a range of microclimates, protection from the elements, and comfortable seating options will make them much more pleasant and inviting. With large amphitheaters and other gathering places, a school can expand its range of community-wide events and comfortably host school celebrations of many kinds. Smaller outdoor classroom spaces entice teachers to connect their curricula to the schoolyard and provide places for individuals and small groups to work on their assignments. The smallest seating areas give students and teachers a few precious moments to relax away from the hustle bustle of the yard. Providing a range of temperature options, from warm and sunny to cool and shady, protection from the wind, and shelter from the rain makes the yard more comfortable in every season.

Cam Collyer

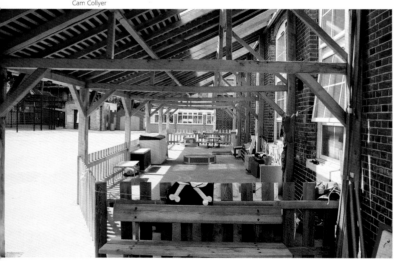

FIGURE 13.43 *A recent addition to the schoolyard at Ravenstone Primary School in England is a covered play area for young children, filled with toys, that connects directly to two classrooms. Translucent skylights let in some light, but the overhanging roof keeps most of it shady.*

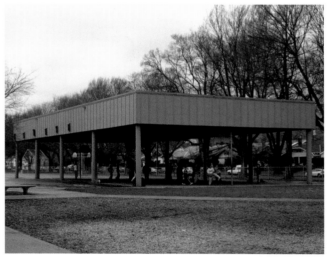

FIGURE 13.44 *Sunnyside Environmental School in Portland, Oregon has a sturdy rain and sun shelter over their basketball court to extend the usefulness of their playground.*[13]

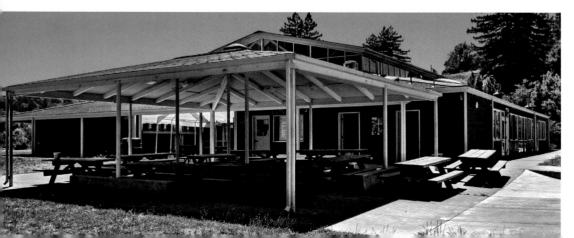

FIGURE 13.45 *The building's roof at Salmon Creek School in Occidental, California, extends over a large picnic table seating area, making the space much more comfortable when it is hot and sunny, or raining.*

14 *Form and Function:*
Key Design Considerations for Well-Organized Green Schoolyards

There is more to a good green schoolyard than a well-rounded list of programmatic features in a beautiful environment. For an ecological schoolyard to run smoothly and function well over time, it has to be arranged in a way that makes it enjoyable for learning and play *and* practical for daily use and maintenance. Well-designed green schoolyards take advantage of the entire school grounds through careful master planning, which allows exuberant ball games and quieter, creative and intellectual pursuits to coexist harmoniously. Successful ecological schoolyards use fences, seat walls, and other attractive structures to create clear boundaries between various uses onsite—and pathways to tie them all together. They also use signs, entry features, and other elements to communicate the purpose of each part of the grounds. This helps the school community to understand and appreciate the green schoolyard's mission, goals, and programming, so that it becomes part of the school's identity.

Defining Spaces and Separating Zones

During the schoolyard design process, many schools choose to create a series of "outdoor rooms," connected by pathways and separated by attractive buffers (walls, fences, or vegetation) that allow more activities to fit into the same space than were there previously. Each space becomes a unique destination, with its own environment, range of activities, and intensity of use that are different from adjacent zones.

Ravenstone Primary School in England, for example, separates active play areas from quieter garden spaces with screens of trees, planters, and low fences that indicate where balls may be thrown and where other activities will take place. The school's edible garden is separated from a lawn by a path and small wooden fence. The lawn, in turn, is separated from the paved playground by a partial screen of trees. (Figure 14.1)

FIGURE 14.1
Ravenstone Primary School in England uses separate zones for different playground functions.

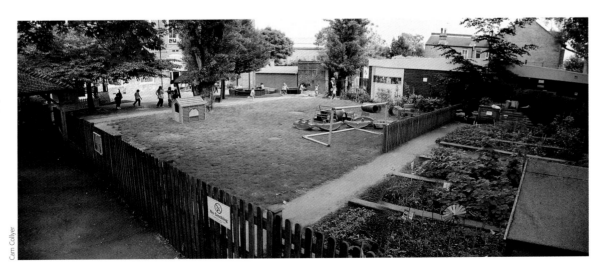

Cam Collyer

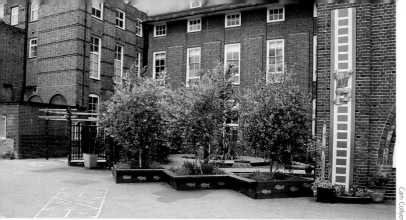

FIGURE 14.2 *The Peace Garden at Ravenstone Primary is separated from the playground's ball play area by a row of trees in bright planter boxes. This visual barrier marks the transition from one space to the other, reminding children to keep the balls out of the garden. The light screen of trees also provides shade and allows visibility between the two spaces.*

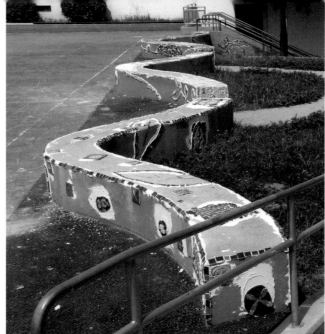

FIGURE 14.3 *A low wall separates two parts of the schoolyard.*

Low walls and fences define boundaries

Low walls, picket fences, and other park-like features are used in green schoolyards to clearly define the edges of each use zone and to make their boundaries easier for children to see as they play.

Some low walls are designed as seats to encourage informal, small group gatherings, and others form the edges of raised garden beds. For example, the undulating concrete seat wall at Bret Harte School in San Francisco, California, visually separates the paved playground from a downward sloping hillside garden. The curving wall is an inviting place for small groups to gather and has become a canvas for an elaborate tile mosaic mural (shown during installation). (Figure 14.3) Horace Mann School in Washington, DC, uses an undulating stone wall to keep balls and running games out of their garden and to clearly define the edges of each space. (Figure 14.4)

FIGURE 14.4

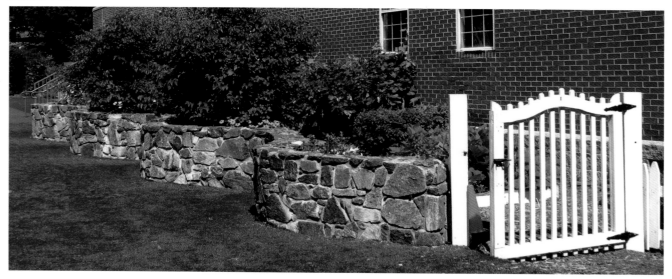

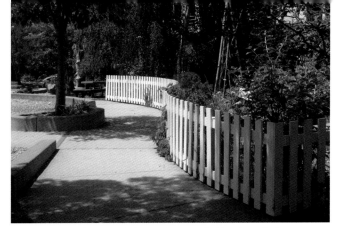

FIGURE 14.5 *The meandering pathway and picket fence help to divide adjacent uses and direct foot traffic through the schoolyard.*

Low fences are also practical solutions for separating schoolyard activity zones. A curving picket fence at Tule Elk Park Child Development Center in San Francisco, California, divides the edible garden from an adjacent tricycle path and play area. (Figure 14.5) The fence creates a clear physical and visual boundary that keeps the young children from inadvertently trampling the garden, but does not disrupt socializing on the playground. Children on each side of the low fence talk to each other as they play.[1]

Fences are sometimes vital to the survival of new plantings on a busy schoolyard because they direct foot-traffic away from sensitive areas as they get established. At Rosa Parks School in Berkeley, California, for example, I worked with the green schoolyard committee to establish plantings in an open area next to the playground. Without a fence, most of the small plants were accidently trampled by vigorous games. (Figure 14.6) After we built a low fence around the space, the plants in the new "nibbling garden" thrived. (Figure 14.7) The fence also turned the space into a destination, giving children another activity "room" at recess. Children now seek out the lemony sorrel, raspberries, and other edibles planted here and have incorporated them into their imaginative games. A kindergarten class created the cheerful sunflowers that adorn the fence.[2]

Pathways direct movement throughout the yard

Schoolyard pathways serve an important role in shaping the school community's experience of the grounds and in directing their movement through and around the site. The design of pathways, and choices made about their form, direction, and materials, subtly influences how the schoolyard will be used.

In traditional schoolyards that are entirely open and paved, the potential paths of travel are infinite, and students can generally see from one side of the yard to the other without many obstructions. This means that "over there" is almost exactly like "over here" so there is little reason for students to bother traveling from one part of the yard to another—despite the ease of movement.

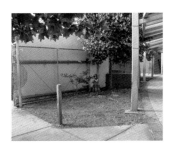

FIGURE 14.6 and 14.7 *A picket fence helps to keep balls out of the schoolyard garden so the plants do not get trampled.*

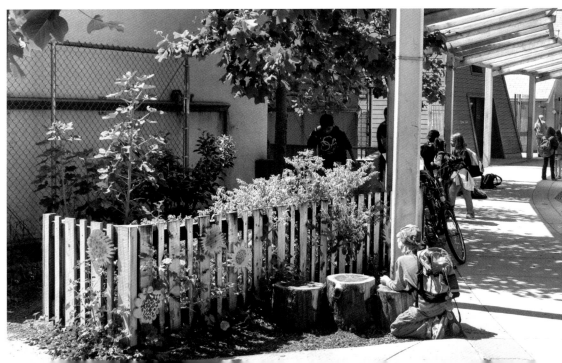

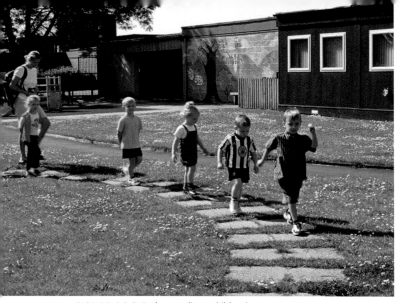

FIGURE 14.8 *Pathways direct children's movement through the schoolyard and influence their behavior.*

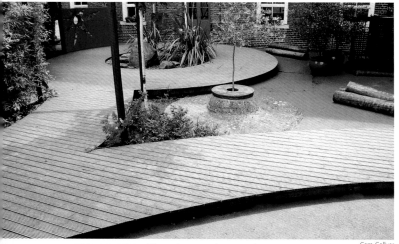

Cam Collyer

FIGURE 14.9 *This pathway makes traveling through school grounds more interesting.*

By contrast, pathways in a green schoolyard *reduce* the potential paths of travel to a relatively small number of interesting and intersecting routes, leading children from one place to another and suggesting places to explore. A path might take them around an interesting corner, over a bridge, through a "forest" and into a sandbox or other intriguing place. Each route should beckon pedestrians to travel its course to see where it leads. Some of the pathways will have clear destinations, while others may be a bit more mysterious with twists and turns that add adventure and fun, making the process of

traveling the path, itself, an activity. (See schoolyard mazes in chapter 10 for more path-traveling ideas.) (Figure 14.8)

Pathway structure. Ideally, pathway networks include both wide primary routes and narrower secondary trails. The primary pathways connect all of the key features—outdoor classrooms and other special points of interest—to the school's main entrances, using wheelchair accessible formats that comply with national standards. These pathways are also useful for children in strollers, for maintenance staff using wheelbarrows, and for moving garden supplies and materials around the site. Primary pathways do not have to be boring and straight—they can curve around corners, climb low hills, pass through archways and arbors, and be constructed from interesting materials. (Figure 14.9)

For wheelchair users, interesting primary pathways may replace ordinary ramps to help them navigate a grade change and have an enjoyable schoolyard experience at the same time. At Alvarado School in San Francisco, California, for example, the main zigzagging pathway through the garden is also intended as a wheelchair accessible ramp that travels from the upper playground to a lower yard. (see chapter 10, Figure 10.40) The main pathway through Sherman School's green schoolyard is also intended as a wheelchair accessible route from the parking lot to the building. (See chapter 5, Figure 5.13)

A secondary network of pathways—varying greatly in form, texture, and material—provides alternative routes to the same schoolyard destinations and may shape children's experiences of the grounds in even more playful ways. For example, pathways with stepping stones encourage children to jump or hop along their length rather than walk. Paths with logs or narrow curbs on each side encourage kids to experiment with balance as they walk. Unusual or natural paving materials—tree rounds, flagstones, multicolored pavers, mosaics, patterned concrete—add texture and color that further enrich the traveler's experience on a particular route. Some schools allow their students to make their own narrow pathways through plantings onsite. Such free-form pathways, off the main trail network, are often among the children's favorites. (Figure 14.10)

Path design shapes experiences. Winding pathways add a sense of mystery and adventure to a schoolyard experience. This is particularly true if they curve in and out of plantings or go

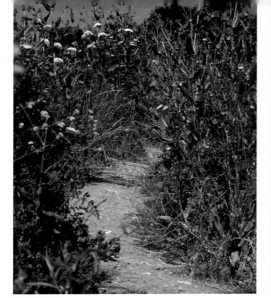

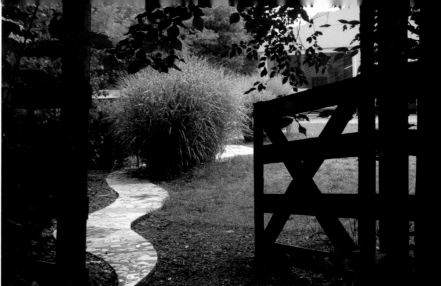

FIGURE 14.10 *This path through the schoolyard "wilderness" was rubbed into the soil by the passage of many pairs of feet.*

FIGURE 14.11 *This winding pathway adds a sense of mystery to the children's play space.*

through tunnels or around features in the yard. If the destination can't be easily seen from the beginning of a path, it will be more fun to get there. (Figure 14.11) Some schools add routes around the perimeter of their schoolyard to lengthen the potential journey for children who enjoy walking on a trail, and to encourage the school community to use the grounds—all the way to the edges. Pathways that travel up and over hills give children an elevated perspective on their schoolyard. Some paths might also provide access to places that would otherwise be inaccessible or hard to reach—such as paths across ponds that give students an opportunity to observe pond life up close. (Figure 14.12)

FIGURE 14.12
This bridge over the water allows children to closely observe the pond life at Sagano Elementary School in Kyoto, Japan.

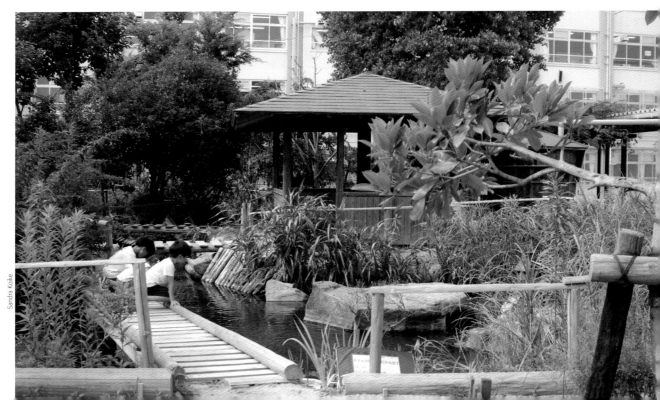

Sandra Koike

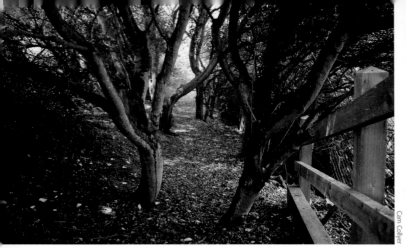

Cam Collyer

FIGURE 14.13 *The onsite forest at the Coombes School in England.*

Child-sized pathways are used to make young children feel more comfortable on school grounds. The Coombes School in England purposely plants some of their trees very close together so that students can easily squeeze between them along a pathway, but adults have to move carefully and bend down to enter their world.[3] (Figure 14.13)

Path design influences behavior. Pathways may be designed as tools that gently guide students toward appropriate behavior by shaping their direction of travel and using path width, form, and texture to influence their speed. At Tokiwano School in Japan, a central pathway edged with small wooden posts and rope shows students where they should walk in order to avoid stepping on sensitive plants. (Figure 14.14) Another pathway made of blue mats shows students where to store their shoes before they enter the classroom building. This slightly raised walkway also stays drier in wet weather and keeps indoor slippers clean after students remove their outdoor shoes. (Figure 14.15)

Narrow pathways, which require children to walk single file, also bring them into close contact with plantings and other elements along the route, so they can observe them closely. Wide paths allow groups of children to move through a space together and interact as they walk.

Thresholds signal transitions and celebrate arrival into special places.

In some schoolyards, movement along the pathway network is punctuated by a series of thresholds that the school community passes through as they enter the school building or make their way around the grounds. These transition points, in the

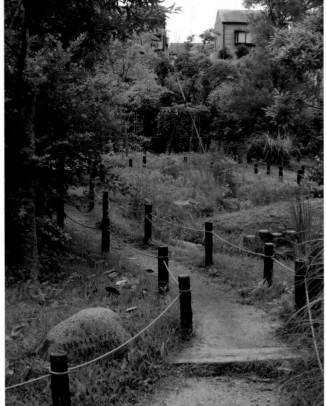

FIGURE 14.14

Sandra Koike

FIGURE 14.15

Sandra Koike

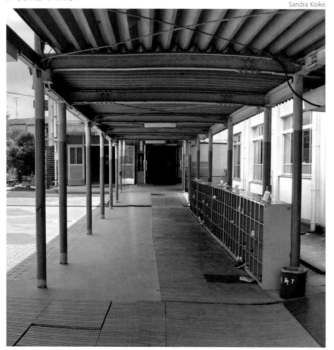

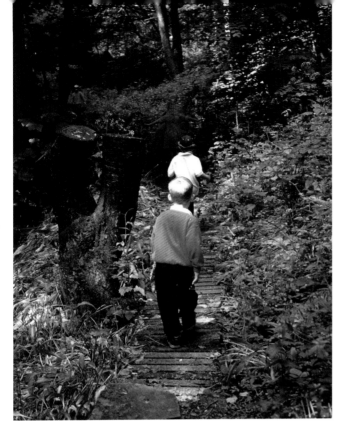

FIGURE 14.16 *Narrow schoolyard trails bring students into close contact with nature on all sides.*

FIGURE 14.17 *This pathway across a pond has low railings for most of its length and no railing closer to shore, which permits students to reach down to touch the water's surface where the pond is shallow.*

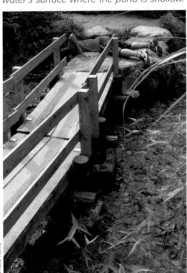

FIGURE 14.18

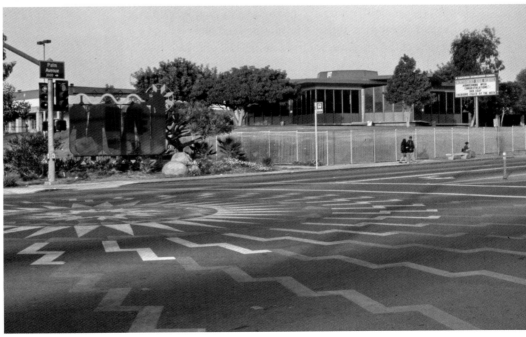

form of entryways, gates, arbors, artful archways or murals, not only can be made from many materials including wood, metal, and living plants, but can also serve as canvases for students' artwork.

Main entrances. Entrances to the school building are often the most prominent transition points on the grounds. Their form and design sets the tone for the surrounding spaces both inside and outside the building, helping to define and convey a unique sense of place. Some schools incorporate themes on their main entrances that speak about community values and local culture or inform visitors about what they will find onsite.

The dramatic artwork at the entrance to Montgomery High School in San Diego, California, reflects cultural themes related to Mexico, which is only five miles away. Designed by students, a pair of 15-foot-tall metal serpents guard the entrance to the student parking lot and watch over an intersection with festively painted geometric designs reminiscent of Central American artwork. (Figure 14.18)

Brightly colored, exuberant murals made from painted wood cutouts adorn Peralta School in Oakland, California, welcoming visitors at every major entrance. The murals were

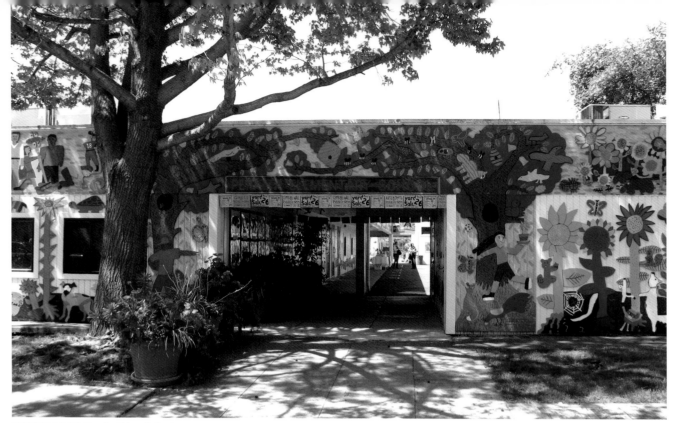

FIGURE 14.19 *Peralta School's lively entrance.*

created by a local artist over the last decade in collaboration with students and the school community.[4] An extensive, nature-themed mural surrounds a side entrance and gives visitors a preview of the vibrant schoolyard onsite. (Figure 14.19)

Schoolyard transitions. Special entryways, arbors and archways mark distinct zones in a schoolyard and set the theme and mood. Some archways frame a special view or entrance, while others convey information about the purpose of the space within. (Figures 14.20–14.23)

Gates. Many entryways have gates that can be opened and closed to shape the "traffic flow" patterns within the school-yard. This allows school staff to restrict children's access to different parts of the yard when needed. Gates like this one near a pond at Suzakudaisan Elementary School in Japan alert students that the environment they are entering requires their attention. (Figure 14.24)

Some gates are designed to more subtly shift students' behavior before they enter a zone that requires special care.

FIGURE 14.20 *This leafy, arched entryway at Edna Maguire School in Mill Valley, California, frames a view of the extensive edible garden beyond the threshold.*

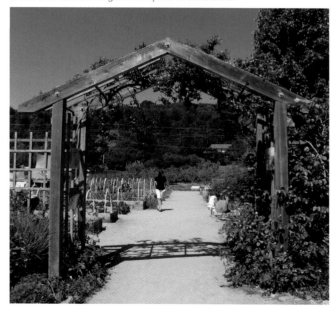

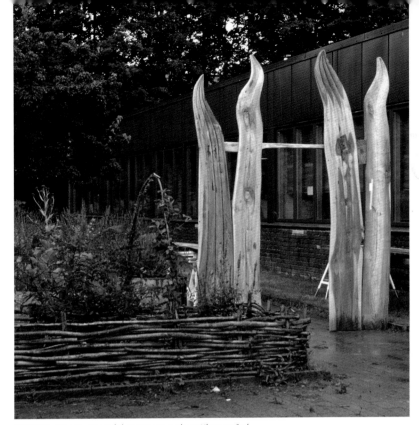

FIGURE 14.21 *An artful entrance arch at Klostergård School in Sweden welcomes visitors to the school garden.*

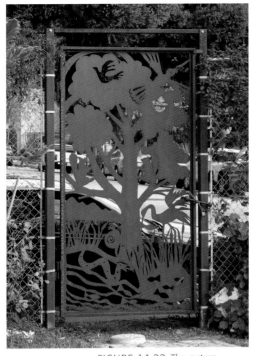

FIGURE 14.22 *The nature-themed steel gate at Peralta School in Oakland, California, was designed collaboratively by two fifth graders and two local artists.*[5]

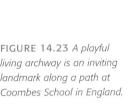

FIGURE 14.23 *A playful living archway is an inviting landmark along a path at Coombes School in England.*

FIGURE 14.24 *Suzakudaisan Elementary School in Kyoto, Japan.*

Sandra Koike

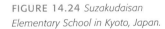

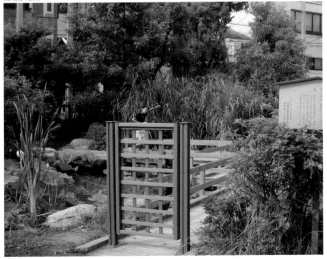

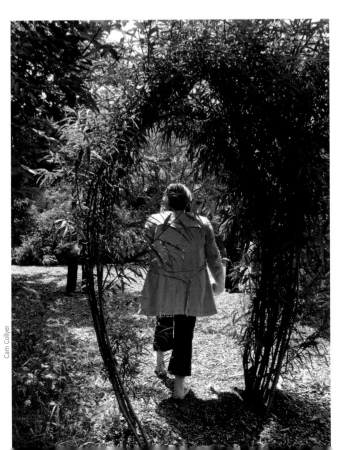

Cam Collyer

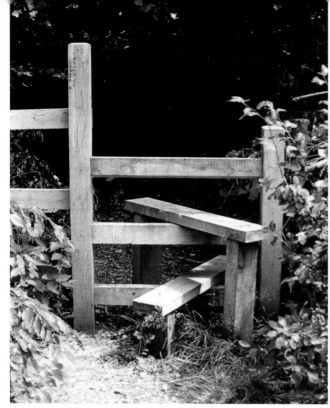

FIGURE 14.25 *This gate is designed to slow down foot traffic.*

FIGURE 14.26 *Boulders are used at this Swedish school to slow pedestrians.*

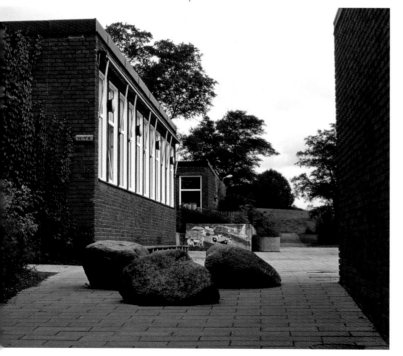

In these cases, gates function as obstacles that require some interaction before students pass through at a more measured pace. St. Paulinus School in England has some "slow" gates along its schoolyard nature trails, designed to require climbing to ensure that everyone who enters the forest is moving at a leisurely pace. This sets the tone for calmer behavior in the forest than on the nearby playfields. (Figure 14.25) Nyvång School in Sweden placed boulders in the middle of a central pathway to encourage students to slow down as they enter and exit the schoolyard. (Figure 14.26) In the United States, laws requiring wheelchair access would make these designs difficult to implement exactly as they are, but the slow gate concept is valuable and can surely be made wheelchair accessible by creative school communities.

Using Signs to Enhance Schoolyard Communication

Because they depend on community involvement, coordination, and enthusiasm, green schoolyards benefit greatly from clear communication. Adding signs to the schoolyard is one way to keep students, teachers, and family members all in the loop about the goals and latest projects for the yard. Signs also help to convey the school's values and philosophy, and they are used to request assistance and cooperation in taking care of sensitive parts of the site.

Welcome signs

Many schools use signs to welcome visitors to their green schoolyard or garden. Like entry arches, welcome signs help to provide a sense of "arrival" to a schoolyard destination. (Figure 14.27)

Signs to explain project history and current events

Schools often use signs in and around the schoolyard to inform visitors and the ever-changing school community of the project's history and purpose. For example, a detailed sign outside the main entrance to Tule Elk Park Child Development Center in San Francisco, California, explains how the project came about and shows dramatic "before" and "after" photographs. (Figure 14.28)

Some schools install bulletin boards to convey current information about the school grounds, and refresh them regularly.

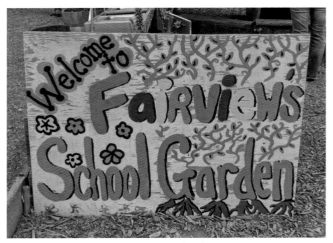

FIGURE 14.27 *A cheerful, hand-painted welcome sign at Fairview School in Oakland, California.*

FIGURE 14.28 *This sign explains the schoolyard's evolution over the years.*

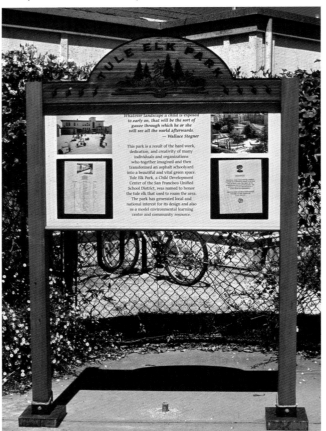

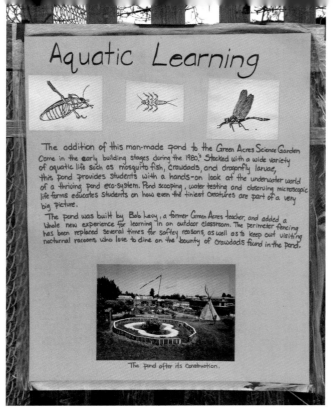

FIGURE 14.29 *This sign at Green Acres Elementary School in Santa Cruz, California, explains how their pond and its curriculum connections have developed over the last thirty years.*

FIGURE 14.30 *The plaque at Ossington/Old Orchard Junior Public School in Ontario, Canada, gives an overview of the school's 20-year history of replacing asphalt with plantings, and asks the community to help take care of the site.*

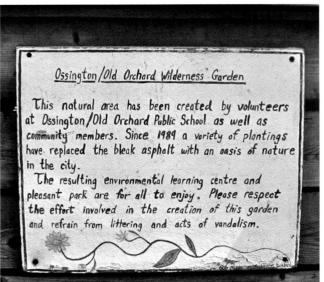

Chapter 14: Form and Function **223**

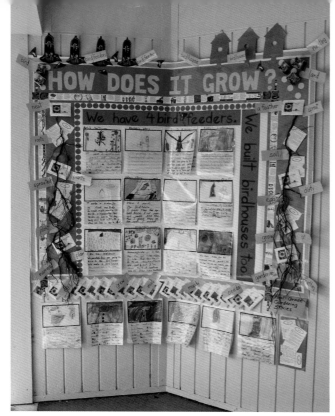

These boards typically describe the newest work in the schoolyard and examples of students' related artwork and writing projects. Most bulletin boards are located outdoors in a protected location or indoors in a central hallway.

Outdoor bulletin boards at Peralta School in Oakland, California, are sheltered by a covered walkway. When I visited in January 2004, one bulletin board displayed students' written reports and drawings about birds and birdhouses (shown, Figure 14.31), and another focused on a first grade study and planting of indigo.

Sunset School in San Francisco, California, uses an indoor bulletin board to display information about its garden. The board changes over time and includes photographs, newspaper articles, student projects, and other related information to share with the school community. (Figure 14.32)

Interpretive signs

Interpretive schoolyard signs serve several purposes: they might explain a specific project or interesting activity in detail or clarify the use of each activity zone. Describing a project's

FIGURES 14.31 and 14.32 *Bulletin boards are useful for sharing information with the school community.*

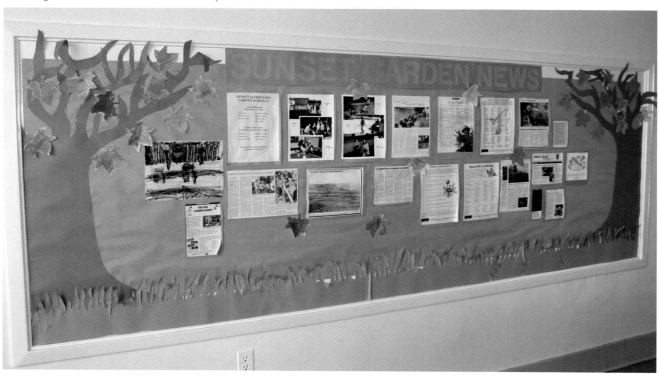

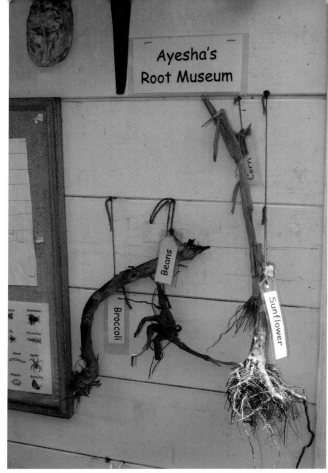

FIGURE 14.33 *Interpretive signs are useful for explaining special schoolyard features.*

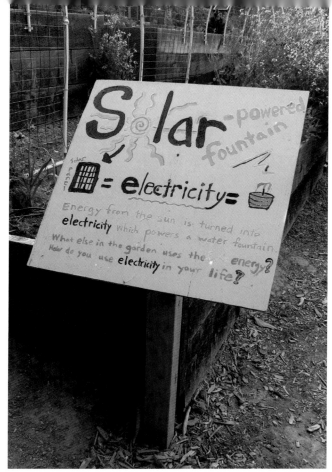

FIGURE 14.34 *Thoughtful interpretive signs throughout the garden at Fairview Elementary School in Oakland, California, explain such elements as the onsite compost bins, greywater system, and plant names. This sign describes the school's portable solar powered fountain.*

FIGURE 14.35 *This sign identifies a portion of the garden used for scientific study at Cobb Elementary School in San Francisco, California.*

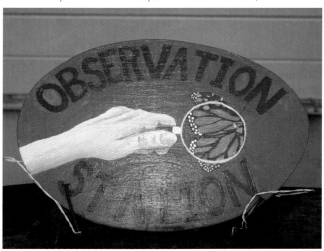

purpose and labeling its key features may not only avoid misunderstandings, but may also help the school community feel included in whatever activities are occurring onsite.

The extensive garden at Tule Elk Park Child Development Center in San Francisco, California, includes a wall-mounted "root museum," developed by garden instructor Ayesha Ercelawn. Ercelawn's tags on each root specimen identify the plant so students and other garden visitors will understand more about what goes on below the soil. (Figure 14.33)

Signs to convey the school's philosophy

Some schools infuse their green schoolyards with inspirational quotations or phrases that express their philosophy and promote good character. Harvey Milk Civil Rights Academy in San Francisco, California, has a vibrant mural that displays the pledge—to be environmentally and socially responsible

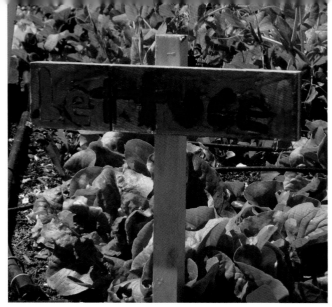

FIGURE 14.36 *Many school gardens use signs like this one to label food crops.*

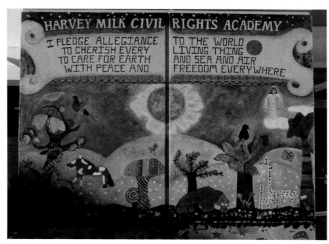

FIGURES 14.37 and 14.38 *Signs can be used to convey the school's philosophy.*

Cam Collyer

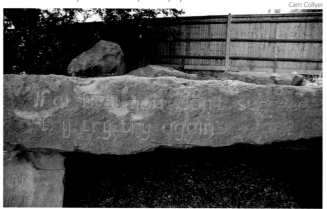

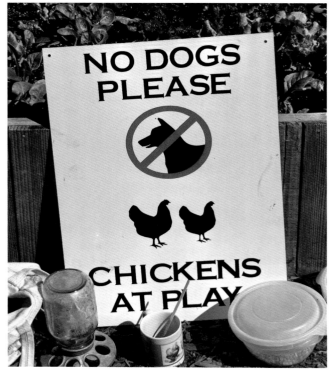

FIGURE 14.39 *This sign protects a schoolyard chicken coop.*

FIGURE 14.40 *The garden at Hennigan School in Jamaica Plain, Massachusetts, uses signs in English and Spanish to explain their policy about sharing garden produce and to request that the community help the school protect the children's gardening efforts.*

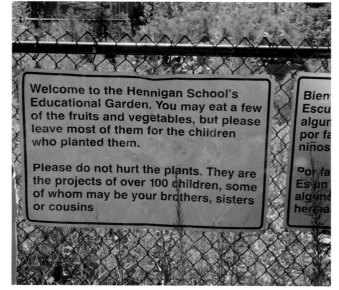

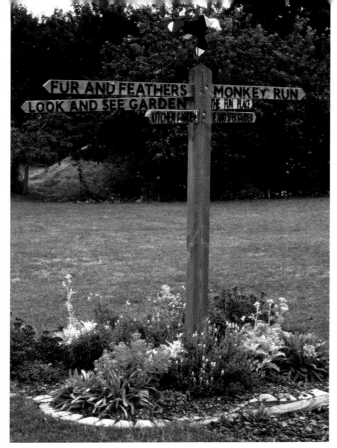

FIGURE 14.41 *This sign post at Cowick First School in England points to many of the schoolyard's important features.*

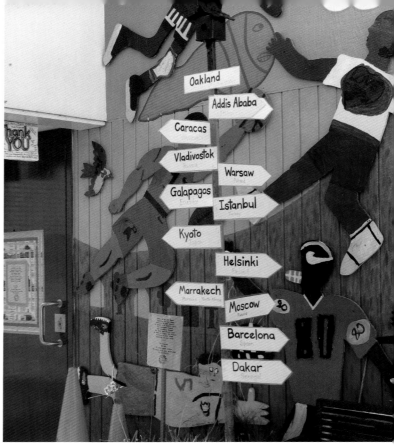

FIGURE 14.42 *Peralta School approaches the topic of giving directions with a bit of humor and a geography lesson. The signpost points out the general directions for many places that are far away from this Oakland, California school.*

people—that students say daily.[6] (Figure 14.37) Coombes School in England engraves small messages on stones throughout their grounds to inspire children and adults. One saying inscribed on a stone playhouse reads, "If at first you don't succeed, try, try, again." (Figure 14.38) Another phrase carved into reused slate asserts "We care for each other."

Signs that request assistance or give directions

Schoolyard signs may communicate directly with the school community to give instructions or directions, describe expected behavior, or request assistance with the schoolyard. (Figures 14.39–14.42)

🍃 Storage and Maintenance Facilities

Unlike indoor spaces, schoolyard environments don't usually come with closets—yet outdoor classrooms, like their indoor counterparts, require storage and other maintenance-related features that help staff run them more smoothly.

To meet their need for secure outdoor storage, most active green schoolyard programs have at least one schoolyard tool shed so they can keep their tools and supplies easily available. Tool sheds are stocked with all manner of gardening hand tools, from shovels and trowels to rakes, hoes, clippers and pruning shears. Also advisable are at least one hand saw for trimming branches, hammers and nails, screwdrivers and screws, a hand drill, and other equipment that can be used for making small repairs. Many schools also stock sets of garden gloves and boots for students who like to protect their hands and feet from mud. All gardens also need hoses and watering cans, plant pots and seeds, and other basic items. If budget and storage space allow, it is a good idea to stock duplicate tools in varying sizes so that children can use smaller shovels and clippers during class time and recess, and adults have access to larger, more powerful tools

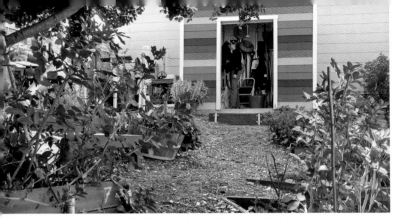

FIGURE 14.43 *The tool shed at Alice Fong Yu School in San Francisco is a brightly colored garden feature.*

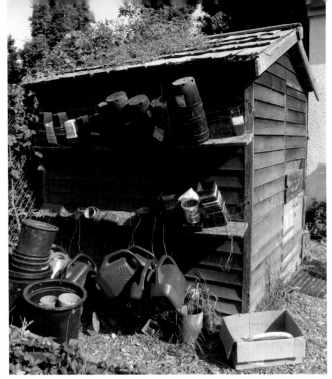

FIGURE 14.44 *Some of the potting and watering supplies at Rosa Parks School in Berkeley, California, are stored on the outside of the tool shed for easy access.*

during community work parties. If the budget only allows for one set, durable children's tools should be the first purchase; volunteering adults can bring their own equipment, if needed.

In addition to tools, many schools find it useful to store educational materials in their sheds. Some have clipboards and paper, pencils and other drawing supplies, magnifying lenses, and durable microscopes, as well as egg cartons or other "collecting boxes" children can use to gather garden treasures. Flora and fauna guidebooks, with photographs and information about local plants, animals, and insects also are useful reference materials to have on hand. Many teachers like to have a portable white board and markers, or chalkboard and chalk, for posting the day's activities or for use during lessons.

Areas set aside as maintenance zones are also helpful. They can be used to store extra mulch, topsoil, and finished compost, and house compost bins, greenhouses, cold frames, and potting tables. Maintenance areas should have access to a water source, such as a hose or a sink, for cleaning tools and dirty hands, watering plants, and washing fresh garden produce. (See additional examples in Chapter 7.) (Figures 14.43–14.45)

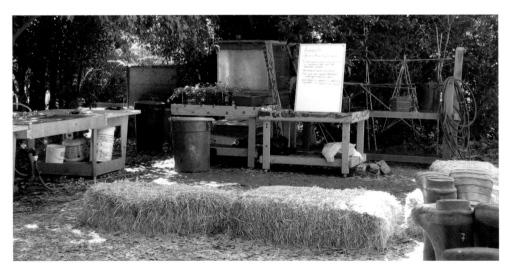

FIGURE 14.45 *The maintenance and potting area at the Edible Schoolyard at Martin Luther King School in Berkeley, California, includes a sink, work tables, and storage containers. It is located next to the school's tool shed and greenhouse for easy access to additional supplies.*

15 *Artful Schoolyards:*
Creating a Unique Sense of Place through Art

Why include artwork in a schoolyard? Not only does art turn an ordinary schoolyard into a memorable place—one that delights the eyes and speaks to the heart—it also signals to students that the school community cares about their environment. Art installations on school grounds reinforce creativity and act as creative outlets. They make the yard more attractive and lively by introducing whimsical, playful elements into spaces that may sometimes feel sterile or institutional. Themes displayed in schoolyard artwork speak to local cultures, showcase the natural environment, instill school spirit, and reflect special programs taught onsite.

Students, teachers, and community members create most playground artwork. In some cases, professional artists, who can visually unify the work or assist with technical aspects of construction, help to guide the project. Complex or substantial works may be commissioned from and created entirely by professional artists.

While various examples of schoolyard artwork are integrated into preceding chapters on ecology, play, and schoolyard function, the following examples showcase additional, distinctive art pieces that reinforce each school's sense of place. These projects use a range of materials—twigs, paint, tile, glass, wood, stone, and metal—to adorn outdoor surfaces from playground asphalt to building walls, garden beds, and play spaces.

🍃 *Ephemeral Artwork on School Grounds*

Some schoolyard art pieces are intended as ephemeral works, constructed from natural materials that will decompose over time or made from durable materials set out for a short-term display. Temporary artwork may grace schoolyards as playful constructions, such as the nature-themed mobile at Church

Crookham School in England (Figure 15.1) or in the artful execution of small projects that show a creative eye and careful attention to detail. (Figures 15.2–15.4)

FIGURE 15.1

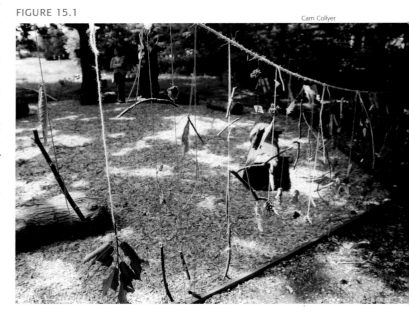
Cam Collyer

FIGURE 15.2 *This beautiful little circle of stones protects a small plant by making it more visible to students as they play nearby at Sloat Elementary School in San Francisco, California.*

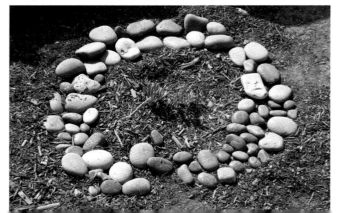

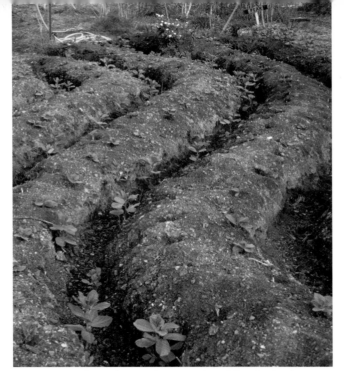

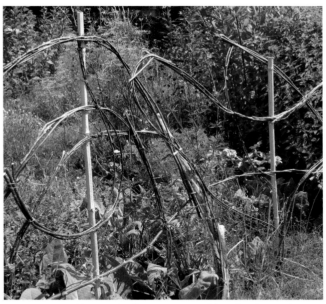

FIGURE 15.3 *The garden coordinators at the Edible Schoolyard at Martin Luther King School in Berkeley, California, shaped their potato planting beds into graceful, curving rows one season, delighting the eye and providing effective growing space for the crop.*

FIGURE 15.4 *This attractive fence, constructed from bamboo stakes and bundles of thin, flexible tree branches tied with twine, adorned the garden at the Edible Schoolyard for a few seasons before decomposing.*

FIGURE 15.5 *Willow branches, living or dried, can be used to create sculptural forms on school grounds.*

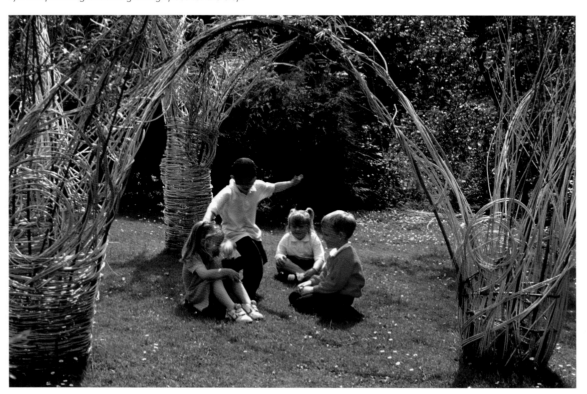

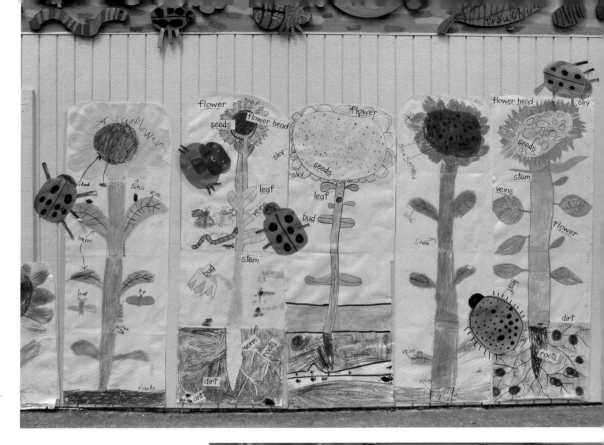

FIGURES 15.6 and 15.7
Students' temporary paper artwork (right) inspired a permanent wooden wall mural (below).

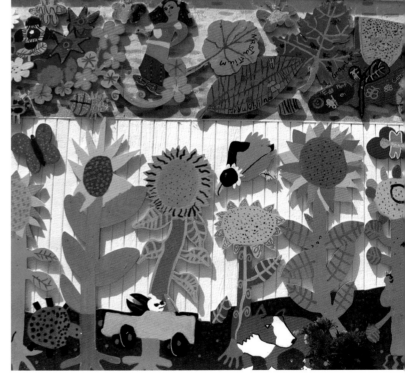

Natural materials, such as willow branches, can be used to create temporary artwork on a larger scale. Young students at Ebchester Church of England Primary School in England worked with local artists in the spring and summer of 2001 to create fanciful, whimsical forms for the children to play in.[1] One project was an airy, open meeting space for informal games and gatherings surrounded by archways and columns in unusual shapes. (Figure 15.5) The tufted columns, built from dried willow whips and vines, were carefully placed around newly planted trees to protect them as they grew. Over time, the woven columns disintegrated to allow the maturing trees to grow unencumbered.

Sometimes temporary art installations are used to test ideas before creating permanent ones. At Peralta School in Oakland, California, students drew giant paper sunflowers, laminated them, and hung them on the building's exterior in 2004 as a cheerful neighborhood artwork display. (Figure 15.6) In 2008, the school worked with a local artist to transform the paper sunflowers into painted wooden cutouts that are now permanently installed in the same place.[2] (Figure 15.7)

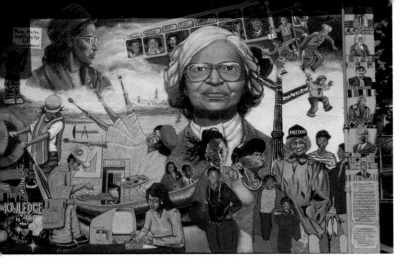

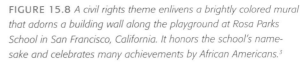

FIGURE 15.8 *A civil rights theme enlivens a brightly colored mural that adorns a building wall along the playground at Rosa Parks School in San Francisco, California. It honors the school's namesake and celebrates many achievements by African Americans.*[3]

🍃 Enlivening Schoolyard Walls, Fences, and Playground Surfaces

The muted colors of many schoolyards are dominated by gray and black pavement and the neutral shades of painted buildings. To brighten and enliven their grounds some schools install murals as vibrant playground backdrops. Murals may be painted directly onto school building walls and pavement or applied to fences using wooden cutouts. Tile mosaics are also a popular medium in many places and their bright colors last for many years. Schoolyard murals may reflect and celebrate

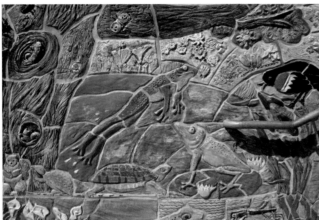

FIGURE 15.9 *Many of the individual creatures shown on this ceramic mural at Alvarado School are labeled so children will learn their names. Students assisted the artists with portions of the project.*[4]

FIGURE 15.10 *This stunning, intricate "jigsaw style" ceramic mural, which adorns a large retaining wall between two of the playgrounds at Alvarado School, illustrates the local natural environment in great detail.*[5]

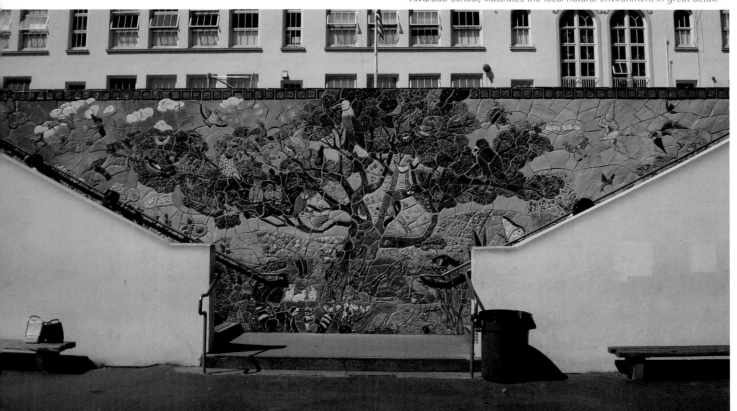

local history, cultures, and customs or the surrounding environment. (Figures 15.8–15.10)

Schoolyard artwork may also incorporate programmatic themes or be purely decorative in nature. César Chávez School in San Francisco, California, has a school program that helps deaf and hard-of-hearing students become bilingual in American sign language and English.[6] A dramatic, brightly colored mural on the outside of the school building beautifully incorporates this theme, while celebrating the cultural diversity of the school and neighborhood at the same time. Twenty-six small panels on the mural, called "Silent Language of the Soul," depict the signs for the alphabet in American sign language. Several larger panels show children signing and participating in activities.[7] (Figure 15.11)

At Tule Elk Park Child Development Center in San Francisco, California, the artist-in-residence and garden instructor worked with a third grade class on a lesson about renewable energy and water systems. The culminating project was a hand-made ceramic triptych that now hangs in the schoolyard. During the lesson, children expressed their ideas about wind, solar, and water energy through drawings, which their artist-in-residence transformed into clay.[8] (Figure 15.12)

Collaborative art projects teach cooperation and result in products that are larger and more complex than individual students can make on their own, instilling in the students a sense of pride and shared "ownership" for an art piece. Individually painted ceramic tiles or individual works of art can be

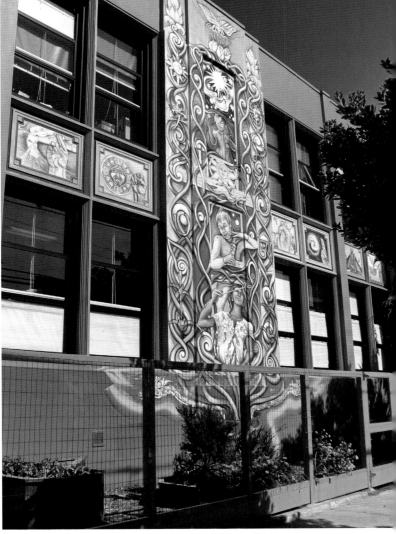

FIGURE 15.11 *César Chávez School in San Francisco, California*

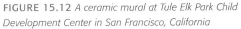

FIGURE 15.12 *A ceramic mural at Tule Elk Park Child Development Center in San Francisco, California*

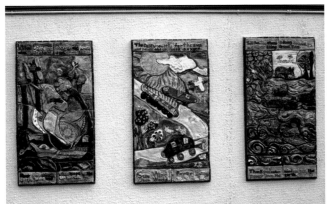

FIGURE 15.13 *Sanchez School in San Francisco, California, brightened their perimeter fence with a series of cheerful, enlarged children's drawings.*[10]

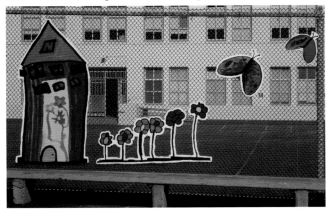

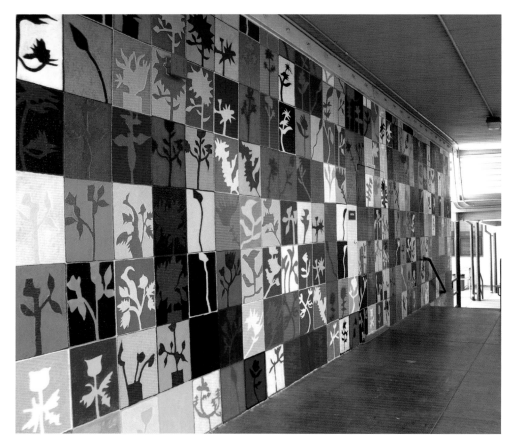

FIGURE 15.14 *A vibrant mural at Sequoia Elementary School in Oakland, California, displays a strong botanical theme that reflects the nearby teaching garden.*[9]

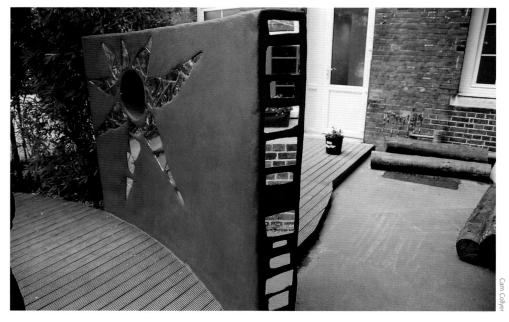

FIGURE 15.15 *Small mirrors in this wall at the edge of a peace garden at Ravenstone Primary School in England reflect light and create an eye-catching decorative backdrop for the garden space.*

Cam Collyer

creatively fused to form composite murals or "ceramic quilts" to adorn school buildings, inside or out. Like all murals, they are most visually effective if they follow a single design vision that is carried consistently through the piece by each contributing artist. (Figures 15.16 and 15.17)

🍃 Three-dimensional Sculptural Pieces on School Grounds

Three-dimensional sculptures, made from a wide range of materials, are usually featured on school entryways, fences, and seating areas, but they can also be incorporated into play elements that children climb on or into. Sculptural pieces may also stand alone as focal points and destinations within the schoolyard, celebrating the community's creativity and showing respect and admiration for the arts.

Artful play elements

Some schools infuse art into the design of their play areas by using memorable characters, close attention to detail, and intriguing designs that add a caring and whimsical touch.

Students at Ebchester Church of England Primary School in England worked with an artist to create a "cat-shaped" domed playhouse using living willow whips (branch cuttings), which grow stronger each year as the trees mature. (Figure 15.18) The cat's head and tail, made from dried branches, adorn the top of the dome. A low door and round windows were woven into the structure at the perfect height for young children to enjoy.

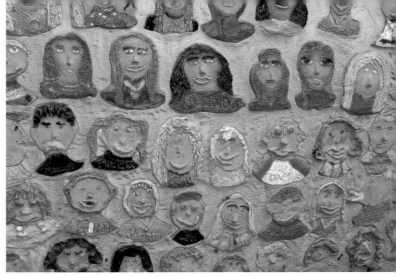

FIGURE 15.16 *This outdoor art piece includes ceramic self-portraits created by the students at Pacific School in Davenport, California.*

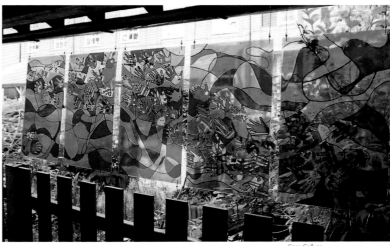

Cam Collyer

FIGURE 15.17 *Students at Ravenstone Primary School in England each contributed a painted handprint "fish" to this luminous, transparent mural. The ocean-themed painting on clear plastic panels hangs at the edge of the schoolyard.*

FIGURE 15.19 *This water play table at Joyful Noise Child Development Center in Portland, Oregon, is filled with interesting textures, colors and patterns for young children to explore as they play with the flowing water. Seashells, artful ceramic tiles, and hand-made concrete frogs are embedded in the surface of the table.*[12]

Aaron Reed

FIGURE 15.18 *A living willow play house at Ebchester School in England.*

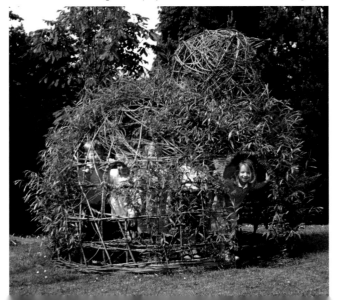

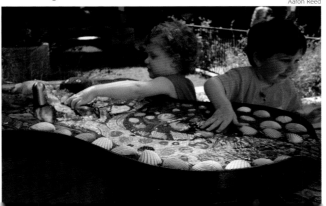

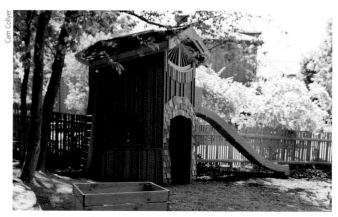

FIGURE 15.20 *This custom-made, whimsical playhouse and slide is one of many artistic touches on the campus at Oslo Steiner School in Norway. The little play structure has ornamental woodwork and colored windows.*

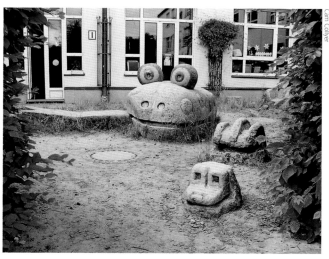

FIGURE 15.21 *Galilei Primary School in Germany has a giant frog sculpture in its playground that makes the schoolyard memorable and inspires children's creative games.*

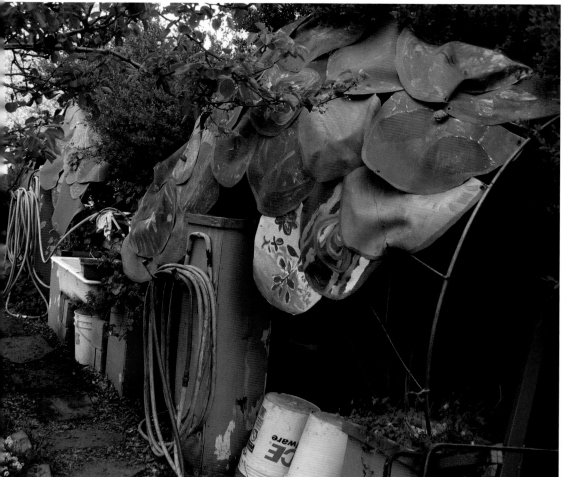

FIGURE 15.22 *A whimsical, serpent-like tunnel weaves through the garden shared by James Denman Middle School and San Miguel Child Development Center in San Francisco, California. This "Living Chinese Dragon Sculpture" incorporates a hedge and a lightweight, bent metal framework, covered with "shingles" made from painted, weatherproof, vinyl sheets.[13]*

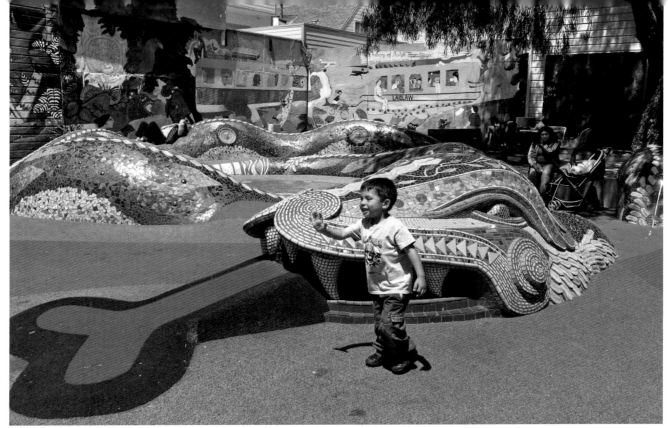

FIGURE 15.23 *The central play element in the 24th and York Street Mini-Park in San Francisco, California, is an exquisitely detailed Quetzal-coatl snake—representing the Mesoamerican feathered serpent god. Children climb the snake, sit on it, and walk along its back as they play. The ground around the serpent is covered with a padded safety surface.*[14]

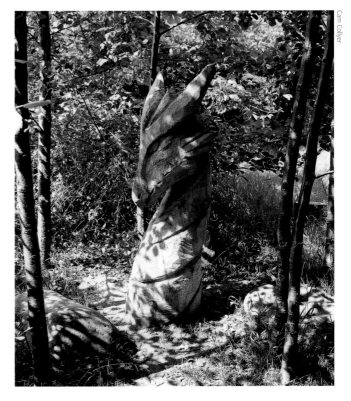

FIGURE 15.24 *This carved wooden dragon's head is at home in a forested clearing at Kløvermarken Nature Workshop in Copenhagen, Denmark.*[15]

Softened by the leaves, the light inside illuminates the interior with a magical yellow and green glow.[11]

Some public parks include playful artwork that would be equally enjoyed on school grounds. (Figures 15.23 and 15.24)

Free-standing sculpture

Whether nestled into quiet corners of the yard or prominent focal points, many art pieces serve as whimsical objects of interest and personal expression in schoolyard landscapes. Some pieces stand on their own while others are clustered into groups to create larger displays. Many of these works of art are large enough to act as destinations within the school grounds.

Scarecrows. Some school gardens use scarecrows as a form of artistic expression. (Figure 15.25) Because their components are often made from clothing, fabric and other materials that are not durable, most scarecrows are ephemeral pieces that change with the seasons. (Figures 15.26–15.27)

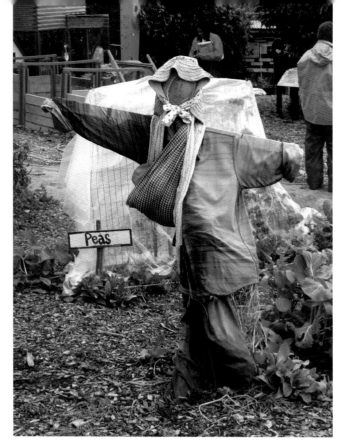

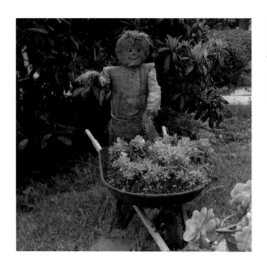

FIGURE 15.25
Scarecrow and potted plants at Pacific School in Davenport, California.

FIGURES 15.26 and 15.27
These fanciful garden scarecrows, dressed in old clothing, pieces of fabric, masks and other materials, were created for the garden at Salmon Creek School in Occidental, California (left) and the Life Lab Garden Classroom in Santa Cruz, California (above).

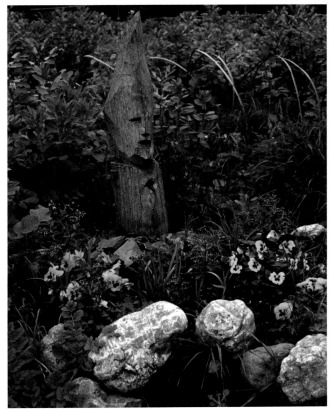

FIGURE 15.28 *A small hand-carved wooden sculpture at the Edible Schoolyard at Martin Luther King Jr. Middle School in Berkeley, California.*

Sculpture gallery

FIGURE 15.30 *The grounds at Waters School in Chicago, Illinois, include an extensive prairie habitat zone and two serene metal "deer" placed among the flowers.*

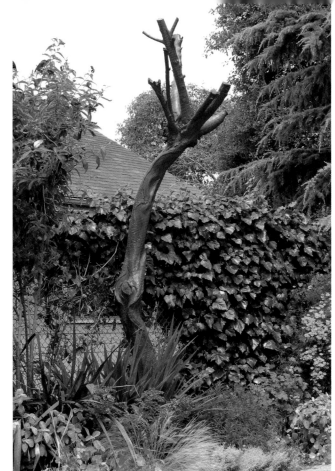

FIGURE 15.29 *When a tree died in the front entry garden at Peralta School in Oakland, California, the school community turned it into an art asset by shortening the branches and painting the sculptural tree trunk blue! It is now a striking landscape feature with an artful presence.*[16]

FIGURE 15.31 *Coombes School in England is home to a dramatic willow sculpture in the shape of a giant. Created by an artist skilled in basket making and fiber arts, the piece was formed from living and dried willow branches. It is approximately 12 feet tall.*[17]

Cam Collyer

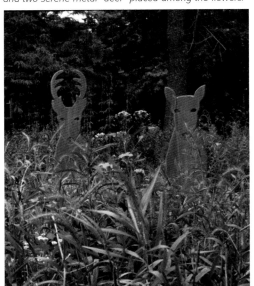

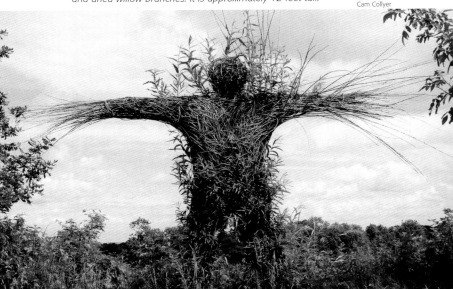

Clustered pieces

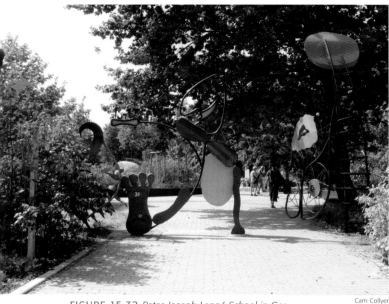

Cam Collyer

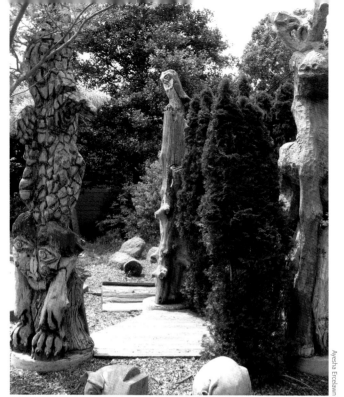

Ayesha Ercelawn

FIGURE 15.32 *Peter Joseph Lenné School in Germany installed many art pieces, with inspiration from artists Joan Miró and Antoni Gaudí, throughout its grounds including this elaborate metal entry gate.* [18]

FIGURES 15.34 *A cheerful sculpture near the front entrance of Wayne Thomas School in Highland Park, Illinois, depicts a circle of dancing children. Students repaint the metal silhouettes each year to vary the sculpture's appearance.* [20]

FIGURE 15.33 *Three totem-pole style pieces at Tule Elk Park Child Development Center in San Francisco were hand-carved with a chainsaw by a local artist. Each piece includes fanciful creatures with undulating surfaces, various textures and brightly colored paint.* [19]

FIGURE 15.35 *Neumark Primary School in Germany displays several clusters of students' artwork. Their collection includes a group of ceramic busts and a "herd" of sculpted giraffes, both situated among leafy vegetation and visible from pathways through the schoolyard.*

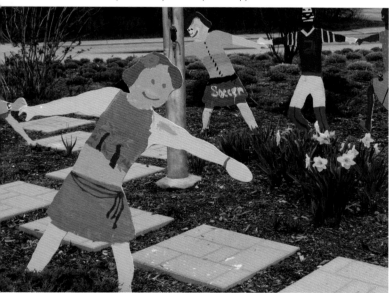

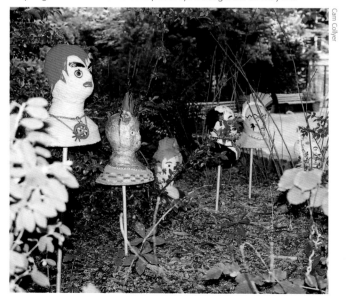

Cam Collyer

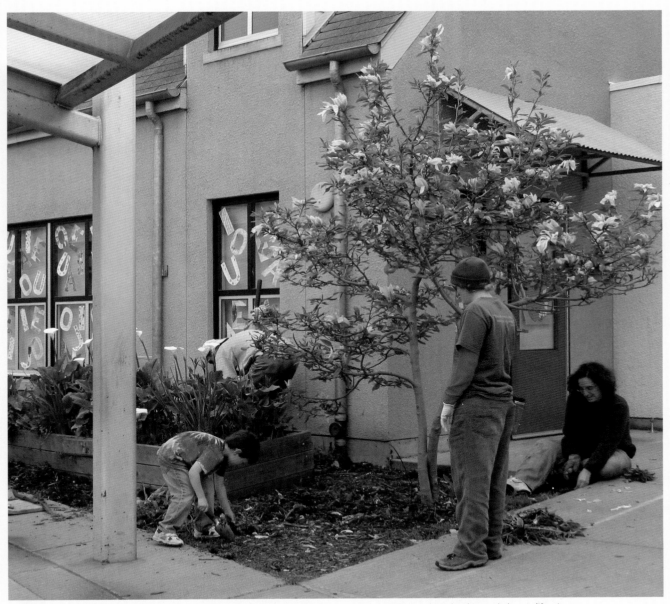

School community members hold work parties to keep the schoolyard looking its best at Rosa Parks School in Berkeley, California.

The school community and visiting volunteers at Oak Grove College in Worthing, England, often participate in school ground stewardship.

16 *Sustaining Ecological Schoolyards*

While it is true that green schoolyards greatly enhance school grounds, enrich learning and play opportunities, schoolyard aesthetics, and local ecology, they are also, without a doubt, more work to maintain over time than traditional school grounds of asphalt and grass. The added maintenance costs and labor needed are, in my view, both manageable and well worth the benefits that they bring to a school. When invited to help shape their schoolyard's transformation, school communities generally rise to the occasion and pitch in with generous donations of their time and money.

🍃 *Schoolyard Stewardship*

When schoolyard "maintenance" is framed as "stewardship" of a neighborhood commons, then it logically becomes the responsibility of schoolyard users—students, teachers, parents, and neighbors—to pitch in to keep *their* space well cared for over time.

Some parts of a green schoolyard take more work than others to look their best and to operate at their full potential. High maintenance areas, requiring stewardship weekly or monthly, include edible and ornamental gardens, ponds and wetland habitats, compost bins, nature play zones, and art play features (with materials that need to be refreshed). Pruning slow growing trees and shrubs, replacing straw bale seating or log stumps, touching up paint or stain on picket fences, and checking schoolyard water and renewable energy systems are all examples of jobs that require maintenance once or twice a year. Some parts of a green schoolyard require very little oversight once installed, including permanent pathways, tile mosaics and murals, most seating areas and shade canopies, schoolyard signage, durable play equipment, and musical play features.

It is essential to have a green schoolyard committee that both spearheads the initial master planning process and takes responsibility for organizing the schoolyard's ongoing stewardship. The committee regularly assesses the yard's maintenance needs and divides the tasks into manageable pieces that can be easily accomplished by various groups within the school community. In some cases, stewardship needs that align closely with the curricula may be accomplished by classes that use those areas of the yard frequently. Tasks that require bigger tools or more skill can be assigned to parents during monthly schoolyard work parties. More complex or dangerous jobs may be saved for professional contractors, for example, maintenance of greywater systems and solar panels or pruning tall trees.

When delegating schoolyard stewardship tasks, do *not* burden the school's janitors or maintenance staff with extra work unless they were part of the design process and volunteered for these roles. Usually, they have sufficient work as part of their daily routine. It pays to stay in close communication with janitors and maintenance staff and to solicit their input, both to make their jobs more pleasant and to give them the respect they deserve.

Children and their teachers as schoolyard stewards

At the heart of the ecological schoolyard philosophy is the concept of raising children to become skilled land stewards. Students practice taking care of their "commons" from an early age when they are entrusted with a modest amount of schoolyard stewardship responsibility. What can a young child do to help sustain and improve the school environment? It is useful to ask students to think about this question, themselves, so they can brainstorm a list of their own ideas. Many people

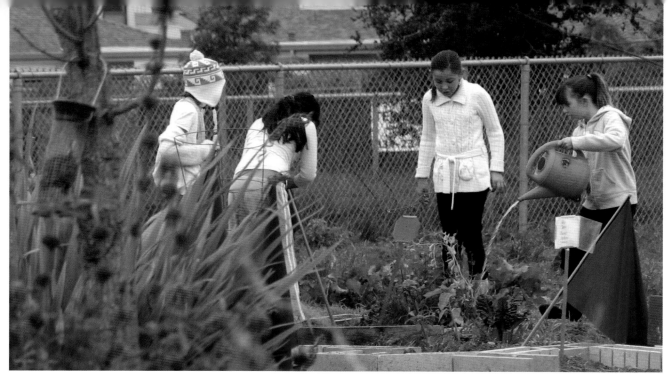

FIGURE 16.1 *Children are very capable of helping to maintain school gardens.*

are surprised to see what children are capable of if they are given the opportunity to be responsible.

Adults enable children's stewardship by breaking tasks into categories that are age appropriate. Most schools should expect that young children, from kindergarten through early elementary school years, can help with straightforward daily schoolyard chores, such as weeding, watering, animal care, raking, sweeping, and composting. (Figure 16.1) They can assist in planting seeds, small shrubs, and small trees, as long as the root balls are not too heavy for them. (Figure 16.2) Older children in upper elementary school and middle school can handle all of these tasks, but they can also take on more complicated roles. Teachers may incorporate research projects or design work into yard stewardship tasks, and give students more power over decisions that are made for a particular area. Ideas used to engage young children may also be scaled up as students get older, so they may continue to participate in schoolyard stewardship in a meaningful way. Middle and high school students are often capable of working with hand tools to build items that are needed in the schoolyard. It is especially important to allow these age groups to think about what needs to be done onsite and decide as a class how to approach a given task. The courtyard "naturescaping" project at Rowe Middle School (see

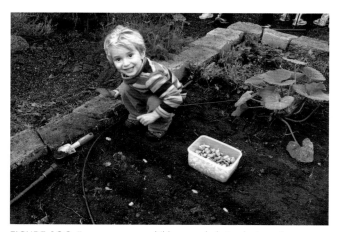

FIGURE 16.2 *Even very young children can help to plant seeds.*

chapters 2 and 4) is a good example of middle school students in the role of schoolyard stewards.

At the elementary school level at Cowick First School in England, students and their teachers developed an "Eco-code" to guide their behavior as school ground stewards. Their code includes ecology-related goals that even the youngest children can follow and establishes a framework for cordial social interactions at the same time:

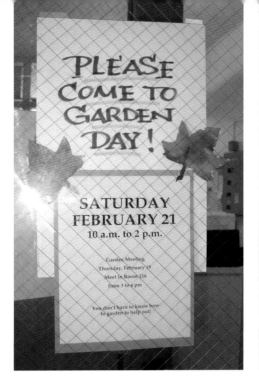

FIGURES 16.3 and 16.4 *Adult members of the school community can participate in seasonal work parties to help maintain the grounds.*

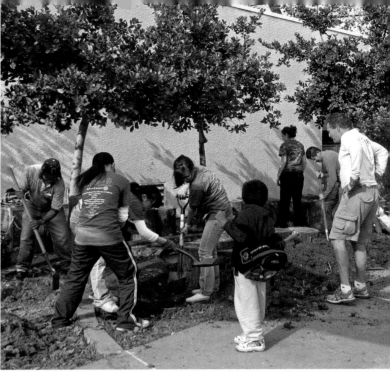

We will look after animals and plants
We will not litter our world
We will only use the water and electricity we need
We will use and reuse materials carefully
Rather than use the car we will walk when we can
We will work peacefully and co-operatively
We have the right to speak and to be heard[1]
—Cowick First School Eco-Code

When I visited Cowick First School in 2001, the Year One classes (five- and six-year-olds) were responsible for taking care of animals in their outdoor pens, rain or shine, all year-round. As they checked on the chickens, guinea pigs and rabbits each day, gave them their food and cared for them, they learned responsible behavior and how to nurture other living beings as stewards of this small part of the yard. Similarly, the Year Two classes (six- and seven-year-olds) were responsible for maintaining the kitchen garden. They helped with crop rotation, planting, harvest, and the garden's compost bins. Year Three children (seven-and eight-year olds) were invited to join an after-school club called "Ground Force" that helped to maintain other parts of the grounds. Over the years, the Ground Force club and their teachers built and installed bird feeders, designed and planted the butterfly garden, planted flowers, improved wildlife habitat zones, cleaned the pond, helped to mulch and weed the yard, and participated in maintaining their living willow playhouse.[2]

PTA and family participation

Adult members of the school community participate as schoolyard stewards by organizing monthly or seasonal work parties to handle larger tasks that require stronger bodies or the use of power tools. (Figures 16.3 and 16.4) It is very helpful if the green schoolyard committee conducts an informal skills inventory to find family members who can build with wood, metal, stone, and other natural materials or who can lay irrigation, install tile, and assemble renewable energy systems. If the school community does not include anyone skilled in these areas of expertise, it may be useful to hire a professional to lead a team of untrained (but enthusiastic) parents to fulfill such tasks. Using a paid professional's skills in this manner will make the school's funding resources go much farther than if a full team of professional contractors is employed.

Professional assistance

There are some tasks that are generally much better to leave entirely to professionals. Hire licensed professionals to help you with dangerous tasks such as pruning tall trees or using chainsaws; tasks that require precision, such as creating code-compliant wheelchair accessible pathways; or tasks that require a permit, such as the installation of a greywater treatment wetland onsite.

It might also make sense for a school to hire a garden or green schoolyard coordinator, full time or part time, to lead garden classes and to be the point person for the green schoolyard committee. The coordinator might also help teachers get the most out of the yard during their regular academic classes, and act as a community organizer to keep the school's families involved. If someone is paid to fill this role, these tasks often become a higher priority within the school and are more likely to be accomplished with regularity.

Some schools also choose to hire a part-time gardener (with no curriculum or community organizing responsibilities) who comes in one day a week, or once or twice a month, to help the school community to keep up with exuberant plant growth. This assistance is particularly useful for schoolyards with an abundance of annual plants or a large site. His or her responsibilities would generally not overlap with the school's janitor or grounds-keeping staff; they would, instead, focus on tasks that require specialized training or plant knowledge (knowing a weed from a garden plant) beyond mowing grass, raking leaves, and other duties that typically fall to a school district's landscaping crew.

🌿 Finding Funding

Fundraising is very important to the longevity and continued vitality of ecological schoolyards. Most schoolyard projects require at least a small amount of funding to build new elements each year, and many require a small annual budget to purchase supplies to make repairs or to replace components that wear out from time to time.

To keep the fundraising needs to a reasonable level, plan for most of the yard to include projects that are fairly simple and inexpensive to maintain. Don't rely on too many expensive paid staff members to assist the project unless the program has a very reliable funding source such as an effective PTA fundraising team, dedicated local business partners or foundations, or similar sources. Projects will be more stable over a long period of time (say, more than 20 years) if they spread stewardship responsibilities throughout the school community rather than rely entirely on paid staff.

Look for funding through the PTA and make direct requests to families in the school community to support their valuable green schoolyard. Local businesses may help schools with in-kind donations of materials, plants, and other supplies. Sometimes community service organizations will provide labor to build a particular project or help with a major "spring clean-up." Grants for schoolyard building projects are available through national, state, and local foundations. Do remember to write thank-you notes for all services, funding, and supplies received from these sources and publicly acknowledge their contributions in some way.

Some school districts go directly to their city's voters to seek earmarked funding through property tax measures or bonds for facilities improvements. These larger funding sources help to spread schoolyard greening throughout an entire school district and to create ecological schoolyard projects on a larger scale.

🌿 Networking and Communication

Networking, though sometimes overlooked, is one of the essential factors of a green schoolyard's long-term success. Visit other schools in your local area that are working on similar projects to learn from their experience and share yours. Connect your project to local, regional, and national organizations and professionals who can give you advice, curriculum ideas, and other types of support that will strengthen your efforts. If your area has many green schoolyard enthusiasts, hold workshops to share gardening, building, and other skills, and to meet other like-minded individuals. Read books, articles, websites, and other sources to find new ideas that may be tailored to the needs of your own project. Chapter 18 includes a resource list to help you begin this effort.

Within the school site, keep the channels of communication open between the green schoolyard committee, garden instructor, teachers, and PTA, so that all of the efforts will be coordinated to achieve the same goals. Meet monthly, if possible, to set small goals, report on progress, and discuss issues as they arise. Keep the school community aware of the green schoolyard's progress and stewardship needs through a school newsletter, website, bulletin board, or other signs onsite. Invite everyone to participate and make the project as inclusive as possible.

17 *Ecological Schoolyards:*
From Grey to Green

🍃 *Where Will Ecological Schoolyards Take Us?*

The movement toward ecological schoolyards represents a paradigm shift in the way we view our school grounds. No longer simply a place to practice sports games and swing on the monkey bars, our school sites now have the potential to teach ecological literacy, invigorate children's bodies, open and inspire young minds, and knit our communities more closely together in the process.

Ecological schoolyards are both a reflection of current trends in environmentally responsible design and a model to teach the next generation how to live more lightly on the earth. By teaching students to explore their environment with their hands, hearts, and minds—whether they are leaping off challenging play structures or into the challenges of the surrounding world—green schoolyards are an important step on the road to building an ecologically literate society.

Successful ecological schoolyards are the product of many hands that harness the cooperative and collaborative potential of their school community. Like the barn raisings of previous generations, this collaboration among community members reinforces interdependence, local self-reliance, and a sense of community as useful, beautiful places get built at very low cost. Parents and teachers working together to improve their school grounds fosters closer relationships between families and their school. Children benefit because parents become more in tune with what they are learning and develop closer relationships with their children's teachers.

The creativity of each school community, as expressed in each schoolyard design, makes each school site unique, which creates greater regional variation in schoolyard aesthetics and reinforces each school's sense of place. Well-designed ecological schoolyards foster children's social and intellectual develop-

ment by providing venues for creative play, exploration, and adventure, while also encouraging playfulness and wonder. All of these qualities help children grow into inquisitive, capable adults.

Ecological schoolyards downplay competitive behavior in favor of cooperation and creativity. They teach collaborative problem-solving techniques while also providing room for individual ideas and personal expression—allowing small voices to be heard and valued along side the opinions of more powerful individuals and groups. These rewarding experiences in the schoolyard provide the social tools that children need to take on larger challenges with skill and grace as they mature and, as adults, to help society address larger environmental issues and community problems.

Green schoolyards are laboratories that students use to observe how ecological systems function on a small scale that they can personally understand. When children are allowed to study, play with, and observe natural systems on an ongoing basis, both during formal class time and on their own, ecological systems thinking becomes a part of their daily lives. In this integrated context, students gain an intuitive understanding of where they fit into the world and how their own actions can influence their surroundings. Students who experience onsite water and energy systems, thriving wildlife habitat zones, or productive edible gardens learn that their own work to improve and sustain the health of the environment is important and makes a difference. They also come to understand that a community, acting together, can make an even bigger difference than an individual, acting alone.

What will children raised in ecological schoolyards demand of tomorrow's world? I hope they will take these ideas with them as they mature and apply them to their own values

❀ Schoolyard Transformation

These images celebrate the accomplishments of the Commodore Sloat School community in San Francisco, California. Your school can achieve this, too![1]

Commodore Sloat School, San Francisco, California

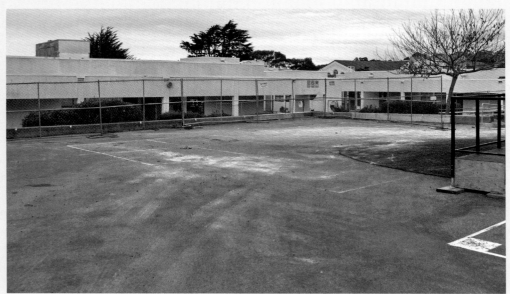

FIGURE 17.1
January 2006—Before schoolyard greening

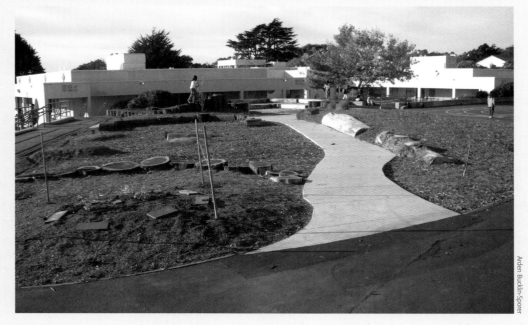

FIGURE 17.2
December 2007—Soon after installation

Arden Bucklin-Sporer

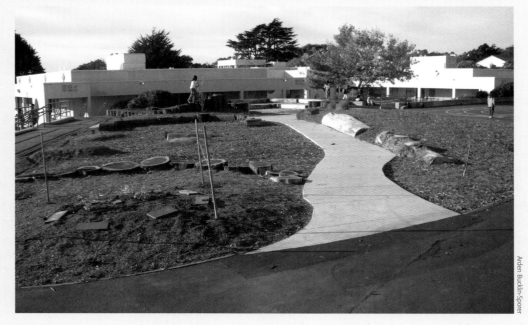

FIGURE 17.3 *April 2009—About a year and a half after installation*

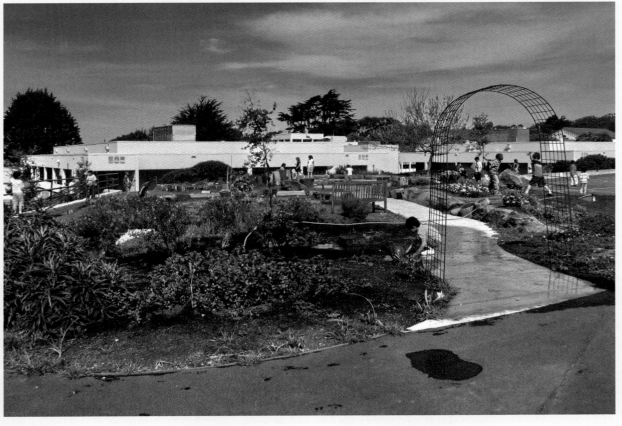

and world view—perhaps one day succeeding in shaping our cities, towns, and settlements along similar ecologically sustainable lines, enriched by interactions with their fellow community members, and enlivened by creativity and art. They may demand sustainable city planning practices, wildlife habitat protection, and buildings that generate their own power, clean their own wastewater, and use green building principles. They may create more places for people to meet their neighbors and enjoy each other's company. Perhaps they will lead their fellow community members in building parks for everyone to enjoy or invest in public art that reflects local culture and context. Maybe they will plant neighborhood orchards to supply fresh produce and build roadside swales to keep their watersheds clean.

Over the last two decades, cities around the world have begun to embrace sustainability goals and green building standards and are increasingly making them a priority. Some are reinvesting in public commons, such as local parks, plazas, and trail systems, and allowing their unique social and physical environment to shape their urban design. Many individual home owners, working on a smaller scale, are responding to the call to plant native species in their backyards, install solar panels on their rooftops, and irrigate with stormwater and greywater. Perhaps, one day we will no longer need the modifier "green" to describe this type of design—if it is assumed to be the only sensible course of action. The green schoolyard movement can only strengthen these efforts as it models ecologically-sound, community-centered, place-based design. Schoolyards can thus be reimagined as microcosms of their community's environmental design philosophy—serving as both a test bed for these ideas and as a blueprint for urban design.

I hope this book has been interesting and useful to you, and that it will help you start or continue on your journey to transform your own school's "asphalt to ecosystems." The examples in this book are intended to help you envision what is best for your school, to help you avoid "reinventing the wheel." Use the book as a springboard to develop your own ideas or tailor those you have read about to reflect your own school community and its geographic location. Dream of the schoolyard you would like to achieve and then help to shape this reality at your school. The schoolyards of tomorrow will be what *you* make them.

> ❧ **Asphalt to Ecosystems in Your Neighborhood**
>
> If this book helps to inspire you to turn your own schoolyard asphalt into ecosystems, please let us know! Visit <www.asphalt2ecosystems.org> or email <info@asphalt2ecosystems.org> for more information.

FIGURE 17.4 *Artwork by secondary school students at Oak Grove College in Worthing, England*

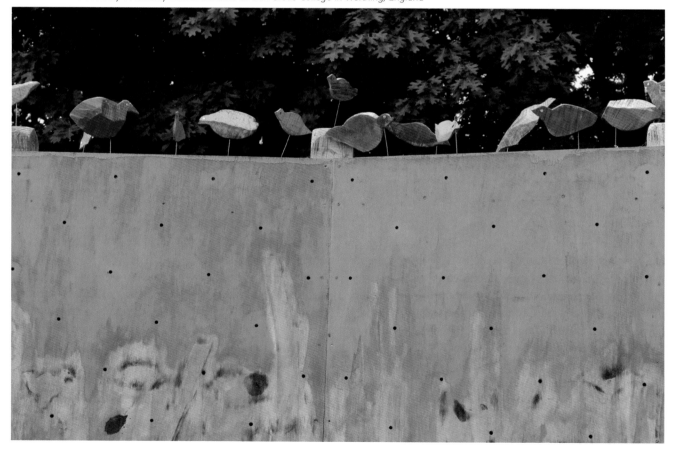

Resources to Help Transform Your "Asphalt to Ecosystems"

Below is a list of organizations in the United States and abroad that are dedicated to helping schools create ecological schoolyards and improving environmental education. Some of these organizations have broad missions; others focus on specific subject areas such as renewable energy systems, school gardens, or play environments. Please see the organizations' websites for more information. Also included below is a list of books that are wonderful resources for developing green schoolyards. Their topics range from children's participation to design, garden management, and green building techniques.

For more information about Sharon Danks's work, or her firm's assistance in transforming your school's "asphalt to ecosystems," please contact her firm:

Bay Tree Design, inc.
<www.baytreedesign.com>
<www.ecoschools.com>

For more information about this book and a listing of related events and information, please visit:

Asphalt to Ecosystems
<www.asphalt2ecosystems.org>

United States

National organizations

Alliance to Save Energy—Green Schools Program
<ase.org/section/program/greenschl>

> **Bay Tree Design, inc.** is a women-owned landscape architecture and planning firm in Berkeley, California. Bay Tree Design works with schools to help them transform their asphalt-covered school grounds into vibrant, multifaceted environments for ecological learning and play. Their work creates beautiful, functional spaces that reflect ecological design principles, green building practices, and edible and native planting palettes. Bay Tree Design offers environmental planning, landscape architecture and horticultural design services for residential, commercial, and educational settings.

American Community Garden Association
<www.communitygarden.org>
Center for Ecoliteracy
<www.ecoliteracy.org>
Center for Environmental Education
<www.ceeonline.org>
Children in Nature Network
<www.childrenandnature.org>
Collaborative for High Performance Schools
<www.chps.net>
Community Built Association
<www.communitybuilt.org>
Energy Star—Program for K–12 School Districts
<www.energystar.gov>
The Foundation for Environmental Education—Solar School Initiative
<www.learnenergy.org>
HarvestH2O
<www.harvesth2o.com>
Life Lab Science Program
<www.lifelab.org>
National Gardening Association—Kidsgardening
<www.kidsgardening.com>
National Wildlife Federation—Schoolyard Habitats
<www.nwf.org/schoolyard>
North American Association for Environmental Education
<www.naaee.org> <www.eelink.net>
Project W.E.T. (Water Education for Teachers)
<www.projectwet.org>
U.S. Environmental Protection Agency
Green Building
<www.epa.gov/greenbuilding/>
Office of Ground Water and Drinking Water
<www.epa.gov/safewater>
Teaching Center
<www.epa.gov/teachers/>
U.S. Green Building Council—Build Green Schools Program

Local, regional, and state-wide organizations

Boston Schoolyard Initiative (Massachusetts)
  <www.schoolyards.org >
California School Garden Network (California)
  <www.csgn.org>
Chicago Botanic Garden—School Gardening Program (Illinois)
  <www.chicagobotanic.org/schoolgarden/index.php>
D.C. Environmental Education Consortium—Schoolyard Greening (District of Columbia)
  <www.dcschoolyardgreening.org>
Earth Partnership for Schools (Wisconsin)
  <uwarboretum.org/eps>
The Green Schools Initiative (California+)
  <www.greenschools.net>
Hawai'i Island School Garden Network (Hawaii)
  <www.kohalacenter.org/HISGN/about.html>
Natural Learning Initiative (North Carolina)
  <www.naturalearning.org>
REAL School Gardens (Texas)
  <www.realschoolgardens.org>
San Francisco Green Schoolyard Alliance (California)
  <www.sfgreenschools.org>

Other related websites

Sustainable Schoolyard Exhibit at the U.S. Botanic Garden
  <www.sustainableschoolyard.org>
Sustainable Communities Network
  <www.sustainable.org>

International Organizations

Eco-Schools
  <www.eco-schools.org>
European Federation of City Farms
  <www.cityfarms.org>
International Play Association
  <www.ipaworld.org>

Australia

Learnscapes
  <www.learnscapes.org>

Canada

Evergreen—Learning Grounds Program
  <www.evergreen.ca>
Green Teacher Magazine
  <www.greenteacher.com>

Germany

Bund der Jugendfarmen und Aktivspielplätze (Federation of Youth Farms and Activity Playgrounds)
  <www.bdja.org>
Grün macht Schule
  <www.gruen-macht-schule.de>
Schulgarten-Forum (School Garden Forum)
  <www.schulgarten-forum.de>

Japan

Association for Children's Environment
  <www.children-environment.org>
ECO-JAPAN Ecosystem Conservation Society
  <www.ecosys.or.jp/eco-japan>

Sweden

Barnens Landskap (Children's Landscape)
  <www.barnenslandskap.com>
Movium–Centrum för miljö-och utomhuspedagogik (Centre for the Urban Public Space at Swedish University of Agricultural Sciences)
  <www.movium.slu.se>
Naturskoleföreningen (Association of Nature Schools in Sweden)
  <www.naturskola.se>
Naturskolan i Lund (Naturskolan in Lund)
  <www.naturskolan.lund.se>

Norway

Levande Skule (Living School)
  <org.umb.no/LevandeSkule/eng/index.html>
Children's Landscapes
  <www.barnas-landskap.org>

United Kingdom

Learning through Landscapes
  <www.ltl.org.uk>
Playlink
  <www.playlink.org>

Useful Books and Articles for Developing Ecological Schoolyards

Bell, Anne C. and Janet E. Dyment. *Grounds for Action: Promoting Physical Activity through School Ground Greening in Canada*. Toronto, Ontario, Canada: Evergreen, 2006.

Bucklin-Sporer, Arden and Rachel Pringle. *How to Grow a School Garden: A Complete Guide for Parents and Teachers*. Portland, Oregon: Timber Press, July 2010 (forthcoming).

California School Garden Network. *Gardens for Learning: Creating and Sustaining Your School Garden*. Irvine, California: California School Garden Network, 2006

Danks, Sharon and Tamar Cooper. "Green Schoolyard Resource Directory for the San Francisco Bay Area." San Francisco, California: San Francisco Green Schoolyard Alliance, 2006. (2008 Revised Edition edited by Marcie Keever and Rachel Pringle).

Danks, Sharon. "Stewardship Begins at School: In England, a Superlative Example of an Ecological Schoolyard." *Landscape Architecture Magazine*. J. William Thompson, editor. Washington, DC: American Society of Landscape Architects, Vol. 93, No. 6 (2003): 42, 44, 46, 48.

Danks, Sharon. "Green Mansions: Living Willow Structures Enhance Children's Play Environments." *Landscape Architecture Magazine*. J. William Thompson, editor. Washington, DC: American Society of Landscape Architects, Vol. 92, No. 6 (2002): 38, 40-43, 93-94.

Danks, Sharon. "Ecological Schoolyards: Design Guidelines." *New Village Journal*. Lynne Elizabeth, editor. Berkeley, CA: Architects / Designers / Planners for Social Responsibility 3 (2002): 74-77.

Danks, Sharon. "Courtyard Oases: Ecology at the Heart of the School." *Landscape Architecture Magazine*. J. William Thompson, editor. Washington, DC: American Society of Landscape Architects Vol. 92, No. 1 (2002): 36-41.

Danks, Sharon. "Ecological Schoolyards." *Landscape Architecture Magazine*. J. William Thompson, editor. Washington, DC: American Society of Landscape Architects, Vol. 92, No. 1 (2000): 42-47.

Denzer, Kiko. *Build Your Own Earth Oven: A Low-Cost, Wood-Fired Mud Oven, Simple Sourdough Bread, Perfect Loaves*. Blodgett, Oregon: Hand Print Press, 2000.

Denzer, Kiko. *Dig Your Hands in the Dirt: A Manual for Making Art out of Earth*. Blodgett, Oregon: Hand Print Press, 2005.

Dunnett, Nigel and Andy Clayden. *Rain Gardens: Managing Water Sustainably in the Garden and Designed Landscape*. Portland, Oregon: Timber Press, 2007.

Evans, Ianto, Michael G. Smith, and Linda Smiley. *The Hand-Sculpted House: A Practical and Philosophical Guide to Building a Cob Cottage*. White River Junction, Vermont: Chelsea Green Publishing Company, 2002.

Evergreen. *All Hands in the Dirt: A Guide to Designing and Creating Natural School Grounds*. Toronto, Ontario, Canada: Evergreen, 2000.

Evergreen. *Nature Nurtures: Investigating the Potential of School Grounds*. Evergreen, 2000.

Evergreen and Banyan Tree. *Bricks of the Earth: A Hands-on Manual, An Innovative Way to Engage Students in Green Building Techniques*. Toronto, Ontario, Canada: Evergreen, 2007.

Grant, Tim and Gail Littlejohn, eds. *Greening School Grounds: Creating Habitats for Learning*. Toronto, Ontario, Canada: New Society Publishers/Green Teacher, 2001.

Hart, Roger A. *Children's Participation: The Theory and Practice of Involving Young Citizens in Community Development and Environmental Care*. New York, New York: Earthscan Publications Ltd./ Unicef, 1997.

Jaffe, Roberta and Gary Appel. *The Growing Classroom: Garden and Nutrition Activity Guide*. Life Lab Science Program and National Gardening Association, 2007.

Keeler, Rusty. *Natural Playspaces: Creating Outdoor Play Environments for the Soul*. Redmond, Washington: Exchange Press, 2008.

Kinkade-Levario, Heather. *Design for Water: Rainwater Harvesting, Stormwater Catchment, and Alternative Water Reuse*. Gabriola Island, British Columbia, Canada: New Society Publishers, 2007.

Life Lab Science Program and Center for Ecoliteracy. *Getting Started: A Guide for Creating School Gardens as Outdoor Classrooms*. Santa Cruz, California: Life Lab Science Program, 1997.

Lyle, John Tillman. *Regenerative Design for Sustainable Development*. New York, New York: Wiley, 1994.

Moore, Robin C. *Plants for Play: A Plant Selection Guide for Children's Outdoor Environments*. Berkeley, California: MIG Communications, 1993.

Moore, Robin C. and Herb H. Wong. *Natural Learning: The Life History of an Environmental Schoolyard*. Berkeley, California: MIG Communications, 1997.

Payne, Binet. *The Worm Cafe: Mid-Scale Vermicomposting of Lunchroom Wastes*. Kalamazoo, Michigan: Flower Press, 1997.

Rahus Institute's Solar Schoolhouse. *Teaching Solar*. Rahus Institute, 2009.

Sobel, David. *Mapmaking with Children: Sense of Place Education for the Elementary Years*. Portsmouth, New Hampshire: Heinemann, 1998.

Stone, Michael and the Center for Ecoliteracy. *Smart by Nature: Schooling for Sustainability*. Berkeley, California: University of California Press, 2009.

Titman, Wendy. *Special Places, Special People: The Hidden Curriculum of School Grounds*. Surrey, United Kingdom: World Wide Fund for Nature/Learning through Landscapes, 1994.

Van der Ryn, Sim and Stuart Cowan. *Ecological Design*. Washington, DC: Island Press, 1996.

Warnes, Jon. *Living Willow Sculpture*. Kent, Great Britain: Search Press, 2001.

Referenced Works

Aguiar, Eloise. "Imu Sizzles Now Even in a Drizzle." *The Honolulu Advertiser* (October 31, 2005).

Alameda County Mosquito Abatement District. "Mosquito Prevention for Fishponds." Hayward, CA (2004).

"A Shady Deal Helps Cool Students." *Los Angeles Times* (June 11, 1998): B4. (author unknown)

The Ashden Awards for Sustainable Energy. "Cassop Primary School, Durham, UK, 2006: Sustainable Energy in Schools," award summary. <www.ashdenawards.org/winners/cassop#>

Bailey, Gary. "Schools—and Students—Brighten in North Carolina." *Schools Going Solar.* Utility PhotoVoltaic Group (April 1998).

Bell, Anne C. and Janet E. Dyment. *Grounds for Action: Promoting Physical Activity through School Ground Greening in Canada.* Evergreen (2006).

Bhattacharjee, Riya. "Willard Students Construct Outdoor Clay Pizza Oven." *The Berkeley Daily Planet* (March 23, 2007).

Braxton-Little, Jane. "Trees Help LA Schools Reduce Energy Use, Increase Community Pride." *California Trees: Exploring Issues in Urban Forestry,* 10.1 (1999).

Buchen, Bill and Mary. "Global Rhythms: Curriculum Guide for Musical Sculptures at Denver's Green Valley Ranch Park." Sonic Architecture brochure (2008).

Buchen, Bill and Mary. "PS 23 Sound Playground." Online article. <www.sonicarchitecture.com/catalogue/ps23%20playground.html>

Cabrera, Yvette. "Cool School: Campus to Echo Nature's Flow." *Los Angeles Times* (June 16,1999): 4

California Department of Education. "School Garden Program Overview." <www.cde.ca.gov/ls/nu/he/gardenoverview.asp>

California Department of Pesticide Regulation. "Fight the bite: A Home and Garden Checklist." California Department of Pesticide Regulation. <www.mosquitoes.org/downloads/Checklist.pdf>

California Energy Commission, Consumer Energy Center, Geothermal Heat Pumps information page. <www.consumerenergycenter.org/home/heating_cooling/geothermal.html>

California Incentives for Renewable Energy, Database of State Incentives for Renewables & Efficiency. <www.dsireusa.org/library/

California Integrated Waste Management Board, Office of Environmental Health Hazard Assessment. *Evaluation of Health Effects of Recycled Waste Tires in Playground and Track Products* (January 2007).

California School Garden Network. *Gardens for Learning: Creating and Sustaining Your School Garden* (2006).

Collaborative for High Performance Schools. "CHPS Fact Sheet." <www.chps.net>

Cornell Lab of Ornithology, All About Birds website article. "The Best Ways to Attract More Songbirds to Your Property." <www.birds.cornell.edu/AllAboutBirds/attracting/landscaping/songbirds/document_view>

Danks, Sharon and Tamar Cooper. "Green Schoolyard Resource Directory for the San Francisco Bay Area." San Francisco Green Schoolyard Alliance, revised ed. (2008).

Danks, Sharon. "Stewardship Begins at School: In England, a Superlative Example of an Ecological Schoolyard." *Landscape Architecture Magazine,* J. William Thompson, ed. Washington, DC: American Society of Landscape Architects, Vol. 93, No. 6 (June 2003): 42, 44, 46, 48.

Danks, Sharon. "Green Mansions: Living Willow Structures Enhance Children's Play Environments." *Landscape Architecture Magazine,* J. William Thompson, ed. Washington, DC: American Society of Landscape Architects, Vol. 92, No. 6 (June 2002): 38, 40–43, 93–94.

Danks, Sharon. "Ecological Schoolyards: Design Guidelines," *New Village Journal,* Lynne Elizabeth, ed. Berkeley, CA: Architects / Designers / Planners for Social Responsibility 3 (May 2002): 74–77.

Danks, Sharon. "Courtyard Oases: Ecology at the Heart of the School." *Landscape Architecture Magazine,* J. William Thompson, ed. Washington, DC: American Society of Landscape Architects, Vol. 92, No. 1 (January 2002): 36–41.

Danks, Sharon. "Ecological Schoolyards." *Landscape Architecture Magazine,* J. William Thompson, ed. Washington, DC: American Society of Landscape Architects, Vol. 90, No. 11 (November 2000): 42–47.

Danks, Sharon. "Ecological Schoolyards," Master's Thesis. Department of Landscape Architecture and Environmental Planning, Department of City and Regional Planning, University of California, Berkeley (May 2000).

Dyment, Janet E. *Gaining Ground: The Power and Potential of School Ground Greening in the Toronto District School Board.* Evergreen (2005).

Earth Partnership Program. "Earth Partnership Gallery." University of Wisconsin-Madison, Wisconsin Arboretum website.

Edible Schoolyard. <www.edibleschoolyard.org>

European Municipal Buildings Climate Campaign. "Durham Cassop School: Integrating Sustainable Energy Technologies with Education." <www.display-campaign.org/rubrique607.html>

Evergreen. *All Hands in the Dirt: A Guide to Designing and Creating Natural School Grounds*. Evergreen (2000).

Evergreen. *Nature Nurtures: Investigating the Potential of School Grounds*. Evergreen (2000).

Farrelly, David. *The Book of Bamboo*. San Francisco: Sierra Club Books (1984).

Fisher, Adrian and George Gerster. *The Art of the Maze*. Seven Dials, Cassell & Co.(2000).

Flemmen, Asbjørn, Real Play—a Socio-Motor Behaviour. Notat 3/2005. Høgskulen i Volda og Møreforsking Volda.

Flemmen, Asbjørn, Volda University College, Norway. "Real Play: A Recognized Sensory-Motor Behaviour in Norway." *Playrights: An International Journal of the Theory and Practice of Play*, International Play Association, Vol. 26, No. 4 (2005).

The Foundation for Environmental Education. "Solar School Initiative." <www.learnenergy.org/solar-school-initiative>

Furger, Robert. "Green Scene: Students Appreciate Sustainable, Eco-Friendly Building Design." *Edutopia Magazine* 1 (Sept. 2004).

Hathaway, Warren, et al. "A Study into the Effects of Light on Children of Elementary School Age: A Case of Daylight Robbery." Alberta Department of Education, Edmonton, Alberta, Canada (1992).

Healthy Schools Network, Inc. Albany, NY. *Daylighting (2005)*.

Heschong Mahone Group/Pacific Gas & Electric. *Daylighting in Schools: An Investigation into the Relationship Between Daylighting and Human Performance (August 20, 1999)*.

Heron, Donna, United States Environmental Protection Agency. "EPA Administrator Christie Whitman Recognizes Philadelphia School District for Achieving Energy Star Designation in 11 Schools—The Philadelphia School District is the Only School District in Pennsylvania to Achieve Energy Efficiency in 11 School Buildings." Press release (December 2, 2002).

Hollywood Beautification Team, Los Angeles Conservation Corps, North East Trees, TreePeople. Professional Consultants: Benshoof/Withers, Landscape Architecture. *Design and Technical Guidelines for Cool Schools, A Campus Greening Project*. Funded by Los Angeles Department of Water and Power for use by the Los Angeles Unified School District (July 15, 1998).

Japan Information Network. "Shiny Mud Balls: Kyoto Professor Taps into the Essence of Play." *Japan Information Network* (October 5, 2001).

Keeler, Rusty. "Play Environments for the Soul." Online article, Planet Earth Playscapes: <www.planetearthplayscapes.com/articles_playenv.html>

Kenton County School District. *Twenhofel Vital Signs Monitoring System*. <www.twhvac.kenton.kyschools.us/GeothermalSystemMain.htm>

King, Rod. "Mason Middle School Environmental Study Area." North American Association of Environmental Educators conference, Convention Center, Cincinnati, Ohio (August 29, 1999).

Kizer, Glen. "Kentucky: High Performance School: Ohio Visitors Tour the School." *Energy Seeds* Blog Archive (September 1, 2006).

Kizer, Katie. "McCracken Middle School: What Came First…the Economic… or the Energy Savings?"*Energy Seeds* blog (September 11, 2008), The Foundation for Environmental Education. <www.energyseeds.com>.

Koike, Sandra. "Sagano Elementary School, Kyoto, Japan." Unpublished case study. (October 2008).

Lemley, Gregory W. "Pressure-Treated Wood: Should I or Shouldn't I Use It?" Fact Sheet, Berkeley Ecology Center. Berkeley, California (November 3, 2000).

Lieberman, Gerald and Linda Hoody. "Closing the Achievement Gap: Using the Environment as an Integrating Context for Learning." Executive Summary, State Education and Environment Roundtable. San Diego, CA (1998).

Louv, Richard, keynote presentation for the San Francisco Green Schoolyard Alliance's *Growing Greener School Grounds Conference*. San Francisco, CA (October 10, 2008).

Lyle, John Tillman. *Regenerative Design for Sustainable Development*. New York: John Wiley & Sons, Inc. (1994).

Maffei, Wesley. "An Abridged Bibliography of Selected Biorational Larvicides for California Mosquito Control, Version 5.1." Alameda County Mosquito Abatement District (June 25, 1997).

Mason Middle School. "Bloom Where You are Planted! Developing an On-Site Environmental Study Area." Mason Middle School, Mason, Ohio (1999).

Maxwell, Lorraine E., Mari R. Mitchell, and Gary W. Evans. "Effects of Play Equipment and Loose Parts on Preschool Children's Outdoor Play Behavior: An Observational Study and Design Intervention." *Children, Youth and Environments*, Vol. 18, No. 2 (2008): 36–63.

Metcalf, Dr. Robert. "Recent Advances in Solar Water Pasteurization," The Solar Cooking Archive. <solarcooking.org/pasteurization/metcalf.htm>

Moore, Robin C. and Herb H. Wong. *Natural Learning: The Life History of an Environmental Schoolyard*. MIG Communications (1997).

Moore, Robin C. *Plants for Play: A Plant Selection Guide for Children's Outdoor Environments*. MIG Communications (1993).

Moore, Robin C. "Before and After Asphalt: Diversity as an Ecological Measure of Quality in Children's Outdoor Environments." *The Ecological Context of Children's Play*. Edited by Block, M.N. and Pellegrini. Ablex (1989).

NASS Sundial Register. <www.sundials.org>

National Wildlife Federation, *Schoolyard Habitats*. Vienna, Virginia: National Wildlife Federation (1995).

Ohio EPA Public Interest Center. "News Release: Ohio EPA Awards $11,665 in Environmental Education Mini Grant to Three Cincinnati-area Organizations." Ohio EPA Public Interest Center (April 30, 2003).

Pacific Gas & Electric. "Net Energy Metering." <www.pge.com/b2b/newgenerator/solarwindgenerators/expandedenet/netenergymetering/index.shtml>

Pacific Gas & Electric, 2008 PG&E Solar Schools Program. *Photovoltaic System Installations: Guidelines and Application.* <californiasolarschools.org/solar-schools/grants/installations>

Perryess, C.S. "Educating the Community: A Watershed Model Project." *Green Teacher Magazine,* Toronto, ON, Canada, Issue 66 (Fall-Winter 2001).

Playlink, Play Policy. <www.freeplaynetwork.org.uk/playlink/exhibition/school/berlin1.htm>

Princeton Energy Resources International, H.Powell Energy Associates, and Alliance to Save Energy. "School Operations and Maintenance: Best Practices for Controlling Energy Costs." (August 2004).

Pushard, Doug. "Oregon School Showcases Demo Rainwater System." *Harvest H2O.* <www.harvesth2o.com/davinci.shtml>

Rauber, Paul. "The Edible Schoolyard: Reading, Writing, Planting, Composting, Slicing, and Dicing." *Food for Thought* (November-December 1997).

The Results Center, Division of IRT Environment, Inc. "School District of Philadelphia: Save Energy Campaign, Profile #114" (1994).

San Francisco Unified School District and Bay Tree Design, inc. "Choosing Materials for a Green Schoolyard." Information Sheet for SFUSD Schools, San Francisco, CA (August 2009).

Sardar, Zahid. "Garden Snake: A Piece of the Bigger Picture, In San Francisco, Mosaic Artists have Retrieved a Playground, Bit by Bit, from Urban Blight." *San Francisco Chronicle* (December 16, 2006): F-1.

Schmidt, Lene. "Outdoor Spaces—Jungle or Exercise Yard? A Study of Facilities, Children and Physical Activity at School." ("Skolegården, jungel eller luftegård?") Norwegian Institute for Urban and Regional Research (NIBR), Oslo, NO, Report (2004):01.

Shimabukuro, Betty. "Steam Bath: At Kailua High School, an Imu Project Helps Students Raise Funds and Study Culture." *Honolulu Star Bulletin* (May 7, 2003).

Skokie School District 73½. "Here Comes the Sun Power." *Community Digest: McCraken—Middleton - Meyer,* Skokie School District 73½ (Winter 2009)

Smith, Doug. "The Greening of L.A. Schools." *Los Angeles Times* (July 21): B2.

Sobel, David. *Mapmaking with Children: Sense of Place Education for the Elementary Years.* Heinemann (1998).

State of California, Division of the State Architect, Department of General Services. "Grid Neutral Schools" PowerPoint presentation posted on their website (December 2008). <www.documents.dgs.ca.gov/dsa/other/Grid-Neutral-Schools-Workshop.pps>

Steen, Athena Swentzell, and Bill Steen, David Bainbridge, and David Eisenberg. *The Straw Bale House.* White River Junction, VT: Chelsea Green Publishing Company (1994).

Stegner, Wallace. *Wolf Willow: A History, a Story, and a Memory of the Last Plains Frontier.* Compass Books (1962). Reprinted by Penguin Classics (2000).

"Students Shine in Daylit Classrooms." *Energy Ideas,* Vol. 4, No. 3 (Spring 1997/Winter 1996). (Author not listed)

Svane, Frode. "The Mini-Mountain at Manglerud Primary School, Oslo: 1999–2000." Children's Landscape, online article. <www.barnas-landskap.org>

Titman, Wendy. *Special Places, Special People: The Hidden Curriculum of School Grounds,* World Wide Fund for Nature/Learning through Landscapes (1994).

Tree People. *Rainwater as a Resource: Report on Three Sites Demonstrating Sustainable Stormwater Management,* Beverly Hills, CA (2007).

United Anglers of Casa Grande High School. "The Results of Our Efforts are Proof Positive," project web page: <www.uacg.org/index.html>

United States Department of Energy, Office of Energy Efficiency and Renewable Energy, Building Technologies Program. "NSBA Endorses EnergySmart Schools," information sheet (January 2008).

United States Department of Energy. "About EnergySmart Schools," and "EnergySmart Schools," website content updated (July 25, 2008). <www.eere.energy.gov/buildings/energysmartschools>

United States Department of Energy. *National Best Practiced Manual for Building High Performance Schools* (October 2007).

United State Environmental Protection Agency, Green Building. <www.epa.gov/greenbuilding/pubs/about.htm>

Van der Ryn, Sim and Stuart Cowan. *Ecological Design,* Washington, DC: Island Press (1996).

Vaughan, Mace and Matthew Shepherd, Claire Kremen, and Scott Hoffman Black. *Farming for Bees: Guidelines for Providing Native Bee Habitat on Farms,* The Xerces Society (2004).

Velle Sea, Linda, Educational Center, Karmøy, Norway. "Skudeneshavn School: The School's Outdoor Areas—An Eldorodo Movement," ("Skudeneshavn skole: Skolens uteområde- et bevegelseseldorado!"), First published in the Danish journal "Skolens rum," Vol. 7 (2001).

Wackernagel, Mathis and William Rees. *Our Ecological Footprint: Reducing Human Impact on the Earth.* Gabriola Island, B.C., Canada: New Society Press (1996).

White Arkitekter AB. *Östratornskolan, Lund, Sweden: A School Built on Ecological Ideas.* 2d. ed. Translated into English from Swedish by Anette Wong Jere. Lund, Sweden (May 2000).

Wilson, Alex. "Cement and Concrete: Environmental Considerations." *Environmental Building News* (March 1, 1993).

Wingman, Karin and Britt Wall-Tydh. "Årstidsträdgården—Barns Föreställningar om Årstider" ("Seasonal Garden: Children's Representation of Seasons"). Excerpt from a project written for Malmö University (1999).

Wisconsin Public Service Corporation. "Schools Participating in Solar-Wise˚ for Schools." (June 2008).

Additional information from site visits, and personal communications with garden educators, artists, and other professionals as noted in the book's text and endnotes.

Endnotes

Preface

1. Professor Lyle visited our campus to give a guest lecture about his work, shortly before he passed away in 1998.
2. This aspect of my approach was strongly influenced by my professors, Randy Hester and Marcia McNally.
3. Bay Tree Design, inc. designed the Sustainable Schoolyard exhibit. Other project partners were members of *Friends of Smart Growth and Sustainable Communities,* including CONCERN, Inc. (project manager), American Farmland Trust, American Planning Association, The Cloud Institute for Sustainability Education, The Conservation Fund, National Association of Counties, National Association of Realtors˙, and Smart Growth Network. The project's website is <www.sustainableschoolyard.org>.

🍂 Part 1

Introduction

1. This is a description of a real schoolyard project I observed in 1999 in Colorado. Text adapted from Sharon Danks, "Ecological Schoolyards," Master's degree thesis for UC Berkeley (Spring 2000), p. 43.
2. Janet E. Dyment, *Gaining Ground: The Power and Potential of School Ground Greening in the Toronto District School Board* (Toronto, Ontario, Canada: Evergreen, 2005), pp. 24–25.
3. This list of benefits was developed from personal observation during site visits over the last ten years, and some of it is also supported by research described in Janet E. Dyment's *Gaining Ground* and Evergreen's publication, *Nature Nurtures: Investigating the Potential of School Grounds* (Toronto, Ontario, Canada: Evergreen, 2000).

Chapter 1

1. Site design by MIG, Inc.
2. Robin Moore, *Plants for Play: A Plant Selection Guide for Children's Outdoor Environments* (MIG Communications, 1993), pp. 29–36.
3. Anne C. Bell and Janet E. Dyment, *Grounds for Action: Promoting Physical Activity through School Ground Greening in Canada* (Evergreen, 2006), pp. 27–28. Bell and Dyment refer to studies on this topic by J. Evens (2001), Robin Moore (1986), Mary Rivkin (1995), and Wendy Titman (1994). Playground aggression is also discussed in Evergreen's *Nature Nurtures*, p. 8, which refers to Robin Moore's work (1989) and Wendy Titman's work (1994).
4. Richard Louv, paraphrased quote from keynote presentation for the *SFGSA 2008 Growing Greener School Grounds Conference*, San Francisco, CA (October 10, 2008).

5. This topic was discussed by author Richard Louv during his presentation at the *SFGSA 2008 Growing Greener School Grounds Conference*. A similar argument about schoolyard aggression on traditional playgrounds is also made by Bell and Dyment in *Grounds for Action*.
6. Robin C. Moore, "Before and After Asphalt: Diversity as an Ecological Measure of Quality in Children's Outdoor Environments," *The Ecological Context of Children's Play*, eds. Block, M.N. and Pellegrini (Ablex, 1989). Wendy Titman, *Special Places; Special People: The Hidden Curriculum of School Grounds*, World Wide Fund For Nature (1994).
7. Richard Louv, op.cit. A similar discussion about the calming effect of playground vegetation, citing the work of many researchers, appears in *Nature Nurtures* (Evergreen), pp. 8–9.
8. I make this observation from my knowledge of schoolyard examples in the United States and abroad. It is also supported in the literature in documents such as: Janet Dyment, *Gaining Ground: The Power and Potential of School Ground Greening in the Toronto District School Board* (Evergreen, 2005), pp. 35–36 and Bell and Dyment, *Grounds for Action*, p. 47.
9. Dyment, *Gaining Ground,* pp. 35–36.
10. Dyment, *Gaining Ground,* pp. 35–36.
11. I say this from anecdotal personal experience through my involvement with the San Francisco Green Schoolyard Alliance and other green schoolyard work, but it is also supported in the literature; Dyment, *Gaining Ground,* p. 43.
12. Wendy Titman, *Special Places, Special People: The Hidden Curriculum of Schoolgrounds*, World Wildlife Fund for Nature (1994).
13. Wallace Stegner, *Wolf Willow* (Compass Books, 1962). Reprinted by Penguin Classic (2000).

Chapter 2

1. This participatory design method blends concepts I learned from my mentors, Professors Marcia McNally and Randy Hester, with techniques I learned from colleagues at the Ecological Design Institute and Trust for Public Land while collaborating on schoolyard design projects. These ideas are also similar to the process described in Evergreen's *All Hands in the Dirt* design manual. Over the last ten years, I have added my own perspective and tailored these approaches to fit my design style as an environmental planner. In the last two years, my design process has also been enriched by ideas from my Bay Tree Design, inc. business partners, landscape architect Lisa Howard and horticulturalist Arden Bucklin-Sporer. Phases 5–6 of this description were originally developed by Lisa Howard and have been adapted for this chapter.
2. *All Hands in the Dirt* is available from Evergreen's Learning Grounds program, <www.evergreen.ca>.

Chapter 3

1. Earlier versions of my design guidelines have been published in three places. This chapter updates and revises previous versions: Sharon Danks, "Ecological Schoolyards," Master's Thesis (MLA-MCP). Department of Landscape Architecture and Environmental Planning, Department of City and Regional Planning, University of California, Berkeley (May 2000), pp. 113–124; Sharon Danks, "Ecological Schoolyards," *Landscape Architecture Magazine*, ed. J. William Thompson, American Society of Landscape Architects, Washington, DC (November 2000), pp. 42–47; and Sharon Danks, "Ecological Schoolyards: Design Guidelines," *New Village Journal*, ed. Lynne Elizabeth, Architects / Designers / Planners for Social Responsibility, Issue 3 (Berkeley: May 2002), pp. 74–77.
2. These four elements are tenets of the Schoolyard Habitats' program run by the National Wildlife Federation.
3. Robin C. Moore, *Plants for Play: A Plant Selection Guide for Children's Outdoor Environments*, (Berkeley: MIG Communications, 1993), p. 29.

Part 2

Introduction

1. Gerald Lieberman and Linda Hoody, "Closing the Achievement Gap: Using the Environment as an Integrating Context for Learning," Executive Summary. State Education and Environment Roundtable (San Diego, CA. 1998), p. 2.
2. Lieberman and Hoody, p. 2.
3. Lieberman and Hoody, pp. 1-2.

Chapter 4

1. National Wildlife Federation, *Schoolyard Habitats* (Vienna, Virginia: National Wildlife Federation (1995).
2. Richard Louv discusses the importance of letting children experience nature throughout his book *Last Child in the Woods: Saving our Children from Nature Deficit Disorder* (Chapel Hill, NC: Algonquin Books, 2006). Many other authors, from Walt Whitman to Robin Moore, discuss this theme in their work, too.
3. Bee nesting block information from Mace Vaughan, Matthew Shepherd, Claire Kremen, and Scott Hoffman Black, *Farming for Bees: Guidelines for Providing Native Bee Habitat on Farms* (The Xerces Society, 2004), pp. 14–17. Garden educator, Laurel Anderson, leads the gardening and green schoolyard efforts at Salmon Creek School.
4. Information for this case study was gathered during visits to the school site (2005 and 2006) and discussions with Salmon Creek School's garden teacher, Laurel Anderson (2009).
5. Site visit to Humber Valley Village School in Canada (May 2001). The beautiful mural was created by students from the Etobicoke School of the Arts, a public high school in Toronto.
6. "The best ways to attract more songbirds to your property," Cornell Lab of Ornithology <www.birds.cornell.edu/AllAboutBirds/attracting/landscaping/songbirds/document_view>
7. Personal communication with Arden Bucklin-Sporer, a local bird expert familiar with this school site (November 2008).
8. Ibid.
9. Ibid.

10. Alameda County Mosquito Abatement District. "Mosquito Prevention for Fishponds," (Hayward, CA: 2004), p.3. <www.mosquitoes.org>
11. Many of these dunks contain a bacteria called BTi (*Bacillus thuringiensis var. israelensis*). See "Fight the Bite: A Home and Garden Checklist," California Department of Pesticide Regulation, <www.mosquitoes.org/downloads/Checklist.pdf> and Wesley Maffei, "An Abridged Bibliography of Selected Biorational Larvicides for California Mosquito Control, version 5.1," Alameda County Mosquito Abatement District (June 25, 1997).
12. The original pair of solar panels on rotating mounts was installed by Hal Aronson of the Rahus Institute's Solar Schoolhouse as part of a workshop for a conference hosted by the San Francisco Green Schoolyard Alliance (October 2002), which I directed. Garden coordinator Arden Bucklin-Sporer built the pond with assistance from the school community.
13. When I visited Cowick First School in 2001, the pond had been successfully in place for more than 20 years without any liability or safety issues. The school has since closed for unrelated reasons. The information for this case study is drawn from research I conducted onsite in 2001 and later updated when I wrote an article about their site, "Stewardship Begins at School," *Landscape Architecture Magazine*, Vol. 93, No. 6 (June 2003).
14. The information for this case study was gathered onsite by my colleague Sandra Koike in July 2008, and will be included in her forthcoming master's degree thesis for the University of Oregon's Landscape Architecture Department. Photographs by Sandra Koike.
15. Personal communication with Linda Myers, garden coordinator, Sherman School over the course of many site visits from 2007-2009.
16. Information from <www.eco-schools.org/countries/news/news_rsa.htm> and <www.epworth.co.za>. Photograph by Mary Jackson.
17. The garden was originally developed by Alice Barrango and Esta Kornfield with assistance from many other volunteers from Ulloa School.
18. Art and ecology teacher David Lochtie started this project and spearheaded its continued development until the project ended in 2002.
19. This case study is an excerpt adapted from Sharon Gamson Danks's master's degree thesis, "Ecological Schoolyards" (May 2000), pp. 43–46.
20. Restoration ecologist and parent Deborah Keammerer spearheaded this project with Rob Layton of Design Concepts. I interviewed Keammerer onsite in Fall 1999, as part of my master's thesis research.
21. Site visit to this school in Tokyo, Japan (August 20, 2008).
22. "Earth Partnership Gallery," University of Wisconsin-Madison, Wisconsin Arboretum, Earth Partnership Program website. Photographs printed with permission from the Earth Partnership Program, granted February 2010.
23. United Anglers of Casa Grande High School's website: <www.uacg.org/index.html> The project was started and is led by teacher Tom Furrer, with the assistance of professional volunteers and a dedicated, ever-changing student body.
24. This case study is an excerpt adapted from Sharon Gamson Danks's master's degree thesis, "Ecological Schoolyards" (May 2000), pp. 27–29. Also from site visit to the school (December 7, 1999).
25. United Anglers of Casa Grande High School, "The Results of Our Efforts are Proof Positive," project web page, : <www.uacg.org/index.html>
26. Site visit to St. Paulinus School in England (July 4, 2001).
27. Site visit to Salmon Creek School in Occidental, California (July 2005) and discussion with garden educator, Laurel Anderson.

20. Site visit to Sankt Hansgården in Sweden, September 7, 2001. I observed the construction process for this wattle and daub structure during a green schoolyard conference onsite.
21. Earthen ovens are not sealed, since they must "breathe" when they are heated.
22. This hands-on workshop, led by Jackson Poretta in October 2002, was part of the *Growing Greener School Grounds Conference* I directed, sponsored by the San Francisco Green Schoolyard Alliance.
23. Garden educator, Rivka Mason, coordinated this project. Architect John Fordice assisted the Malcolm X School community with the greenhouse's design and the technical aspects of the cob construction process.
24. This tool shed was designed by architect David Arkin, for a UC Berkeley class co-taught by Arkin and Professor Randy Hester in 2000.
25. Personal communication with landscape architect, Frode Svane, September 17, 2001, during a site visit to the school in Norway. Svane designed this project and worked with this school to build it.
26. This bench was created by garden instructor Matt Tseng and middle school students at Willard Middle School.
27. Many sources report these environmental impacts of cement, including: Alex Wilson. "Cement and Concrete: Environmental Considerations." *Environmental Building News*, March 1, 1993. Reprinted online at: <www.buildinggreen.com/auth/article.cfm?fileName=020201b.xml>
28. These urbanite walls were created during a hands-on workshop led by artist Josho Somine, in October 2004, as part of the *Growing Greener School Grounds Conference* I directed, sponsored by the San Francisco Green Schoolyard Alliance. I created the initial concept plan and design guidelines for this project, for the Trust for Public Land, in 2001. The project was later implemented by their landscape architects who created the construction drawings for the wall.
29. Personal communication with teacher Theresa Accero onsite at Montgomery School in San Diego, CA, Nov. 1999 and June 2001. This information was originally gathered for use in my master's thesis, *Ecological Schoolyards*.
30. Metal gate created by artist Josho Somine.
31. Information from a site visit to Cowick First School on July 9, 2001, and from subsequent correspondence with teacher Steve Smith in the course of writing an article about this school for *Landscape Architecture Magazine* in spring 2003. The tile mosaic mural was created by artist Elaine Goodwin.
32. Sidwell Friends School's website: <www.sidwell.edu/about_sfs/greenbuilding_ms.asp>
33. Information from a site tour given by Sidwell Friends School's Plant Manager, Steve Sawyer, July 17, 2008. The building's architect was Kieran-Timberlake Associates, LLP.
34. Sharon Gamson Danks. *Ecological Schoolyards*. Master's degree thesis, UC Berkeley. Berkeley, CA: May 2000. pp. 85–86.
35. This project was coordinated by garden educator, Tanya Stiller
36. San Francisco Unified School District and Bay Tree Design, inc., "Choosing Materials for a Green Schoolyard," information sheet for SFUSD school. Information on this point was gathered through phone conversations with a plastic lumber producer.

Chapter 9

1. Site visit to Royston High School in England, June 2001; site tour given by teacher Ken Dunn.

2. Nuala Creed, artist-in-residence at Tule Elk Park Child Development Center, created this work with students. Site visit to the school (August 2007) and information from the artist's website, <www.nualacreed.org>
3. Site visit to Manglerud School (September 2001); tour given by landscape architect Frode Svane and the school's principal. Additional information and photograph from Cam Collyer, who visited the school in July 2008.
4. This mural was created between 1996 and 1998 at Redding Elementary School in San Francisco, California. This school has since been re-named Tenderloin Community School. Artist Martha Heavenston Nojima helped 200 students in kindergarten through fifth grade create this project. Information from wall mounted interpretive signs, observed during my visit to the school site (December 2003).
5. Mural by artist Josef Norris and Bret Harte School's students.
6. Site visit to Lampton School in England (July 2, 2001); tour and personal communication with Deputy Headteacher Les Carswell.
7. This playground was designed by Leathers & Associates. Photographs by Leathers & Associates.
8. Photograph by Kirk Meyer, Boston Schoolyard Initiative: <www.schoolyards.org/education.htm>
9. This sundial was designed by Gelfand Partners Architects and installed when the school was modernized and expanded in 2002. Personal communication with Chris Duncan and Ken Rackow of Gelfand Partners Architects (December 2008).
10. Site visit to Hennigan School in Jamaica Plain, Massachusetts (August 7, 2002); tour led by the Boston Schoolyard Initiative.
11. There is a comprehensive list of solar calendar sites at <www.solarcalendar.org/03_edu_sky.html>; and another informative list at: <solar-center.stanford.edu/AO>
12. Information from the NASS Sundial Register website, <www.sundials.org>. Photograph by Analy High School.
13. Teachers Karin Wingman and Britt Wall-Rydh from Vega School in Lund, Sweden, developed this sun-based calendar. This information is from my site visit to Vega School (September 10, 2001); tour given by Anders Kjellson, and from the written project summary: "Årstidsträdgården - Barns Föreställningar om Årstider" ("Seasonal Garden: Children's Representation of Seasons"). Excerpt from a project written for Malmö University (1999). I reproduced and translated the hand-sketched diagram that accompanied an article about this project (using an online translation program), written by Karin Wingman and Britt Wall-Rydh.
14. Information from personal experience as the green schoolyard coordinator at Rosa Parks School. I designed this project in collaboration with Suzanne Ingley, Rosa Parks School's science teacher.
15. The geology trail at Coombes School was the inspiration for our geology walk at Rosa Parks School.
16. Artist Euan McEuan carved the face on this rock at the Coombes School: <www.thecoombes.com>
17. Information about The Coombes School is from a lecture I attended, given by longtime Headteacher Susan Humphries (September 6, 2001) at a schoolyard conference in Lund, Sweden. Some information is also from their website: <www.thecoombes.com> Additional information and photographs are by Cam Collyer, who visited this school site (July 2008).
18. Information from personal observation of the exhibit on the National Mall, and from the program's website: <voyagesolarsystem.org> "Voyage is a program of the National Center for Earth and Space Science Education."

19. Photograph by the Boston Schoolyard Initiative: <www.schoolyards.org/education.htm>

20. Information about Tule Elk Park Child Development Center's garden and art projects from garden instructor, Ayesha Ercelawn (September 2008). Photos by Ayesha Ercelawn.

21. Information is from Skudeneshavn School's website. Photograph by Frode Svane.

22. Information from personal communication with Cam Collyer, after his visit to Ravenstone Primary School (July 2008). Photograph by Cam Collyer. Additional information from the school's website, <www.ravenstoneschool.co.uk/school_facilities>. The Rose Amphitheater was designed by Chloe Cookson and Rory McNally and built by Tobie Arnott.

🍃 Part 3

Introduction

1. Playlink Play Policy: <www.freeplaynetwork.org.uk/playlink/exhibition/school/berlin1.htm>

2. Some of these organizations include the Children and Nature Network, Evergreen, the Free Play Network, the International Play Association, Children's Landscape, Norway (Barnas Landskap), Grün macht Schule, and the Natural Learning Initiative.

3. One example of play categories is described in this article: Lorraine E. Maxwell, Mari R. Mitchell, and Gary W. Evans, "Effects of Play Equipment and Loose Parts on Preschool Children's Outdoor Play Behavior: An Observational Study and Design Intervention," *Children, Youth and Environments* 18(2) (2008), pp. 36–63.

4. Robin C. Moore and Herb H. Wong, *Natural Learning: The Life History of an Environmental Schoolyard,* MIG Communications (Berkeley, CA. 1997), pp. 247–248 and Robin C. Moore, *Plants for Play: A Plant Selection Guide for Children's Outdoor Environments*, MIG Communications (Berkeley, CA. 1993), pp. 29–36.

5. Asbjørn Flemmen, Volda University College, Norway. "Real Play: A Recognized Sensory-Motor Behaviour in Norway," *Playrights: An International Journal of the Theory and Practice of Play*, Vol. 26, No. 4 (International Play Association: 2005).

Chapter 10

1. I am on the board of directors for the Community Built Association. Their website is: <www.communitybuilt.org>

2. Information from personal communication with Kyle Cundy, Leathers & Associates (May 2009) and <www.leathersassociates.com>.

3. The playground at Skaneateles Early Childhood Center was designed by Planet Earth Playscapes.

4. Asbjørn Flemmen: Real Play—a Socio-Motor Behaviour. Notat 3/2005. Høgskulen i Volda og Møreforsking Volda.

5. Ibid.

6. Information in this case study from the school's website, <www.karmoyped.no/lek/eng/teksteng.htm> and from information presented in an article by Linda Velle Sea of the Educational Center in Karmøy, Norway, *Skudeneshavn School: The School's Outdoor Areas—An Eldorodo Movement* (*Skudeneshavn skole: Skolens uteområde- et bevegelseseldorado!*); first published in the Danish journal "Skolens rum," Vol. No. 7 (2001) and also posted on the internet in Norwegian at: <www.skole.karmoy.kommune.no/wskud/karmoy-ute.htm>

7. Skudeneshavn School's website: <www.karmoyped.no/lek/eng/teksteng.htm>

8. Linda Velle Sea, op.cit.

9. This quote is from Skudeneshavn School's website: <www.karmoyped.no/lek/eng/teksteng.htm>

10. Lene Schmidt, "Outdoor spaces—Jungle or Exercise Yard? A Study of Facilities, Children and Physical Activity at School," ("Skolegården, jungel eller luftegård?") Norwegian Institute for Urban and Regional Research (NIBR), Oslo, Norway (Report 2004:01), <www.nibr.no/publikasjoner/rapporter/116/>

11. Boulder structure designed by Planet Earth Playscapes and built by a local rock sculptor.

12. Personal communication with landscape architect Frode Svane and with Manglerud's school principal, Tom Moen (September 17, 2001); Information also from an article by Frode Svane, "The Mini-Mountain" at Manglerud Primary School, Oslo: 1999–2000" on his website, Children's Landscape: <www.barnas-landskap.org>.

13. Murergården Daycare Center's playground was designed by Helle Nebelong.

14. This definition is based on references found in *The Art of the Maze* by Adrian Fisher and George Gerster (Seven Dials, Cassell & Co, 2000) and online materials from *Labryinthos: The Labyrinth Resource Centre*: <www.labyrinthos.net>.

15. The boulder "mini-mountain" at Manglerud School was designed by Frode Svane, 2000. Photograph by Frode Svane.

16. This labyrinth was created during a workshop led by Stephen Shibley and Kiko Denzer at the Community Built Association's conference, Pacific Grove, California (March 2008).

17. Personal communication with Frode Svane (September 2001).

18. Site visit to Leadgate Infant School in England (June 25, 2001).

19. This information and insight was given to me by Cam Collyer, who visited Ravenstone School and spoke with school staff in 2008.

20. Information from and photographs by Frode Svane.

21. The nature play schoolyard at Mercy Care for Kids was designed by Planet Earth Playscapes.

22. Information from personal communication with Rusty Keeler (May 2009). Photos by Rusty Keeler, Planet Earth Playscapes.

23. *Evaluation of Health Effects of Recycled Waste Tires in Playground and Track Products,* California Integrated Waste Management Board, Office of Environmental Health Hazard Assessment (January 2007).

Chapter 11

1. This section about living willow play structures is an adapted excerpt from a longer article I wrote: Sharon Danks, "Green Mansions: Living Willow Structures Enhance Children's Play Environments," *Landscape Architecture Magazine*, Vol. 92, No. 6 (June 2002), pp. 38–43, 93.

2. Site visit to Palett School in Sweden (September 12, 2001); tour and discussion with teacher Ann Olsson.

3. The school grounds at Cowick First School are no longer used as an elementary school, for reasons unrelated to the schoolyard design.

4. Teacher Barbara Heath, Gorsemoor School's Assistant Headteacher, members of the British Trust for Conservation Volunteers and the Cannock

District Rangers helped to organize the project and train the school's students and teachers.

5. Gorsemoor County Primary School, School Grounds webpage: <www.gorsemoor.staffs.sch.uk/> and information from teacher Barbara Heath, Gorsemoor School's Assistant Headteacher.

6. Weidenhof Primary School's playground was designed by Dietzen + Teichmann Landschafts Architekten.

7. Our firm, Bay Tree Design, inc., designed the Sustainable Schoolyard exhibit, including the playhouse, and helped to install it. Other partners who helped to produce this exhibit were members of *Friends of Smart Growth and Sustainable Communities* including: CONCERN, Inc. (project manager), American Farmland Trust, American Planning Association, The Cloud Institute for Sustainability Education, The Conservation Fund, National Association of Counties, National Association of Realtors®, and Smart Growth Network. The project's website is: <www.sustainableschoolyard.org>.

8. Information from The Coombes School website <www.thecoombes.com> and from Cam Collyer who visited the site in July 2008.

9. Information from Skudeneshavn School's website: <www.karmoyped.no/lek/eng/teksteng.htm> Photograph by Skudeneshavn School.

10. Photograph by Mary Jackson from her site visit to Brungle Public School in Australia (2003).

Chapter 12

1. Personal communication with Tule Elk Park Child Development Center's garden educator, Ayesha Ercelawn (May 2009).

2. "Shiny Mud Balls: Kyoto Professor Taps into the Essence of Play," *Japan Information Network*. (October 5, 2001), <web-japan.org/trends01/article/011005sci_r.html>

3. Personal communication with teacher Shinobu Suzuki at Little Lamb Kindergarten, Wakoshi, Saitama, Japan (August 21, 2008).

4. Planet Earth Playscapes <www.planetearthplayscapes.com>

5. Rusty Keeler, "Play Environments for the Soul," online article, Planet Earth Playscapes's website <www.planetearthplayscapes.com/articles_playenv.html> Reprinted with permission from Rusty Keeler.

6. Information about this project is from personal communication with Bill and Mary Buchen (May 2009) and from: Sonic Architecture's brochure: "Global Rhythms: Curriculum Guide for Musical Sculptures at Denver's Green Valley Ranch Park." Artist/musicians: Bill and Mary Buchen (2008); and <www.sonicarchitecture.com> "Global Rhythms" playground at Green Valley Ranch Park was completed in 2009.

7. "Global Rhythms: Curriculum Guide for Musical Sculptures at Denver's Green Valley Ranch Park." Artist/musicians: Bill and Mary Buchen (2008). This park was commissioned by the Public Art Program of Denver's Commission on Cultural Affairs.

8. Information and photographs from Bill and Mary Buchen of Sonic Architecture (May 2009). This project was commissioned by the NYC Public Schools, the NYC School Construction Authority, and the NYC Department of Cultural Affairs, Percent for Art Program. It was completed in 1996.

9. Bill and Mary Buchen's Sonic Architecture website, "PS 23 Sound Playground," overview, <www.sonicarchitecture.com/catalogue/ps23 playground.html> This schoolyard was designed by artists Bill Buchen and Mary Buchen of Sonic Architecture and completed in 1992. Photo by Paul Warchol.

10. Personal communication with Bond Anderson, Sound Play, Inc. (May 2009) and <www.soundplay.com>.

11. The site design was created by Leathers & Associates of Ithaca, New York, and was built by the community. The instruments were created by Sound Play of Parrott, Georgia. Information from personal communication with Bond Anderson, Sound Play, Inc. (May 2009) <www.soundplay.com>.

12. This instrument was made by Tree of Us in Van Etten, NY, <treeofus.net> The playground was designed by Planet Earth Playscapes, <www.planetearthplayscapes.com>

13. This instrument, by Sound Play, also includes a panel with a dedication to a teacher who passed away.

14. Playground design by Planet Earth Playscapes.

15. The concept for the outdoor music therapy space at Alternatives for Children was conceived by Dr. Petra Kern. The Sound Garden was designed and implemented by Rusty Keeler of Planet Earth Playscapes with the help of the school community. Photograph by Ingrid Spiotto.

16. This sound play structure was created by Freya van Dien, with help from other Adventure Playground staff members, and visiting children.

17. This playground was designed by Leathers & Associates and built with the assistance of more than a thousand local community members. <www.frogpark.org>

18. Personal communication with Bond Anderson, Sound Play, Inc. (May 2009). Photograph by Bond Anderson.

🍃 Part 4

Introduction

1. Detail from "A Peaceable Kingdom" tile mosaic mural by 4th graders at Rooftop School in San Francisco, California, led by artist Josef Norris of Kid Serve.

Chapter 13

1. Architect Jean Lemanski of Lemanski Rockwell helped the school community design and build this amphitheater.

2. Photograph by Mary Jackson from her site visit to Meadowbank School in New Zealand (2003).

3. Artist Lauren Elder designed this amphitheater and then collaborated with artist Gitty Duncan to make hand glazed, low relief cast tiles with the students. Personal communication with Lauren Elder (July 2009).

4. This project at Peralta School was created by teacher Calvert Hand and his first grade class.

5. Artist Josho Somine worked with Salmon Creek School to build this cob bench.

6. The Ecology Center of San Francisco led this cob bench-building project at West Portal School.

7. Work by artist Shane Eagleton.

8. This space was designed by Lauren Elder with input from the school community.

9. This garden seating area was built by parent volunteers, Hisao Yokota and Joshua Eden.

10. This gazebo at Salmon Creek School was designed and built by local artist Josho Somine, with the assistance of the school community.

11. Peter Joseph Lenné School's playground was designed by Dietzen + Teichmann Landschafts Architekten.
12. Photograph by Mary Jackson from her site visit to Middle Swan Primary School in Australia (2003).
13. Site visit to Environmental Middle School in Portland, Oregon (December 1999). The school's name is now Sunnyside Environmental School.

Chapter 14

1. Personal communication with garden educator, Ayesha Ercelawn (May 2009).
2. I founded the green schoolyard at Rosa Parks School and organized the fence building project. I also helped teacher Michelle Contreras's kindergarten class to make the wooden sunflower cutouts.
3. Information from personal communication with Cam Collyer (Spring 2009) after his visit to the Coombes School (Summer 2008).
4. Artist Jamie Morgan made enlarged plywood cutouts from students' drawings and returned them to the children to paint. Morgan attached the painted cutouts to the building's walls on top of vibrant murals he painted as a backdrop.
5. Artist Lauren Elder designed this piece collaboratively with two students and it was fabricated by artist Amy Blackstone following their drawings. Personal communication with artist Lauren Elder (July 2009).
6. The "Pledge of Allegiance to the Earth" mural was created by K–5th grade students at Harvey Milk Civil Rights Academy and artist Tiffany Graham.

Chapter 15

1. Artists Kath Bedingfield, Jane Gower, Paul Denton and Tony Scandrett of Makers and Shakers participated in this project at Ebchester Primary School. I visited this school in 2001 and wrote an article describing these features: Sharon Danks, "Green Mansions: Living Willow Structures Enhance Children's Play Environments," *Landscape Architecture Magazine* (June 2002), pp. 38, 40–41, 43–44, 93.
2. Peralta first grade students created the temporary sunflower display. The permanent wooden cutouts were created by artist Jamie Morgan, based on student drawings, and later painted by the students.
3. This mural at Rosa Parks School in San Francisco, California, was designed by artists from "Culture on the Corner" in 1996.
4. This ceramic mural was designed and created by artists Paul Lanier and Nancy Thompson in 2008. Students helped the artists with portions of the project.
5. Ibid.
6. Information from San Francisco Unified School District's website, <www.sfusd.edu/schwww/sch603/DEAFED.HTM>
7. This mural at Cesar Chavez School was created by artists Juana Alicia and Susan Cervantes of the Precita Eyes Mural Arts Center in 1990.
8. The triptych at Tule Elk Child Development Center was created by artist-in-residence, Nuala Creed, with the help of garden educator, Ayesha Ercelawn, and children at the school; information from personal communication with Ayesha Ercelawn (May 2009).
9. Artist Debbie Koppman worked with Sequoia students to make this mural.
10. Artwork created by students at Sanchez School with the assistance of artist Ellen Rogers.
11. Artists Kath Bedingfield, Jane Gower, Paul Denton and Tony Scandrett of Makers and Shakers participated in this project at Ebchester Primary School. I visited this school in 2001 and wrote an article describing these features: Sharon Danks, "Green Mansions: Living Willow Structures Enhance Children's Play Environments," op.cit.
12. Water play table created by artists Ann and Marvin Rosenberg. The natural playground that surrounds it was designed by Leon Smith of Planet Earth Playscapes.
13. This metal sculpture was welded by a local artist, and the painted vinyl "dragon scales" were added by students from both schools, under the direction of Bonnie Ora Sherk of A Living Library and Life Frames, Inc.
14. The Quetzalcoatl sculpture was fabricated by Interplay Design; handmade tile by Aileen Barr and Mark Roller; mosaics by Colette Crutcher and Mark Roller; under the auspices of The Precita Eyes Muralists, with help from dozens of volunteers.
15. The grounds at Kløvermarken Nature Workshop were designed by Helle Nebelong.
16. This art piece was created by teacher Calvert Hand, Principal Rosette Costello, and Peralta parents.
17. Information from personal communication with Cam Collyer (Spring 2009) after his visit to the Coombes School (Summer 2008). Photograph by Cam Collyer.
18. Information from personal communication with Cam Collyer (Spring 2009) after his visit to the Lenné School (Summer 2008). Photograph by Cam Collyer.
19. These sculptures were created by artist John Abduljaami of Oakland, California.
20. Information from Wayne Thomas School.

🍃 Part 5

Chapter 16

1. "Cowick First School Eco-Code" on a sign posted inside the school near the front entrance when I visited the site in July 2001. This school site has since been closed for reasons unrelated to its school grounds.
2. Information from my site visit to Cowick First School (July 2001) and from subsequent communications while writing an article about this school in 2003: Sharon Gamson Danks, "Stewardship Begins at School: In England, a Superlative Example of an Ecological Schoolyard," *Landscape Architecture Magazine*, J. William Thompson, editor (Washington, DC: American Society of Landscape Architects, June 2003), pp. 42, 44, 46, 48.

Chapter 17

1. I was involved in the early stages of the design process for this project in 2005 and 2006, as part of the 2003 Proposition A Bond's Green Schoolyard Program for San Francisco Unified School District. I also collaborated with landscape architect Chris Ford of Chris Ford Landscape Architecture and the Sloat School greening committee on the general layout for this portion of the yard. Ford further developed the plan with the Sloat School greening committee and created the construction drawings and planting plan for the project. Sloat's green schoolyard committee and garden coordinators spearheaded the impressive plantings, implementation, and site stewardship, with some additional assistance from other community organizations including the San Francisco Green Schoolyard Alliance.

Acknowledgments

This book, like an ecological schoolyard, has come about as the result of countless helping hands. I am grateful to my colleagues and friends for generously sharing their time and expertise with me over the years, helping to make this book a reality.

A warm, special thank you to all of the garden educators, teachers, principals, school district staff, and school community members who shared their insights with me, gave me tours of their school grounds, and allowed me to observe their schoolyard projects in action. Your help was invaluable and will now inspire readers to green their own school grounds around the world. Thank you for the work you do everyday, for all of our children.

A heartfelt thank you to my friends and colleagues who generously contributed photographs, text, and information to this book from their own research travels and inspiring work: Analy High School, Bond Anderson, Hal Aronson, Gary Bailey, Tamar Barlev, Jared Blumenfeld, Boston Schoolyard Initiative, Susan Boyd, Bill and Mary Buchen, Arden Bucklin-Sporer, Beth Bythrow, Cam Collyer, Michelle Contreras, Kyle Cundy, Rebecca Drayse, Earth Partnership Program, Kimberlee Eggers, Ayesha Ercelawn, Asbjørn Flemmen, Leanne Gargett Gelfand Partners Architects, Lori Hardenbergh, Barbara Heath, Todd Hendricks, Lisa Howard, Innovative Design, Mary Jackson, Abby Jaramillo, Rosey Jencks, Lynne Juarez, Rusty Keeler, Melinda Kelley, Glen Kizer, Anders Kjellsson, Sandra Koike, Leathers and Associates, Montgomery Watson Constructors, Linda Myers, Judy Neuhauser, Precita Eyes, Rachel Pringle, Doug Pushard, Aaron Reed, Steve Ruelli, San Francisco Green Schoolyard Alliance, Steve Sawyer, Beth Schwartz, Lori Shelton, Shrewsbury School, SHWGroup, Skudeneshavn School, Leon Smith, Ingrid Spiotto, Shinobu and Shunji Suzuki, Frode Svane, Tokiwano Elementary School, TreePeople, Twenhofel Middle School, United Anglers of Casa Grande High School, Brit Wall-Rydh, Judy Walsby, Paul Warchol, Clare Watsky, White Arkitekter AB, and Karin Wingman—I greatly appreciate your contributions to this book. It is a much richer volume today, because of your help.

Where would I have been without patient readers who took the time to review my draft chapters and give me feedback about the book's content and style? Thank you so much Tor Allen, Carla Barros, Arden Bucklin-Sporer, Carol Danks, Debra Gamson, Lisa Howard, Rosey Jencks, Glen Kizer, and Tali Reicher. A special thanks to Tamar Barlev for reviewing so much of the book and helping me to overcome writer's block at key points in the writing process.

Thank you Randy Hester, Marcia McNally, Tim Duane, and Michael Southworth for helping me many years ago with my master's thesis, which became the springboard for this book. Thank you UC Berkeley Department of Landscape Architecture and Environmental Planning for the incredible opportunity to visit schoolyards abroad on the Geraldine Knight Scott Traveling Fellowship; a trip on which I gathered many examples for this book.

Thank you Cam Collyer, Mary Jackson, Anders Kjellsson, Julie Mountain, Shunji and Shinobu Suzuki, and Frode Svane for taking me on wonderful schoolyard tours and helping to shape my perspective about school grounds in your countries.

Thank you, San Francisco Unified School District—Tamar Barlev, Wazi Chowdhury, Nik Kaestner, Lori Shelton, and Leonard Tom—for believing in green schoolyards and being leaders in this emerging field. I am greatly enjoying my work with you; it has helped to inspire and test many of the ideas presented in these pages.

Thank you Cam Collyer, for taking the time to write the foreword for this book and for sharing so many beautiful photographs and inspiring stories with me that are included here.

Thank you Lisa Howard for being so patient with my never ending project, and for contributing your wisdom and expertise to our collaborative green schoolyard work.

Thank you New Village Press for the wonderful opportunity to write and publish this book, and for your skillful guidance and patience through the many years it took me to put it on paper. I am deeply grateful for Lynne Elizabeth's interest in my work and her wise, guiding hands throughout the book's development; Nancy Bauer's sage advice as my editor, helping me to articulate my thoughts in the clearest manner; Karen Stewart Kearney, Erin Burns, Julie Miller, Sylvie Schmid and Leigh McLellan's assistance with business, marketing, and graphic design; and Amanda Bensel, Stefania DePetris, Terri Northcutt, Janice Sapigao, and Megan Whiteford's work on the book's production process.

To my husband Mark, children Maia and Ayden, and other family members—thank you so much for your patience through the years as I worked long days and nights. We can go out and play now that I'm finished!

Index

🍃 Index of Places Mentioned in the Book

The letter *f* following a page number denotes a figure

United States

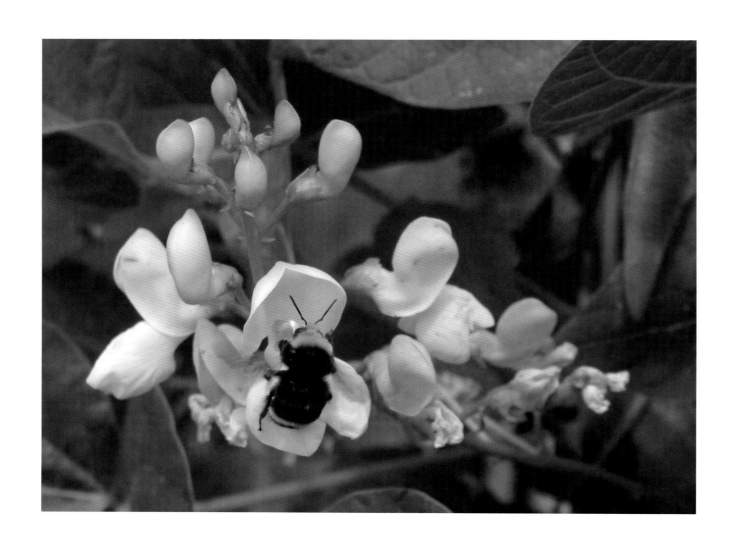

About the Author

Sharon Gamson Danks is an environmental planner and founding partner of Bay Tree Design, inc. in Berkeley, California, a women-owned landscape architecture and planning firm that collaborates with clients to develop lively outdoor spaces including ecological schoolyards.

Sharon's schoolyard ecology background includes research, writing, and hands-on design and planning with school communities in the San Francisco Bay Area and beyond. She has visited and documented approximately 200 green schoolyard projects in North America, Europe, Great Britain, and Japan over the last ten years. This has helped her develop design guidelines and best practices for green schoolyards and informs her work as an author and designer. Since 2001, Sharon and her firm, Bay Tree Design, have assisted over three dozen schools, using a participatory master planning process to help them transform their grounds from ordinary asphalt into vibrant ecosystems for learning and play. The green schoolyard master plans that Bay Tree Design creates follow ecological design principles and reflect each school's unique community, curricula and site-specific ecology.

Sharon Gamson Danks and Bay Tree Design are currently working with San Francisco Unified School District on their cutting-edge green schoolyard program. Ms. Danks has directed three hands-on schoolyard ecology conferences for the San Francisco Green Schoolyard Alliance and serves on their advisory board. She also serves on the national board for the Community Built Association. In 2008, Sharon and Bay Tree Design designed a Sustainable Schoolyard exhibit for display at the US Botanic Garden

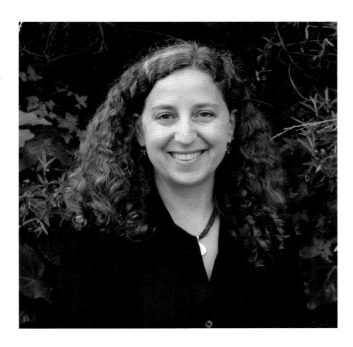

in Washington DC. Sharon has written a number of green schoolyard-themed articles that have appeared in *Landscape Architect Magazine, Orion, New Village Journal*, and *Green Teacher*. She is also the lead-author of the *Green Schoolyard Resource Directory* for the San Francisco Bay Area. In addition to a MLA-MCP from University of California, Berkeley, Sharon holds a Professional Certificate in Natural Resource Management from U.C. San Diego Extension and a BA from Princeton University.

Sharon is also the mother of two expert playground testers, ages 7 and 10.

About New Village Press

The book you are holding was brought to you by New Village Press, the first publisher to serve the emerging field of community building. Subjects we cover include social justice, urban ecology, and community-based arts and culture. In particular, our publications focus on the "good news" of community development—spreading the word about inspirational examples and replicable models emerging from the creativity and inventiveness of self-organized communities.

If you enjoyed *Asphalt to Ecosystems* you may be interested in other books that explore how a healthy connection with nature can promote vibrant communities and social change:

- *Building Commons and Communities,* by Karl Linn, details several grassroots projects inspired by visionary leader Karl Linn, a pioneer of community building who for more than forty years brought life to economically disenfranchised neighborhoods in nine American cities, from Boston to Berkeley.

- *Works of Heart: Building Village through the Arts*, edited by Lynne Elizabeth and Suzanne Young, describes seven inspiring community-based arts projects. Examples range from murals realized by Oregon students using natural materials gathered in their schoolyard to a garden refuge built by cancer patients, neighbors, and staff in the courtyard of a San Francisco hospital.

- *Awakening Creativity: The Dandelion School Blossoms*, by Lily Yeh, describes the innovative efforts by internationally renowned artist and community activist Lily Yeh to transform a school for the children of migrant workers on the outskirts of Beijing, China. Lily Yeh shows how arts and creativity allow students to express their feelings, heal their wounds, and envision a better future for themselves.

- *Doing Time in the Garden: Life Lessons through Prison Horticulture*, by James Jiler, offers an engaging personal account of a highly succesful horticultural job-training program at Rikers Island, the largest jail complex in the United States. The book shows how vocational education and interaction with nature can transform the lives of men and women caught in the American prison system.

New Village Press is a public-benefit project of Architects/Designers/Planners for Social Responsibility, an educational nonprofit working since 1983 for peace, environmental protection, social justice, and the development of healthy communities (www.adpsr.org).

You can order our books and browse our catalog at www.newvillagepress.net.